The AIDS Crisis

THE AIDS CRISIS

A Documentary History

Edited by DOUGLAS A. FELDMAN
and JULIA WANG MILLER

Primary Documents in American History and Contemporary Issues

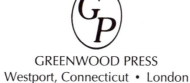

GREENWOOD PRESS
Westport, Connecticut • London

Library of Congress Cataloging-in-Publication Data

The AIDS crisis : a documentary history / edited by Douglas A. Feldman
and Julia Wang Miller.
    p. cm.—(Primary documents in American history and
contemporary issues series, ISSN 1069–5605)
   Includes bibliographical references and index.
   ISBN 0–313–28715–5 (alk. paper)
   1. AIDS (Disease)—History. I. Feldman, Douglas A. II. Miller,
Julia Wang. III. Series.
RA644.A25A3554   1998
362.1'969792'009—dc21   97–26891

British Library Cataloguing in Publication Data is available.

Library of Congress Catalog Card Number: 97–26891
ISBN: 0–313–28715–5
ISSN: 1069–5605

First published in 1998

Greenwood Press, 88 Post Road West, Westport, CT 06881
An imprint of Greenwood Publishing Group, Inc.

Printed in the United States of America

The paper used in this book complies with the
Permanent Paper Standard issued by the National
Information Standards Organization (Z39.48–1984).

10 9 8 7 6 5 4 3 2

Copyright Acknowledgments

The editors and publisher are grateful to the following for granting permission to reprint
from their material:

Excerpts taken from abstracts appearing in the CDC NCHSTP Daily News Update, Copyright, Information, Inc., Bethesda, MD, appear courtesy of the CDC NCHSTP Daily News
Update©Information, Inc.

This book is dedicated to the memory of my good friend William Browne (1968–1994), who was infected with HIV as a teenager and died from complications of AIDS a few days before his twenty-sixth birthday. He will always be remembered for his humor, intelligence, creativity, and concern for others.

Douglas A. Feldman

Contents

Series Foreword

This series is designed to meet the research needs of high school and college students by making available in one volume the key primary documents on a given historical event or contemporary issue. Documents include speeches and letters, congressional testimony, Supreme Court and lower court decisions, government reports, biographical accounts, position papers, statutes, and news stories.

The purpose of the series is twofold: (1) to provide substantive and background material on an event or issue through the texts of primary documents that shaped policy or law, raised controversy, or influenced the course of events; and (2) to trace the controversial aspects of the event or issue through documents that represent a variety of viewpoints. Documents for each volume have been selected by a recognized specialist in that subject with the advice of a board of other subject specialists, school librarians, and teachers.

To place the subject in historical perspective, the volume editor has prepared an introductory overview and a chronology of events. Documents are organized either chronologically or topically. The documents are full text or, if unusually long, have been excerpted by the volume editor. To facilitate understanding, each document is accompanied by an explanatory introduction. Suggestions for further reading follow the document or the chapter.

It is the hope of Greenwood Press that this series will enable students and other readers to use primary documents more easily in their research, to exercise critical thinking skills by examining the key documents in American history and public policy, and to critique the variety of viewpoints represented by this selection of documents.

Acknowledgments

We would like to thank Dr. Ralph Bolton (Pomona College), Dr. Norris G. Lang (University of Houston), Dr. William L. Leap (The American University), Dr. Peggy O'Hara (University of Miami), and Dr. Michael D. Quam (State University of Illinois at Springfield) for their excellent editorial reviews in the early stages of this book. We would also like to thank June Seldin for her secretarial services, Dr. Barbara Rader of Greenwood Press for her patience and encouragement, and—most especially—Jean Dingee for her tireless research assistance.

Introduction

Imagine a disease that was usually fatal and could spread each and every time two people have sex. Now imagine that that disease progressed so slowly that it took an average of ten years from the time of infection until the infected person's death, sometimes as much as twenty years. Let's also imagine that the disease was caused by a virus so small, a mere 130 millionth of a millimeter in diameter, that if it was magnified several times, it still could not be seen with the naked eye. And what if the disease affected mostly people in the prime of their lives, rather than at the end of their years? And what if the disease produced hideous symptoms like purplish blotches on the skin, extreme fatigue, and severe weight loss? And imagine that disease was new and spreading around the world at an alarming rate, infecting tens of millions of people.

There is no need to imagine such a disease, because that disease is very real; it is called AIDS (acquired immunodeficiency syndrome). Since it was first mentioned in the medical literature in 1981, AIDS has spread into nearly every nation on earth and has caused more widespread panic, fear, and concern than any other medical catastrophe in the twentieth century. A new class of drugs, called protease inhibitors, appears to be prolonging the lives of most of those in the developed nations who are taking them. But whether they will remain effective is not yet clear. For the tens of millions of persons with HIV (human immunodeficiency virus) or AIDS in the developing world who cannot afford their prohibitive cost, the new drugs are not available. For them, AIDS is usually fatal, though we now have good reason to believe that a small proportion of those infected with the virus that causes AIDS will never develop symptoms and will not die from it. We also now know that some people who are repeatedly exposed to the virus will never become infected. But there is no easy way of knowing at this point who is immune and who is not, nor to yet harness that immunity for developing an effective vaccine for others.

AIDS AND HIV

The virus that causes AIDS is called HIV and is visible only with an electron microscope. It was first discovered by Dr. Louis Montagnier of France in 1983 and was called LAV. The following year, it was called HTLV-III by Dr. Robert Gallo of the United States, and then widely recognized as the cause of AIDS. It was renamed HIV two years later. The virus initially infects the body, sometimes producing flu-like acute symptoms, then remains dormant in the infected person's body for anywhere from two to twenty years (averaging about eight or nine years) before noticeable illness occurs. Since HIV breaks down the immune system of the infected person, almost anything can happen, and the person with AIDS is susceptible to developing serious illness from even the most commonplace microorganisms.

Symptoms include purplish or brownish blotches on the skin (caused by a cancer called Kaposi's sarcoma), severe coughing (caused by a deadly form of pneumonia called *Pneumocystis carinii* pneumonia, or by tuberculosis), vomiting, diarrhea, memory loss and senility (often called AIDS dementia), severe weight loss (often called the wasting syndrome), trembling (caused by toxoplasmosis), chronic tiredness, chronic fever, blindness (caused by cytomegalovirus retinopathy), swollen lymph glands, night sweats, white patches in the mouth and throat (called thrush), white bumps on the tongue (called oral hairy leukoplakia), and rows of painful blisters (called shingles or herpes zoster). Of course, few people with AIDS will have all of these symptoms. But clearly, experiencing the symptoms of AIDS is difficult and very unpleasant.

There are two distantly related viruses that cause AIDS: the more prevalent and more deadly HIV-1, which is found throughout the world, and the rarer and not nearly as lethal HIV-2, found mostly in West Africa. Unless indicated otherwise, when we refer to HIV in this book, we are referring only to HIV-1.

THE ORIGINS OF AIDS

It is still not known how and where AIDS originated. Most probably HIV (that is, HIV-1) evolved naturally by mutating from either another, less lethal human virus or from a virus in an animal closely related to humans, such as an ape or monkey. In the mid-1980s it was thought that HIV mutated from the type of simian immunodeficiency virus (SIV) found in African green monkeys in central Africa. Today we know that is not true. Others have thought that HIV was brought to central Africa through mass polio inoculations conducted in the 1950s. The evidence for this is believed to be inconclusive at best. Others continue to believe that HIV is not natural at all, but was somehow concocted in the 1950s at a biological warfare lab, purposely to infect gay men, Africans, Haitians, injecting drug users, and others that the "government" did not like. However, those who are familiar with the capabilities of biological warfare labs in the 1950s believe that biotechnology at that time was not advanced enough to intentionally develop something as complex as HIV.

Some critics, such as virologist Dr. Peter Duesberg and the *New York Native* (a former gay weekly publication in New York City), have gone so far as to argue that HIV does not cause AIDS. They have claimed that AIDS may be caused by some other unknown pathogen (a disease-causing agent), or by too many drugs and too much sex overburdening the immune system. But today the evidence that HIV is the cause of AIDS is overwhelming. While it is true that other biological and socio-cultural cofactors may influence the susceptibility to and the trajectory of HIV in producing AIDS, the fact that HIV is the cause of AIDS is unquestionable.

Some researchers believe that wild chimpanzees in central Africa, humans' closest relatives in the animal kingdom, are the source of HIV, but the evidence has not yet been established. Recently, work by researchers in Zambia suggests a possibility that a less deadly AIDS-like human illness common in parts of Zambia, Malawi, and maybe elsewhere in central Africa may be the source from which HIV mutated a few decades ago. More research is needed to determine whether there is any truth to this. If we find out where HIV originated, it may help in developing a vaccine and be useful in better understanding the pattern of disease spread.

In any event, it is very likely that HIV did start somewhere in sub-Saharan Africa, because there are more subtypes of the virus on that continent than anywhere else in the world, and it is likely that the presence of these ten subtypes (also called clades) suggests a more diverse pattern of viral evolution that occurred over a long period of time. There is also reason to believe that AIDS affects a greater proportion of women and children through heterosexual transmission in Africa than in North America and Europe because of the nature of these more diverse subtypes, some of which may be more readily transmissible through semen and vaginal secretions. Only subtype B is common in North America and Europe, but as the other subtypes spread throughout the world, it is possible that the same pervasiveness of heterosexual transmission that is currently seen in Africa, India, Thailand, and other developing regions may become more visible in North America and Europe. The worldwide spread of AIDS is far from over. As frightening as it sounds, we may be only at the beginning of the epidemic as the various subtypes of HIV begin to enter new geographic areas.

From the very beginning, the question of where HIV came from has been very politically charged. Bigots have used the question of the origin of AIDS to attack gays, Haitians, and Africans in order to promote their own racist or homophobic (gay-hating) agendas, attempting to have others believe that those who were first infected by the virus are somehow responsible for causing the virus. But viruses have no political agendas. They will spread and occasionally mutate when the opportunity arises, and their first casualties are no less innocent than their last casualties. Using the question of where AIDS originated to point the finger of blame at Africans or others is very destructive, mean-spirited, and absurd.

There is virtually no question, however, where HIV-2 came from. It came from the type of SIV found in sooty mangabey monkeys in West Africa, and originally spread through people's eating infected monkey meat or skinning monkeys for their pelts and handling their infected blood. HIV-2 may have spread to humans even before HIV-1 did. Although HIV-2 can readily cause AIDS, evidence suggests that many, perhaps most, persons infected with it never develop any AIDS-related symptoms. HIV-2 has found its way to Brazil, France, and other countries. But, since it is much weaker than HIV-1, it is unlikely that its impact will be comparably significant.

HOW HIV IS SPREAD

There has been a lot of misinformation about AIDS and HIV over the years. Some of this misinformation has been spread through lack of knowledge about the disease, through fear of the unknown, and even intentionally by people with certain political or religious views who would have us believe things about AIDS that are not true. Here is what we do know:

1. HIV is not easily spread.
2. The various forms of hepatitis, which spread much as HIV does, are much more contagious than HIV.
3. Although hepatitis can cause severe illness, in most instances, unlike HIV, it does not lead to death.

HIV is spread mainly in two ways:

1. Through vaginal, anal, or oral sexual intercourse with an HIV-infected person.
2. By sharing a needle with an HIV-infected person to inject (shoot) drugs, such as heroin, cocaine, speed, or anabolic steroids.

HIV can also be spread from an infected mother to her baby before, during, or after birth. Infection after birth can easily occur through breast-feeding. At the beginning of the epidemic, many persons with hemophilia (a genetic blood disorder) and people who had a blood trans-fusion were also at high risk for becoming HIV-infected. Today, how-ever, this is extremely rare in developed nations, since blood donors are carefully screened and donors' blood and blood products are tested be-fore being used.

There are other, much less common ways that HIV can be spread. It is possible, or at least theoretically possible, to become infected through the following ways:

- Directly handling blood or vomit of an HIV-infected person without wearing gloves, and having an open wound or cut on your hand.

- Joining blood with another person's blood through a blood oath, if one of the two people is HIV-positive (which means that the person has HIV).

- Biting or being bitten by someone if the person doing the biting has bleeding gums (which is common with habitual crack users) and the bite is deep enough to draw blood.

- Getting an organ transplant from an HIV-infected donor, if the organ has not been screened.

- Using a needle, drill, or other sharp implement that was previously used by or on an HIV-infected person and was not disinfected—as when getting a tattoo, or an ear pierced, or undergoing dental work or surgery. Today, however, it is routine at health care settings in developed nations for all needles, drills, and other sharp implements to be disinfected, sterilized, or disposed of.

- Failure of health care professionals, such as dentists, dental hygienists, and surgeons, to routinely use gloves and masks to prevent HIV infection from their patients.

In developing nations (most of Africa, Asia, and Latin America), HIV is more easily spread because blood products often are not screened, and needles used for inoculations or treatments by doctors, nurses, and tra-ditional healers (herbalists and shamans) may not be adequately disin-fected. There is excellent evidence from Africa that uncircumcised men who do not use condoms during sexual intercourse are twice as likely to become HIV-infected as circumcised men who do not use condoms. In tropical climates, such as parts of sub-Saharan Africa and India, where there is a greater variety of infectious microorganisms in the environ-ment, it is likely that these microorganisms may weaken the immune system, thus making persons more susceptible to HIV infection in the first place, and persons with HIV more likely to develop serious illness more quickly. And, as indicated earlier, the wider variety of HIV subtypes found in developing countries may explain the greater apparent ease of HIV transmission among heterosexuals.

HOW YOU CANNOT GET AIDS

We know that you cannot get AIDS through nonsexual physical contact. HIV is not passed through casual contact or through the air (by coughing, or sneezing). You cannot become infected with HIV by doing any of the following:

• Sitting next to someone at work, at school, on a bus, or elsewhere.

• Touching or shaking hands.

• Eating in a restaurant or a cafeteria.

• Sharing food, plates, cups, or utensils.

• Using rest rooms, water fountains, or telephones.

• Caring for a person with AIDS, as long as you follow the proper procedures.

• Donating blood (in developed nations).

• Being bitten by mosquitoes or any other insect (Department of Health and Rehabilitative Services 1988).

You can approach, touch, shake hands, hug, or kiss a person with AIDS, and have absolutely no fear of becoming HIV-infected. You can even deep-kiss a person with AIDS and not become infected with HIV, since there is an enzyme in saliva that instantly kills the virus. It is important for everyone to learn exactly what one should do and what one should not do to remain healthy and free from HIV infection.

UNPROTECTED SEX IS THE MAJOR REASON FOR THE EPIDEMIC

Sexual intercourse is the major way that HIV has spread around the world. The vast majority of persons with AIDS in the United States and in every other nation have become infected through unprotected sex. An important point to keep in mind is that most people infected with HIV look and feel perfectly healthy. People with HIV infection usually do not become noticeably sick until nearly a decade after they are first infected, yet during this period they are potentially infectious to others. Two of the times that HIV-infected persons are most infectious to others are a few weeks after they are exposed to the virus and many years later, just before developing full-blown AIDS symptoms. At such times, the infected person will appear healthy and, unless he or she has been tested for HIV, will not know that he or she is HIV-infected and infectious to others. Your sex partner or needle-sharing partner does not have to look sick to pass the virus to you. A pregnant woman may carry HIV and pass it to her baby even though she does not show any signs of illness. The best strategy is to assume that anyone you have sex with is HIV-positive, unless you are in a mutually faithful and totally monogamous relationship where both partners have been tested for HIV at the beginning and at the end of a six-month period, and remain HIV-negative. If you find a person so attractive or good-looking that you would like to have sex with her or him, remember that that person may have had unprotected sex with an HIV-infected individual who found her or him to be just as sexy.

ABSTINENCE IS A CHOICE

The surest way for teenagers to avoid HIV infection is to delay having sex. A couple of generations ago, before the birth control pill was developed, teenagers in North America and Europe usually had sex by fondling their partner (often called petting) and rarely had sexual intercourse with or without a condom, or at least the male withdrew just before ejaculating. By the 1970s and 1980s, too many teenagers were having unprotected (without a condom) vaginal (penis to vagina) and anal (penis to rectum) intercourse at earlier and earlier ages. Unwanted pregnancies and a rise in a wide array of sexually transmitted diseases were the result. Even today, with the AIDS epidemic raging, too many teenagers continue to have unprotected vaginal and anal intercourse. Studies show that only about half of all sexually active teenagers use condoms when having intercourse. Research reported in 1997, however, shows a downturn in the percentage of teenagers in the United States who have sex and an increase in the percentage of teenagers who are using condoms when they do engage in sex.

AIDS, however, is a very deceptive disease. While very few teenagers develop AIDS (0.5 percent), more than one out of six persons with AIDS are in their twenties (17.7 percent) (Centers for Disease Control and Prevention 1996). The sad reality is that most of the people with AIDS (often called PWAs) who are in their twenties were infected with HIV when they were teenagers. Pedro Zamora, of MTV fame, was a typical example: he became infected in his midteens, then became sick and died in his early twenties. Every year that you can put off starting sexual intercourse delays the possibility of your having an unwanted child, syphilis, gonorrhea, chlamydia, herpes, venereal warts, pubic lice (crabs), or HIV infection. Abstinence (not having sex) during your teen years is something to think about seriously. Even if you are already sexually active, you can become abstinent by making up your mind to do it, and sticking to it in spite of pressure from your friends. While sex is a wonderful thing, is nothing to be ashamed about, can be a very rewarding experience (especially when done with someone you love), and feels good, you should not be pressured by your partner or friends into having sex. It requires both responsibility and knowledge.

The sexual revolution of the late 1960s and early 1970s was a liberating experience for many in our society, but in this age of AIDS you should not be the youngest one on your block to be having sex. It is your decision when to start having sex, though you need to consider the views of your parents and your religion. A reasonable choice after examining all the facts might very well be to wait a few years.

THE POWER OF SAFER SEX

If you choose to have sex, you must know what you are doing and how to have safer sex. It is called "safer sex" instead of "safe sex" because there is still a small element of risk with these methods. If you have vaginal, oral (mouth to penis), or anal sex, you must always use a condom. There is a remote chance that the condom may break, fall off, or not be properly constructed, but studies have repeatedly demonstrated that condoms do work and are highly effective, and making sure that they are worn is the single most important thing a sexually active person can do to avoid becoming infected by an HIV-infected partner. (Always assume that your partner is HIV-infected!) Condoms, when used properly,[1] are also effective in preventing pregnancies and sexually transmitted diseases.

AIDS AMONG GAY MEN

From the beginning of the AIDS epidemic, gay and bisexual men in the United States and other developed nations have been much more likely to become HIV-positive than heterosexual men and women or lesbians. This was not necessarily because gay and bisexual men were having more sex than unmarried, sexually active heterosexuals or lesbians. AIDS probably spread so rapidly in the late 1970s and early 1980s in the gay male community because gay men were more likely to have unprotected sex with a different partner each time they had sex. An easy and quick way to spread a sexually transmitted disease is to have unprotected sex with a large number of different partners. Heterosexual men during that period were probably likely to have sex as often, but with far fewer different partners.

Another factor for the early spread of AIDS in the gay community is that the subtype B of HIV, which is found in North America and Europe, appears to be somewhat more easily spread through anal than through vaginal intercourse. The lining of the rectum is very delicate and more likely to undergo trauma than the vaginal wall. Today, most gay men routinely practice safer sex by using condoms during anal sex, and (to a much lesser extent) oral sex. As a result, the rate of new HIV infections among gay men has declined dramatically. However, safer sex skills need to be continually reinforced, so that gay men do not become complacent and take risks. Gay and bisexual male teens are at very high risk for HIV infection, since they may have poor self-esteem and often are not as knowledgeable about safer sex than are older gay and bisexual men. In one study of male prostitutes in Miami, many of whom are runaway youths, 62 percent tested HIV-positive. If you are a gay or bisexual male teenager and are sexually active, it is especially important for you to learn how to practice and negotiate safer sex. If there is a gay youth group in your community, find out what they are doing. Some black and Latino gay men may be less informed about safer sex practices and thus at greater risk for HIV infection.

It is not who you are, but what you do, that makes you become HIV-infected. A gay man who has one completely faithful, truly HIV-negative, totally monogamous partner can have as much sex as he wants, even without a condom, and never worry about becoming HIV-infected. Even a gay man who has many different partners, some of whom may be HIV-infected, and carefully practices safer sex each and every time, can significantly reduce his chances of ever becoming infected with HIV. Being gay does not put you at risk for AIDS; what you do puts you at risk. Lesbians who have sex only with other lesbians who do not inject drugs are at extremely low risk for acquiring HIV.

The effect of the epidemic upon gay communities throughout the world has been profound. Many gay men have watched most of their gay friends sicken and die of AIDS. Gay communities have undergone rapid social and political change in the face of the epidemic. ACT-UP is a political organization created to support AIDS activism. The gay marriage debate of the mid-1990s was fostered in part by a desire for legally recognizing monogamous unions among gay men and among lesbians. Gay men have played an important role in the arts, literature, the entertainment industry, and other creative domains. There is no way to determine what effect the loss of so many gay men to AIDS will ultimately have upon our society.

AIDS AND INJECTING DRUG USERS

After gay men, the second largest group of people infected with HIV in most developed nations is injecting drug users. They become infected not from the drugs themselves but from using needles and syringes that contain HIV-infected blood from a previous user. In states where it is illegal to buy a needle or syringe without a prescription, drug users resort to renting their "works" (the needle, syringe, cooker, and cotton) at "shooting galleries" or "get-off houses" (places where people go to shoot drugs and get high). In those states where clean needles and syringes are not generally available, HIV infection rates tend to be much higher than in those states where they are legal and available.

Again, it is not being an injecting drug user that makes you susceptible to HIV. The risk comes from using infected needles and syringes when shooting drugs. It is not who you are, but what you do and how you do it that causes AIDS. An injecting drug user who is sexually abstinent and shoots drugs with his or her own uninfected equipment every day may die of an overdose or some other health-related problem, but will not get AIDS. If you shoot drugs, seek help to stop. Go to a drug treatment center. If you cannot stop at this time, make certain that your needle, syringe, cooker, and cotton are clean (not used by anyone else or disinfected with bleach). If there is a needle exchange program in your area, use it.

HETEROSEXUAL TRANSMISSION OF HIV

Although they are still a minority of those infected with HIV in the United States, heterosexual men and women are becoming infected today at a more rapid pace than either gay men or injecting drug users. Inner-city African-Americans, Caribbean blacks, and some Latino populations have been most affected. HIV-positive men infect their female sex partners, who in turn infect their newborn infants. About one-fourth of all children born to HIV-infected mothers will remain HIV-positive, unless the pregnant mother is treated with AZT (a common drug that attacks HIV). Virtually all new HIV infections spread heterosexually (between men and women) occur from not properly wearing a condom during vaginal or anal sex.

The problem of heterosexual AIDS transmission in the United States is nowhere near the level that it has reached in parts of the developing world, and it is unlikely that it will become so in the near future. Indeed, in rural parts of the upper Midwest and Great Plains states, heterosexually transmitted HIV remains very rare. But for heterosexuals who live in places like New York City, northeastern New Jersey, South Florida, Baltimore, Washington, D.C., Puerto Rico, and several other metropolitan areas in and around the United States and even some rural areas of the southeastern states, safer sex practices (including condom use) are an absolute must. More than one in twelve AIDS cases (8.6 percent) are the result of heterosexual contact. An additional 1.3 percent of AIDS cases are among children under the age of thirteen (Centers for Disease Control and Prevention 1996).

Heterosexual transmission of HIV is extremely common in central and eastern Africa. In some of the major cities of Uganda, Rwanda, Burundi,

Zambia, and Malawi, three out of every ten adults are infected with HIV. Death and funerals have become an everyday occurrence. AIDS has had a profound effect upon the social fabric of central and eastern African daily life. Millions of men, women, and children have already died from the disease. Millions more remain ill because the kinds of expensive treatments available in North America and Europe are not available to most in Africa. And millions of children born to HIV-infected parents, but who themselves are HIV-negative, have become orphaned and often homeless, living in the streets of large African cities.

Unlike some of the developed nations, where the HIV epidemic appears to have stabilized at a constant growth rate in the mid-1990s, the epidemic in developing nations shows no signs of peaking or stabilizing in the near future. Indeed, in places like India and elsewhere in Asia, it appears to be on the verge of exploding, making the devastating numbers of infected that we have seen in Africa pale by comparison.

HIV TESTING

If you are sexually active and have not yet been tested for HIV, you should consider being tested. If it turns out that you are HIV-negative, it will give you some peace of mind and confirm that your safer sex practices have been successful. While there are a very few people who appear to be immune from getting infected with HIV, do not assume that you are one of them. It is more likely that you are HIV-negative because of your safer sex practices or because you are lucky. Learning that you are HIV-negative is not a reason for you to let your guard down.

If it turns out that you are HIV-positive, here are some things that you will need to do:

- Give yourself time to work through your feelings.
- Learn all you can about living with HIV and about treatments.
- Find a support group—there are many people who can help.
- You are not alone—turn to your parents, partner, friends, and AIDS organizations.
- Stay healthy: eat healthy foods, get enough rest, exercise regularly, reduce stress, avoid using alcohol and other drugs, be active.
- Find a doctor or clinic experienced in treating people with HIV (Department of Health and Rehabilitative Services 1995).

Today, people with HIV and AIDS in developed nations are living longer than ever before. Today, the search for better treatments and possibly even a cure seems very promising. The new protease inhibitors are unquestionably prolonging lives of many who would have died without them. Newer drugs are likely to be even more effective. AIDS is becoming less of a terminal illness and more of a chronic illness, like diabetes. Remember, your life is not over until it's over! The good news today is that an HIV-positive diagnosis is no longer necessarily a death sentence.

AIDS, ETHICS, AND VALUES

The emergence of AIDS at the end of the twentieth century has tested the humanity of humankind. The results so far have been mixed. Some have used the epidemic to perpetuate their prejudices against groups of people that they never liked. Some have used AIDS to justify their discrimination against certain people. Some have opportunistically claimed that AIDS is the product of God's wrath, second-guessing God's true intentions.

Others, however, have demonstrated their compassion for persons with AIDS by giving generously of their time, effort, and money to support funding for AIDS research and assisting with AIDS care. They have participated in a wide variety of fund-raising events; have become AIDS buddies (helping and befriending a PWA); have manned HIV hot lines; have marched in AIDS walks; have called, written to, and visited their political representatives to convince them to support AIDS programs funded by the federal, state, and city governments; have demonstrated with ACT-UP and other political groups for AIDS-related issues; have served as caregivers for a family member, spouse, or loved one with AIDS; have kept themselves fully informed about HIV and AIDS; have delivered meals to needy PWAs; have seen the spectacular AIDS quilt firsthand; and have joined in World AIDS Day events and candlelight vigils. They are the true heroes of our time; you can become one, too, by getting involved with your local AIDS organization.

ABOUT THIS BOOK

The AIDS Crisis: A Documentary History is designed to give the reader a comprehensive perspective of the social, cultural, psychological, historical, political, economic, and biomedical aspects of AIDS in the United States and on a global level, by presenting the original texts from primary documents and key secondary sources. This book can either be read from cover to cover or used as a reference tool, by using the table of contents and the index. Each chapter begins with a short introduction, followed by edited passages from various sources. Each passage is introduced with a header note that describes what the passage will be about or sets the scene for some of the issues highlighted in the passage. The edited passages come from primary documents, such as government publications, or from secondary sources, such as newspaper and magazine articles. Ellipses indicate that some of the original text of the document or article has been deleted. A word or phrase in square brackets means that the text in a reading was changed for greater clarity or to make it easier to read. The source of the reading is given at its end. It is important to note the publication year of the source in order to determine how current the information is. Some documents are mostly of historic interest. Additional suggested readings are included at the end of each chapter. A glossary of common AIDS terms, a resource directory of selected AIDS organizations, and an index are included at the back of the book.

Chapter 1 ("The History of HIV/AIDS") includes readings on the origin of HIV and AIDS, how the epidemic emerged in society, and how public opinion was shaped through the media. Chapter 2 ("The Impact of the Epidemic") describes the situation in the United States and globally, and has readings on the way in which the epidemic has been taking its toll. Chapter 3 ("HIV/AIDS Within Communities and Populations") discusses HIV/AIDS among teenagers, women, children, injecting drug users, gay men, commercial sex workers (prostitutes), the homeless, prisoners, and persons with hemophilia.

Chapter 4 ("AIDS in the Developing World") describes the growing crisis in sub-Saharan Africa, much of Asia, and Latin America and the Caribbean. Chapter 5 ("The Human Side of AIDS") discusses HIV/AIDS from the perspective of persons with HIV/AIDS; the psychosocial needs of PWAs; the role of their families, partners (spouses and lovers), and friends; and the role of health care providers and caregivers. Chapter 6 ("The Politics of AIDS") details how communities have responded to AIDS, and how both activism and apathy have affected the politics of AIDS.

Chapter 7 ("Education and Behavioral Change") includes readings on how to promote awareness of and education about HIV prevention and AIDS, and how to produce desired behavioral change among people at risk for HIV infection. Chapter 8 ("Legal and Ethical Issues") discusses AIDS, the workplace, and the law, as well as important ethical issues for HIV/AIDS policy. Chapter 9 ("The Future of AIDS") looks ahead to see what we might anticipate about HIV/AIDS in the coming years.

THE GLOBAL PERSPECTIVE

About 90 percent of the people in the world who are HIV-positive live in the developing nations, mostly poor countries where anti-viral drugs for AIDS usually do not exist. While most of this volume is focused on AIDS in the United States, only about 4 percent of persons with HIV live in the United States. In Africa and Asia, where most of the people with AIDS reside, HIV has been transmitted primarily through heterosexual sex. Unmarried women become infected by having unprotected sex with HIV-positive men. These infected unmarried women have sex, sometimes for small amounts of money or token gifts, with married men, who also become infected. The married men then have sex with their wives, who become infected and sometimes pass the virus on to their children. Since the late 1970s, tens of millions of men, women, and children throughout the world have become infected this way.

Today, in remote villages in Uganda, Thailand, Senegal, Botswana, and elsewhere, people are learning how to use condoms and how to care for a relative dying of AIDS. Some governments have been very progressive about HIV education, putting public health concerns first, while more politically repressive governments have been very reluctant to induce any kind of behavioral change among their populace, since it might adversely impact upon traditional values and culture. Some governments have respected the rights of people with HIV/AIDS and have prevented discrimination; other governments have condemned people with HIV/AIDS as criminals and sinners, denying them their basic human rights.

Much has been done to promote HIV education, stop AIDS discrimination, and assist with AIDS-related health and support services on an international level. The World Health Organization, the United Nations Children's Fund, AIDSCAP (funded by the United States Agency for International Development), and other public agencies and private foundations have spent many hundreds of millions of dollars fighting AIDS in Africa, Asia, and Latin America. Yet, the total amount spent on AIDS in the developing (poorer) nations is a small fraction of what has been spent in the developed (richer) nations. Very often, the programs that have been put into place have not been developed with either the leadership or the assistance of applied or medical anthropologists (professionals trained in cross-cultural applied health research), and frequently have been ineffective or wasteful as a result.

THE SOCIAL ASPECTS OF AIDS IN THE UNITED STATES

This volume looks closely at the social, political, psychological, economic, cultural, and historical aspects of AIDS and HIV, especially in the United States. Other books are available that focus upon the biological, clinical, and medical aspects of AIDS and HIV. The topics in this volume are quite diverse, to interest the reader in a wide variety of questions about AIDS. For example, how did the media shape public opinion about AIDS? What are the ten principles of AIDS in the workplace? Should marijuana be legalized for medicinal use in the treatment of AIDS? If education is necessary but not sufficient to change risky sexual behavior, what will work? Did ACT-UP have any effect on changing AIDS policies?

What is the purpose of an AIDS service organization? What rights are guaranteed under the Americans with Disabilities Act for persons with AIDS? What is it like to be gay and HIV-positive? Should free condoms be given out in the high schools? What is the prospect for an AIDS vaccine in the near future? What can injecting drug users do to prevent HIV infection? What are the psychosocial needs of persons with AIDS? What are the economic costs of AIDS? When did political activism against AIDS reach a peak in the United States? Why? What should be done about AIDS in our prisons and jails? Are the homeless at greater risk for AIDS? What can be done? What is an AIDS buddy? Is a health care professional obligated to care for a person with HIV? How has AIDS changed and affected our society? What would America be like today if AIDS never happened? These are just some of the questions that this volume will attempt to answer.

A strong focus of this book will be upon the historical development of AIDS from its first recognition in 1981 to the present. The edited selections use the original words of various authors to give you a sense of the issues, and sometimes the drama, about AIDS facing the world at the time they were written. Looking back, we can perhaps see within these thoughts a concise blueprint for where we now need to be heading.

NOTE

1. To use a condom properly: use a water-based (not an oil-based) lubricant; hold the tip of the condom when putting it on to ensure that no air gets into it; use a lubricated condom with nonoxydol-9 spermicide for vaginal or anal sex; use a non-lubricated or flavored condom for oral sex; never reuse a condom; do not store condoms in a hot location; and hold on to the condom at the base when withdrawing the penis after sex.

REFERENCES CITED

Centers for Disease Control and Prevention. *HIV/AIDS Surveillance Report*, 8 (2): 1–39. Atlanta: U.S. Department of Health and Human Services, 1996.
Department of Health and Rehabilitative Services, State of Florida. *About AIDS and Shooting Drugs*. South Deerfield, Mass.: Channing L. Bete, 1988.
Department of Health and Rehabilitative Services, State of Florida. *About Living with HIV*. South Deerfield, Mass.: Channing L. Bete, 1995.

The AIDS Crisis

1

The History of HIV/AIDS

THE ORIGIN OF HIV/AIDS

No one knows for certain how AIDS, or HIV, first began. From the very start of the epidemic, there has been considerable speculation about where the disease, and the virus, originated. Some people have theorized that it began in rural Haiti and spread to urban Haiti, and then to gay men in the United States and to Africans in Kinshasa, Zaire (the capital of that central African nation), where many Haitians were living. This theory is no longer accepted, since HIV research in rural Haiti shows that HIV was very rare there, and that it has been spreading from urban Haiti to rural Haiti, not the other way around. HIV in the late 1970s and early 1980s was more likely to have spread into Haiti from gay men coming from the United States to bisexual male Haitians, and from HIV-infected Haitian men and women returning from Zaire to persons living in Haiti.

There have been a lot of unusual theories attempting to explain the origin of AIDS. Some have argued that AIDS and HIV have been around for thousands of years and we are simply seeing a reemergence of the scourge. We know from reading the hieroglyphics (pictorial words) on the temple and pyramid walls of ancient Egypt that the Egyptians of nearly five thousand years ago had a similar epidemic where people mysteriously died of immunosuppressive (weakening the immune system) disorders very much like what we see today in AIDS patients. But today we know that HIV mutates very rapidly, changing about 1 percent each year. It is likely that throughout human history, infectious diseases that were highly virulent and immunosuppressive emerged, killing many thousands, and then subsided. A virus that weakens the immune system opens the way for the same kinds of opportunistic infections and cancers that occur in people with AIDS. In other words, the disease would be AIDS-like but not AIDS itself, caused by an HIV-like agent but not HIV itself.

Some have claimed that HIV was artificially created in a biological warfare laboratory and purposely released in the population to kill off gay men, injecting drug users, Haitians, and Africans. Near the end of the Cold War in the mid-1980s, the then Soviet Union went so far as to claim that HIV was invented and released just for that purpose from a biological warfare lab in Maryland. The United States Department of State spent much time and effort to counter that argument around the world, insisting there was no truth to the allegation. But could it have happened? The evidence makes it appear highly unlikely. We know for certain that HIV has been around since at least the 1950s, maybe even earlier. While today there are perhaps a dozen nations in the world with biological warfare laboratories, in the 1950s there were only four countries with such labs: the United States, France, Great Britain, and the Soviet Union.

At the height of the Cold War in the early and mid-1950s, both the United States and the Soviet Union were doing things that placed large segments of their own populations at serious risk. For instance, in the early 1950s a virus was purposely released into the New York City subway to see how it would affect the commuter population. Fortunately, the study failed; few people, if any, were affected. Thousands of Soviet soldiers were killed by intentionally exposing them to nuclear radiation during atomic bomb testing. However, experts agree that while there may have been the desire to do so, no one had the technological sophistication at that time to artificially create a retrovirus anything like HIV and then intentionally and successfully release it into the population, targeting specifically high-risk populations. A remote possibility exists that HIV may have been accidentally created during failed research with simian immunodeficiency virus (SIV), a retrovirus that affects some apes and monkeys, and unintentionally released into the population through infection of one of the biological researchers who may have been gay. But there is no way of proving this to be either true or untrue over forty years later, and the evidence for a natural origin of HIV in Africa appears to be much stronger.

Some have argued that HIV was introduced to Africa during massive vaccinations against polio in Africa during the 1950s. The problem with this theory is that if that were so, we would expect to find HIV extremely prevalent in stored blood samples from Africa in the 1950s. In one very well-documented study of stored blood from the then Belgian Congo (now Zaire) in 1959, out of a sample of 818 blood samples, only one had confirmed HIV. While this tells us that HIV was clearly in Africa in the late 1950s, the massive polio vaccination theory does not hold up because more people were not infected at that time. Research reported in 1998 confirms that at least one person had already died from AIDS in 1959.

Others have argued that HIV is not the cause of AIDS at all, and that billions of dollars have been wasted trying to understand a virus that does not cause AIDS. The very earliest explanation, in 1981, of why gay men were becoming ill with this new syndrome was the "overload theory." This theory stated that sexually active gay men had been infected with so many different microorganisms that their immune systems were overloaded, causing them to break down or "overload." Indeed, throughout the late 1970s and early 1980s gay men increasingly were developing intestinal parasites through sexual exposure, and it is now known that some of these pathogens will weaken the immune system.

In 1983, a year before HIV was first reported as the cause of AIDS, there were many other theories attempting to explain what might be causing this emerging and rapidly spreading epidemic. One of the many theories espoused at the time was put forward by Jane Teas, a microbiologist, who said AIDS was caused by African swine fever virus (not to be confused with African swine flu virus, which is different). African swine fever virus (ASFV) is spread through pigs and goats in central Africa and Haiti. The pattern of its spread seems to closely parallel the spread of HIV where it has occurred. The largest and most influential gay newspaper in New York City during the 1980s, the *New York Native*, ran major editorials insisting that ASFV, not HIV, is the real cause of AIDS, and accused the Centers for Disease Control and Prevention (CDC) and the National Institutes of Health (NIH) of a massive cover-up.

In the late 1980s, Peter Duesberg, a prominent researcher, argued that HIV is not the cause of AIDS. Instead, sexual "promiscuity" and recreational drug use were the causes. This explanation was similar to, but different from, the overload theory, arguing that many behavioral factors, instead of biological factors, were responsible for the epidemic. Some people argued that poverty was directly responsible for spreading AIDS, and that environmental factors (rather than a virus) explained the rapid spread of AIDS in poor areas of the world such as central Africa. Those who claim that HIV is not the cause of AIDS often point to the erratic trajectory of HIV in the world, to the fact that the disease spreads more rapidly in some areas of the world and more slowly in other areas, and to the slow pace of the retrovirus (it does not proliferate rapidly throughout the human body).

However, the nature of a retrovirus such as HIV is that it does proliferate slowly throughout the body and that it is not necessary for the virus to be found in large quantities in organs and human tissue for it to do its damage. The major reason why we know for certain that HIV is the cause, or at least the primary cause, of AIDS is that throughout the world all (or at least nearly all) of those who develop AIDS-related illness are HIV-positive. In other words, HIV is (with a few rare exceptions) a necessary condition occurring before the onset of AIDS. Where HIV appears, AIDS usually follows. The global occurrence of HIV and of AIDS is virtually identical.

Certainly, more research is needed to find out what cofactors may be responsible for making people more likely to become infected with HIV following exposure, and more likely to develop symptoms sooner once they are HIV-infected. It is possible that ASFV, other viruses, intestinal parasites, bacteria, or other pathogenic (disease-producing) agents may be responsible for making some people more susceptible to HIV or for making HIV-infected people sicker sooner. Recent research suggests that HIV may not cause immunosuppression itself, but may cause nutritional deficiencies that cause the immune system to weaken. Also, some people may have stronger immune systems than others because of genetic differences.

Some theologians and politicians from the political right have asserted that HIV is not the reason why people get AIDS. They get AIDS because they have sinned, and this is God's punishment against them. They maintain that homosexuality is a sin and that AIDS is a sign of God's wrath. But other theologians have pointed out that if that were true, it would mean that God must then favor lesbians above all others, since among sexually active populations they are the least likely to contract AIDS or other sexually transmitted diseases. These other theologians also argue that God placed AIDS in the world to test our compassion and willingness to care for our fellow human beings. From a scientific view, there is no question today that HIV causes AIDS and that it is spread through unprotected sexual activity, through blood, and during birth.

The most prevalent theory has been that AIDS and HIV started naturally in Africa. In the mid-1980s it was thought that the common African green monkey was the culprit, infecting humans through bites, scratches, being skinned, and being eaten by some African populations. We now know that the African green monkey is not the cause of HIV, since the monkey retrovirus that it carries (SIV) is only very remotely related to HIV found in central Africa. Actually, as we have already discussed in the Introduction, there are two kinds of HIV in Africa: HIV-1, the more common AIDS-related virus found throughout the world, including central Africa; and HIV-2, found mostly in West Africa. Recent research shows that the SIV found in sooty mangabeys (a kind of monkey in West Africa) is virtually identical to HIV-2 in humans in West Africa. There is also some speculation that the virus found in wild chimpanzees in central Africa may be closely related to HIV-1.

There are ten clades (families of viral strains) of HIV-1 in the world today. While the United States has only one predominant clade, Africa has all ten. This suggests either that the virus is mutating more rapidly in Africa, or that it originated there and has had more time to become diversified. More research is needed in the microevolution of HIV clades. The rapid proliferation of AIDS throughout central Africa appears to have occurred during the 1970s, and those who have argued that AIDS is an ancient, very common disease throughout Africa are clearly wrong. Studies of stored blood, interviews with traditional healers, and medical chart reviews from health clinics demonstrate without doubt that AIDS as a widespread phenomenon is new to Africa. However, recent evidence from Zambia indicates that a local sexually transmissible disease called *kaliondeonde* may have been an AIDS-like precursor for generations in Zambia and Malawi, possibly caused by a milder, less lethal virus that was the precursor to HIV-1. Research is needed to find out if this is true. Though it is likely that HIV began naturally somewhere in the vast continent of Africa, the evidence has not yet been found. The origin of HIV and AIDS still remains a mystery.

The question of the origin of AIDS has been a very sensitive one. Some maintain that even suggesting that it originated in Africa is racist. They point to the discrimination that has occurred against Africans and Haitians, who were stigmatized as the source of HIV and blamed for its spread. Indeed, much of the early speculation in the popular press about the origin of AIDS in Africa and Haiti was very racist. There was nonsensical talk about Africans having sex with monkeys and "promiscuity" as the reasons why it was spreading in Africa. The truth is that if it did begin in Africa, Africans cannot be held responsible for its spread. There is no reason to believe that the average African is any more sexually active than the average American, and Africans certainly do not have sex with monkeys. If AIDS began in Africa, the tropical and subtropical climate there is likely to be to blame, since we know that diseases tend to proliferate in such climates more easily than they do in more moderate climates.

Even if we can pinpoint the first person to have become infected with HIV, it is certain that that person had no idea that he or she had become infected or how it had happened. It could have happened to anyone. Blaming the sufferer is not going to solve the problem. However, the search for the origin of HIV may be useful, since it may lead us to an effective vaccine to combat the illness. Africa is a huge continent covering 20 percent of the Earth's land surface, with hundreds of human cultures and over 900 million men, women, and children.

By 1997, 20 million of the 900 million Africans had become infected with HIV. Pointing the finger of blame either at all Africans or at those who have become HIV-positive makes no sense at all.

DOCUMENT 1: AIDS Is Perfectly Natural

Writing at a time when it was seriously thought that AIDS might infect virtually everyone and cause the deaths of about 1.5 billion humans (now we believe that the pandemic has the capacity to cause the deaths of perhaps 200 or 300 million people around the globe in the early twenty-first century), famed biologist Stephen Jay Gould places AIDS within the context of natural processes and biological evolution.

AIDS represents the ordinary workings of biology, not an irrational or diabolical plague with moral meaning. Disease, including epidemic spread, is a natural phenomenon, part of human history from the beginning. . . . AIDS must be viewed as a virulent expression of an ordinary natural phenomenon. . . . Yes, AIDS may run through the entire population, and may carry off a quarter or more of us . . . but there will still be plenty of us left and we can start again. Evolution cares as little for its agents . . . as physics cares for individual atoms of hydrogen in the sun. But *we* care. These atoms are our neighbors, our lovers, our children and ourselves. AIDS is both a natural phenomenon and, potentially, the greatest natural tragedy in human history.

Source: Stephen Jay Gould, "The Terrifying Normalcy of AIDS," *The New York Times Magazine* 136, p. 32 (April 19, 1987).

DOCUMENT 2: AIDS as an Emerging Infection

The discoverer of HIV, French scientist Luc Montagnier, suggests that HIV is merely the first of many viruses to plague humankind in the present and near future. Clearly, we need to be on the lookout for these new viruses, against which (like HIV) we would have no immunity.

The AIDS virus's complexity shows that it has undergone an arduous process of selection. With nine genes, it's the most complex retrovirus known to man. . . . I would have to say [that I was surprised by the emergence of AIDS.] But epidemiologists have known for a long time that we're vulnerable to new epidemics. The same civilization that created the AIDS epidemic could create others, with infectious agents even more virulent. We haven't exhausted all the germs in our tissue capable of being transmitted by sexual relations. The greatest danger lies in nonconventional viruses that produce no immune reaction. . . . Our civilization is in the process of selecting the successful germs of the future— those capable of escaping detection by the immune system. . . . If any time remains for me after AIDS, this is what I hope to work on next.

Source: "Interview: Luc Montagnier," *Omni* 11(3): 102ff–134 (December 1988).

DOCUMENT 3: Just Another Great Plague?

Epidemics are certainly nothing new in human history. Plagues have altered the course of world history, and have had a profound effect upon the cultural evolution of humankind. Jonathan E. Kaplan places AIDS within this context while emphasizing the particularly insidious nature of HIV.

To those under thirty, AIDS must seem a wholly new phenomenon, but epidemics have always been with us. In our early history, smallpox decimated Indian populations, and in colonial times, yellow fever and cholera periodically wreaked havoc in the cities. Influenza killed 500,000 in the United States in the winter of 1918/19; and in the early 1950's polio increased . . . before the Salk vaccine effectively halted the epidemic at mid-decade. Other infectious diseases have played important roles in world history: typhus determined the outcomes of military campaigns; plague killed one-fourth of the population of Europe in the late fourteenth century.

AIDS . . . has already proved itself a formidable member of this elite group of epidemic diseases. AIDS destroys the immune system and renders the victim susceptible to a variety of unusual infections and tumors. . . . [In addition, there are] special properties of the virus that set it apart from other epidemic-causing agents in history. . . . [It] appears extraordinarily well adapted to human blood lymphocytes, specifically to a subpopulation of these cells called T-helper cells, which serve as orchestrators of the immune system . . . it does not appear to be confined to blood lymphocytes . . . [but] finds its way into the brain . . . [and] it does not lend itself easily to the creation of a vaccine.

Source: Jonathan E. Kaplan, "A Modern-Day Plague," *Natural History* 95(2): 28–33 (February 1986).

DOCUMENT 4: The Origins of the AIDS Virus

If HIV did mutate naturally from animals to humans, monkeys and apes are the most likely candidates because they are so closely related to humans. HIV-2, the less widespread of the two AIDS-related viruses, found mostly in western Africa, is now known to be virtually identical to SIV of one species of monkeys. An understanding of the natural history and possible origins of HIV-1 and HIV-2 is potentially important for vaccine development.

One way to begin searching out the origin of HIV is to look for similar viruses in nonhuman primates. . . . Monkeys and apes are often the only animal species . . . that are infected with important human viruses. . . . The search for monkey viruses related to HIV had a precedent in the discovery of a primate counterpart of another human retrovirus. . . . The simian virus was found to infect both Asian and African Old World monkeys and apes. . . . [W]e [were successful] in finding . . . antibodies— and hence evidence of the presence of a monkey virus related to HIV—in blood samples from Asian macaques [but subsequently learned] that SIV did not naturally infect Asian monkeys in the wild. . . . [Our research ultimately found that] people in West Africa were infected with a retro-virus different from the one infecting people in central Africa, Europe and the U.S., and that the West African virus was more closely related to SIV than to HIV. . . .

[I]t appears likely that some species of monkeys, and perhaps some people, have already evolved protective mechanisms that keep certain HIV's and SIV's from causing lethal disease. . . . [T]he origin and history of the AIDS viruses themselves may provide the very information that is critical to the prevention and control of AIDS.

Source: Max Essex and Phyllis J. Kanki, "The Origins of the AIDS Virus," *Scientific American* 259, pp. 67–71 (1988).

DOCUMENT 5: AIDS Is a Product of the "Global Village"

Susan Sontag correctly points out that the world is getting smaller and that viruses can be transmitted around the world very easily. Whatever social and physical isolation of human populations existed in the past is now largely gone.

Like the effects of industrial pollution and the new system of global financial markets, the AIDS crisis is evidence of a world in which nothing important is regional, local, limited; in which everything that can circulate does, and every problem is, or is destined to become, worldwide. Goods circulate (including images and sounds and documents . . .). Garbage circulates: the poisonous industrial wastes of . . . [European cities] are being dumped in the coastal towns of West Africa. People circulate, in greater numbers than ever. And diseases. From the untrammeled intercontinental air travel for pleasure and business of the privileged to the unprecedented migrations of the underprivileged from villages to cities and, legally and illegally, from country to country—and this physical mobility and interconnectedness with its consequent dissolving of old taboos (social and sexual), is as vital to the maximum functioning of the advanced . . . economy as is the easy transmissibility of goods and images and financial instruments. But now that heightened modern interconnectedness . . . is the bearer of a health menace. . . . AIDS is one of the . . . [products] of the global village.

Source: Susan Sontag, *AIDS and Its Metaphors* (New York: Farrar, Straus, Giroux, 1989), pp. 92, 93.

DOCUMENT 6: The Evolution of AIDS

This article argues that AIDS may be an old disease that has recently become more widespread and more lethal. It is possible that the disease existed in a relatively remote population for decades or centuries, and then (with the rise of modern transportation, increasing urbanization, and other factors that promote the spread of sexually transmitted diseases) began to infect people outside of its ecosystem with no resistance to it.

HIV may not be a new and inherently deadly virus . . . but an old one that has recently acquired deadly tendencies. . . . Paul Ewald, an environmental biologist at Amherst College, argues that HIV may have infected people benignly for decades, even centuries, before it started causing AIDS. He traces its virulence to the social upheavals of the 1960's and '70's, which not only sped its movement through populations but rewarded it for reproducing more aggressively within the body. . . . Starting in the 1960's, war, tourism and commercial trucking forced the outside world on Africa's once isolated villages. At the same time, drought and industrialization prompted mass migrations from the countryside into newly teeming cities. . . . [The newly created urban environment brought increases in prostitution, venereal disease, and the use of hypodermic needles.] Did these trends actually turn a chronic but relatively benign infection into a killer? The evidence is circumstantial, but it's hard to discount.

Source: Geoffrey Cowley, "The Future of AIDS," *Newsweek* 121(12): 46–52 (March 22, 1993).

DOCUMENT 7: HIV: Natural or Man-made?

The author briefly explores two popular theories to explain the origin of AIDS. While it may prove very beneficial to learn how the virus originated, no group of people should be blamed for being the source of the virus.

We do not know where and how AIDS originated . . . [b]ut let us briefly explore two possible scenarios. Scenario one: it is the 1950's and we are in a biological warfare laboratory. . . . An experimental retrovirus, later to be named human immunodeficiency virus . . . is manufactured using an existing animal retrovirus as a model. Something goes terribly wrong. The virus escapes and gradually makes its way through sexual relations, infected needles, and blood transfusions to diverse at-risk populations in different parts of the world.

In scenario two, simian immunodeficiency virus (SIV) mutates into human immunodeficiency virus, type two (HIV-2), perhaps from blood contamination while skinning an infected monkey, possibly in a remote West African village many decades ago. This now human retrovirus rapidly evolves, and as it inadvertently spreads through sexual transmission into new tribal populations . . . it takes on a more aggressive and lethal character. . . . [T]he virus spreads rapidly from city to city throughout central Africa, into Haiti and among gay men in North America.

Perhaps there are other equally viable scenarios. One can always speculate. But speculation . . . has already caused much consternation, distress, and harm . . . AIDS is a stigmatized and stigmatizing disease and . . . is perceived to pollute everyone and everything. . . . The truth . . . however, is . . . [that] [r]etroviruses do not have morals. They move through human populations without conscious intent. If HIV-1 did originate somewhere in Africa, or North America, or Europe, or Asia, or elsewhere, it spread from person to person without anyone aware of its lethal direction. There is no blame to share for the early spread of the disease because no one is guilty.

Source: Douglas A. Feldman, "Introduction," in D. A. Feldman, ed., *Culture and AIDS* (Westport, Conn.: Praeger, 1990), pp. 1–7.

DOCUMENT 8: The Evidence That HIV Causes AIDS

Since what is now known as HIV was publicly proclaimed the cause of AIDS in 1984, skeptics have attacked this idea. They argue that we have been fighting the wrong cause of AIDS all these years. However, today the evidence that HIV causes AIDS is overwhelming and unquestionable.

- Before the appearance of HIV, AIDS-like syndromes were rare; today, they are common in HIV-infected individuals.
- AIDS and HIV infection are invariably linked in time, place and population group.
- The main risk factors for AIDS—sexual contact between men and between men and women, transfusions, treatment for hemophilia and needle-sharing during injection-drug use—have existed for years, increasing only in a relative sense in recent years.
- Many studies agree that only a single factor, HIV, predicts whether a person will develop AIDS.
- Numerous serosurveys [blood-testing surveys] show that AIDS is common in populations where many individuals have HIV antibodies [test positive for HIV]. Conversely, in populations with low seroprevalence [blood-tested rates] of HIV antibodies, AIDS is extremely rare.
- In cohort studies [research with groups of similar people], severe immunosuppression [weakening of the immune system] and AIDS-defining illnesses occur exclusively in individuals who are HIV-infected.
- The specific immunologic profile [characteristics of a person's immune system] that typifies AIDS—a persistently low CD4+ T cell count [the helper cells that fight off infections]—is extraordinarily rare in the absence of HIV infection or other known cause of immunosuppression.
- Nearly everyone with AIDS has antibodies [a blood protein produced as a response to a molecule introduced into the body] to HIV.
- HIV can be detected in virtually everyone with AIDS.
- HIV fulfills Koch's postulates as the cause of AIDS. Koch's postulates of disease causation [say] that an infectious agent must be found in all cases of the disease, the agent must be isolated from the host's body, the agent must cause disease when injected into healthy hosts, and the same agent must once again be isolated from the newly diseased host.
- Newborn infants have no behavioral risk factors, yet [thousands of] children in the United States developed AIDS. . . .

- The HIV-infected twin develops AIDS while the uninfected twin does not.
- Since the appearance of HIV, mortality [the death rate] has increased dramatically among [persons with hemophilia].
- Studies of transfusion-acquired AIDS cases have repeatedly led to the discovery of HIV in the patient as well as in the blood donor.
- Sex partners of HIV-infected [persons with hemophilia] and transfusion recipients acquire the virus and develop AIDS without other risk factors.
- HIV infects and is responsible for the death of CD4+ T lymphocytes [the helper T cells] *in vitro* [in laboratory studies] and *in vivo* [in studies with human subjects].
- HIV damages the body's sources of CD4+ T cells and centers of immune activity.
- Studies of HIV-infected people show that increasing amounts of HIV in the body correlate [are associated] with the progression of the immunologic processes [the weakening of immune system] that leads to AIDS.
- HIV is similar in genetic structure and morphology [form] to other lentiviruses [slow-acting viruses] that often cause immunodeficiency in their animal hosts in addition to slow, progressive wasting disorders, neurodegeneration [weakening of the functions of the brain and nervous system] and death.
- Baboons develop AIDS after inoculation with [HIV-2]. . . .
- Asian monkeys develop AIDS after infection with the simian immunodeficiency virus (SIV), a virus closely related to [HIV-2].

Source: The Evidence That HIV Causes AIDS, booklet (Bethesda, Md.: National Institute of Allergy and Infectious Diseases, National Institutes of Health, July 1995).

DOCUMENT 9: A Cofactor Cause of an AIDS-Related Cancer?

Kaposi's sarcoma (KS) is a disfiguring cancer that shows up in purplish or brown blotches on some persons with AIDS. It usually occurs on the arms and legs, but can appear on the face or other parts of the body. It may even become extremely invasive, attacking the internal organs. Untreated, KS can be very deadly to persons with AIDS. For many years, it was suspected that nitrite drugs ("poppers")—an inhalant aphrodisiac drug used frequently by some gay men—might play a role in causing KS. But this association has never been causally established. Now there appears to be new evidence that the reason gay men are more likely to develop KS than women or heterosexual men is a sexually transmissible virus called human herpesvirus 8. This theory would certainly explain why some gay men with KS do not have HIV. However, even if this is a causal factor in promoting KS, it does not necessarily rule out the possibility that "poppers" may play a contributory role in the development of this deadly cancer.

Kaposi's sarcoma (KS) is the most common neoplasm [cancer] among AIDS patients and is 20,000 times more common in this group than in the general population. Incidence of KS varies widely among those infected with HIV, however, and it is also found in some HIV-negative groups, suggesting the disease is not caused only by HIV. A sexually transmitted cofactor is thought to be involved in the disease's pathogenicity [deadly spread], but efforts to link KS with recognized sexually transmitted agents have been unsuccessful. Don Ganem, of the University of California at San Francisco and the Howard Hughes Medical Institute, and colleagues used an immunofluorescence assay [testing method] they developed to evaluate serum samples from 913 patients for the presence of an antibody for human herpesvirus 8 (HHV8), a virus identified in KS tissues. They report that the distribution of HHV8 they found is strongly suggestive of sexual transmission and that within different HIV-infected groups, the distribution of HHV8 seropositivity parallels the relative risk for KS. The authors say their results support the theory that HHV8 is the sexually transmitted cofactor involved in the epidemiology of KS.

Source: Dean H. Kedes, Eva Operskalski, Michael Busch et al., "The Seroepidemiology of Human Herpesvirus 8 (Kaposi's Sarcoma-Associated Herpesvirus): Distribution of Infection in KS Risk Groups and Evidence for Sexual Transmission," *Nature Medicine* 2(8): 918 (August 1996); CDC National AIDS Clearinghouse (Bethesda, Md.: Information, Inc., 1996).

AN EPIDEMIC EMERGES

American physicians with predominately gay male patients began to notice that something unusual was happening in 1979. Some of their patients were showing up with a form of cancer called Kaposi's sarcoma (KS), which produces purplish or brownish blotches on the body. Before then, in the United States, KS usually was seen only in elderly men, and was a fairly chronic condition. Now it was occurring in younger gay and bisexual men, spreading rapidly through their bodies and often killing them. Other patients were coming down with a previously rare form of pneumonia called *Pneumocystis carinii* pneumonia (PCP for short), which is often fatal and is known to occur only in people with weakened immune systems. Some patients had both KS and PCP.

In June 1981, the first report in the medical literature appeared in the *Morbidity and Mortality Weekly Report (MMWR)*, the main publication for the Centers for Disease Control and Prevention (CDC). It simply stated that five gay men in Los Angeles had developed PCP for no known reason and two of them had died. A month later, *MMWR* reported that ten more cases of PCP had occurred in California and that there were also twenty-six cases of KS in gay men. Seven weeks later, *MMWR* reported an additional seventy persons with KS and/or PCP throughout the United States, mostly in New York City and California. The disease was spreading rapidly. By the end of 1981, 150 adults (mostly, but not entirely, gay men) and nine children in the United States were dead of this new mysterious illness.

At first, it was unclear what was spreading it. Could it be spread through the air? Or a handshake? No one knew for sure. Hospitals were beginning to use extreme precautions to protect health care workers from becoming infected by this mystery disease, including masks and gloves when touching or even standing near a patient. And no one knew quite what to call the new disease. Some called it gay-related immune deficiency (or GRID), others termed it KSOI (for Kaposi's sarcoma and opportunistic infections), and others coined the term "gay plague." By September 1982, the term "acquired immunodeficiency syndrome" (AIDS) had become popular and widely accepted.

There was growing concern within the gay communities of large American cities; the first community-based organization to fight AIDS was established in New York City in 1982 and named the Gay Men's Health Crisis (GMHC). Similar organizations were set up soon after in San Francisco, Los Angeles, and Miami. There was considerable fear among gay men at that time about this new disease; one study shows that gay men in New York City were already changing their sexual behavior, reducing by half their number of sex partners.

Subsequent articles in *MMWR* made it increasingly clear that AIDS was affecting not only gay men but also persons with hemophilia, injecting drug users, and Haitian-Americans. Though it was assumed by many people that AIDS was sexually transmitted, the evidence was not certain until July 1982, when the *MMWR* reported a cluster of AIDS cases among gay men who had sex together in Orange County, California. As the additional evidence grew that AIDS could not be transmitted through the air by a sneeze or a cough, like a cold or tuberculosis, the fear and extreme precautions used by health care workers treating persons with AIDS gradually subsided. By the end of 1982, over five hundred men, women, and children had died of AIDS in the United States.

By 1983, the first report in the medical literature indicated that AIDS was found in wealthy Africans seeking medical treatment in Europe. It was quickly learned that AIDS had been spreading rapidly through parts of central Africa. Reports of AIDS were coming in from Zaire, Rwanda, Uganda, and Zambia. Increasingly, AIDS was being seen as an international epidemic.

In 1983, Dr. Luc Montagnier of the Pasteur Institute in France discovered the virus that causes AIDS, which he called LAV. He sent his findings to Dr. Robert Gallo of the National Institutes of Health in Maryland to have him examine them. Although what exactly transpired still remains debatable, Dr. Gallo maintains that he independently discovered the AIDS virus, which he named HTLV-III, in 1984. By 1986, the AIDS virus had been renamed "human immunodeficiency virus," or HIV. In April 1984, a month after Dr. Gallo announced that he "discovered" the AIDS virus, Secretary of Health and Human Services Margaret Heckler held a press conference where she predicted that a cure for AIDS would be found in a few months. Unfortunately, her prediction proved untrue; no cure has been found.

A commercial test to detect antibodies (proteins produced by the body that react specifically with a foreign substance in the body) to HIV first became available in early 1985, and people were encouraged to be tested for HIV. It was then learned that thousands of blood transfusion recipients and persons with hemophilia had become infected with HIV through infected blood or blood products. Mass screening of all donated blood for HIV began. By the middle of 1985, however, nearly one thousand Americans were dead from AIDS.

The definition of what is considered AIDS changed in 1987 and again in 1993, becoming more accurate as we learned more about the opportunistic diseases that affect persons with HIV. The number of reported AIDS cases grew with each change in definition. By the end of 1997, there were an estimated 30.6 million persons with HIV in the world, mostly in Africa, and at least one million persons with HIV in the United States. By December 1995, a total of 513,486 people had been reported to the CDC as AIDS patients, of whom 319,849 (including 3,921 children) had died. Of those adults and teenagers with AIDS, 51 percent were men who had sex with men, 25 percent were men and women who injected recreational drugs, 7 percent were men who had sex with men and injected recreational drugs, 4 percent were men and women who had heterosexual sex with an injecting drug user, 4 percent were men and women who had heterosexual sex with someone other than an injecting drug user (or the behavior of their partner was unknown), 1 percent were men and women who received a blood transfusion, 1 percent were men and women with hemophilia, and 7 percent were men and women whose risk was not reported or identified.

By the middle of the 1990s, HIV had become truly pandemic, spreading throughout the globe. In spite of the new treatments available in the developed nations, it was clear that the best hope to slow the spread of the disease was still through education and behavioral change.

DOCUMENT 10: The First Medical Report About AIDS

This is the first report in the medical literature on what we now know is AIDS. While this news came as a surprise to most people, a few public health researchers and behavioral scientists saw this as a continuation of the growth in dangerous sexually transmitted diseases that were increasingly affecting all Americans throughout the 1970s, particularly within the gay community.

In the period October 1980–May 1981, 5 young men, all active homosexuals, were treated for biopsy-confirmed *Pneumocystis carinii* pneumonia at 3 different hospitals in Los Angeles, California. Two of the patients died. All 5 patients had laboratory-confirmed previous or current cytomegalovirus (CMV) infection and candidal mucosal infection. [This historic announcement was followed by case reports of the five patients.]

The diagnosis of *Pneumocystis* pneumonia was confirmed for all 5 patients. . . . The patients did not know each other and had no known common contacts or knowledge of sexual partners who had had similar illnesses. The 5 did not have comparable histories of sexually transmitted disease. . . . Two of the 5 reported having frequent homosexual contact with various partners. All 5 reported using inhalant drugs. . . .

Editorial note [which immediately followed this announcement]: *Pneumocystis* pneumonia in the United States is almost exclusively limited to severely immunosuppressed patients. The occurrence of *Pneumocystosis* in these 5 previously healthy individuals without a clinically apparent underlying immunodeficiency is unusual. The fact that these patients were all homosexuals suggests an association between some aspect of a homosexual lifestyle or disease acquired through sexual contact and *Pneumocystis* pneumonia in this population.

Source: "*Pneumocystis* Pneumonia—Los Angeles," *Morbidity and Mortality Weekly Report* 30(21): 250–252 (June 5, 1981).

DOCUMENT 11: The Second Medical Report: More Evidence of an Emerging Epidemic

The first report in *MMWR* brought in a flood of reports of gay men with unexpected illnesses. This second report, one month later, shows the growing awareness that an epidemic was brewing. Kaposi's sarcoma is a form of cancer that produces purplish or brownish blotches on the skin and mouth and affects internal organs. *Pneumocystis carinii* pneumonia is a particularly deadly form of pneumonia that produces difficulty in breathing, coughing, chills, high fever, and vomiting.

During the past 30 months, Kaposi's sarcoma (KS), an uncommonly reported malignancy in the United States, has been diagnosed in 26 homosexual men. . . . Eight of these patients died. . . . all 8 within 24 months after KS was diagnosed. . . .

Since the previous report of 5 cases of *Pneumocystis* pneumonia in homosexual men from Los Angeles, 10 additional cases (4 in Los Angeles and 6 in the San Francisco Bay area) of biopsy-confirmed PC pneumonia have been identified in homosexual men in the State. Two of the 10 patients also have KS. This brings the total number of *Pneumocystis* cases among homosexual men in California to 15 since September 1979. Patients range in age from 25 to 46 years.

Editorial note [following this report]: . . . That 10 new cases of *Pneumocystis* pneumonia have been identified in homosexual men suggests that the 5 previously reported cases were not an isolated phenomenon. . . . Although it is not certain that the increase in KS and PC pneumonia is restricted to homosexual men, the vast majority of recent cases have been reported from this group. Physicians should be alert for Kaposi's sarcoma, PC pneumonia, and other opportunistic infections associated with immunosuppression in homosexual men.

Source: "Kaposi's Sarcoma and *Pneumocystis* Pneumonia Among Homosexual Men—New York and California," *Morbidity and Mortality Weekly Report* 30 (25): 305–307 (July 3, 1981).

DOCUMENT 12: A "Gay Plague"?

Seven weeks later, it was clear that an epidemic was emerging. Nevertheless, there was very little publicity about this in the media. Only the gay newspapers were reporting what was happening. At that time, it was wrongly thought that only gay or bisexual men were susceptible to the new disease. We now know that while gay and bisexual men remain at potentially very high risk for HIV, most of the people in the world who are currently infected with HIV acquired the virus through sexual intercourse with a member of the opposite sex. The editorial note points out that Kaposi's sarcoma was usually found in elderly men and was rarely fatal; now it was being found in young men and was often fatal.

Twenty-six cases of Kaposi's sarcoma (KS) and 15 cases of *Pneumocystis carinii* pneumonia (PCP) among previously healthy homosexual men were recently reported. Since July 3, 1981, CDC has received reports of an additional 70 cases of these 2 conditions in persons without known underlying disease. . . . The majority of the reported cases of KS and/or PCP have occurred in white men. Patients ranged in age from 15–52 years; over 95% were men 25–49 years of age. Ninety-four percent . . . of the men for whom sexual [orientation] was known were homosexual or bisexual. Forty percent of the reported cases were fatal. Of the 82 cases for which the month of diagnosis is known, 75 . . . have occurred since January 1980, with 55 . . . diagnosed from January through July 1981. Although physicians from several states have reported cases of KS and PCP among previously healthy homosexual men, the majority of cases have been reported from New York and California.

Editorial note [which followed this report]: KS is a rare, malignant [disease] seen predominantly in elderly men. . . . [It is] manifested by skin lesions and [ongoing symptoms]; it is rarely fatal. In contrast, the persons currently reported to have KS are young to middle-aged men, and 20% of the cases have been fatal. . . . The occurrence of *Pneumocystis carinii* pneumonia in patients who are not immunosuppressed due to known underlying disease or therapy is also highly unusual.

Source: "Follow-up on Kaposi's Sarcoma and *Pneumocystis* Pneumonia," *Morbidity and Mortality Weekly Report* 30(33): 409–410 (August 28, 1981).

DOCUMENT 13: Physicians Are Frustrated

This was one of the first major articles in the national media about AIDS. At that time, it was assumed that a cure for AIDS would just be a matter of time. While articles like this one alerted the public to a deadly disease that was spreading rapidly, it also helped to produce the first wave of AIDS hysteria, which resulted in persons perceived to be at risk for AIDS being shunned or losing their jobs.

Since it came into public view in 1981, derisively called "The Gay Plague," AIDS (Acquired Immune Deficiency Syndrome), which ravages the body's immune system, has stricken 1,300 Americans, more than half of them in the last year. And there is no cure in sight. "In my professional career, I have never encountered a more frustrating and depressing situation," says Dr. Peter Mansell of Houston's M.D. Anderson Hospital and Tumor Institute. "People who you know are likely to die ask what they can do to help themselves, and you are forced to say, more or less, 'I have no idea'." ... "As the months go by, we see more and more groups," says Dr. Anthony Fauci of the National Institute of Allergic and Infectious Diseases. "AIDS is creeping out of well-defined, [epidemiologic] confines." ... "It has caught everybody by surprise," says Dr. Abe Macher of the National Institute[s] of Health. "Textbooks are being rewritten. We're observing the evolution of a new disease." ...

"We don't know" remains the frustrating answer to almost all questions about AIDS. We don't know what causes the disease, we don't know how to treat it and we don't know whether the epidemic is about to level off or race through the population like a forest fire. ...

Source: Jean Seligmann, Mariana Gosnell, Vincent Coppola, and Mary Hager, "The AIDS Epidemic: The Search for a Cure," Newsweek 101(16): 74–79 (April 18, 1983).

DOCUMENT 14: An Early Perspective on the Future of AIDS

By January 1985, we had learned much about AIDS and HIV, but we still had much more to learn. We now know that most people infected with HIV will develop symptoms of AIDS nearly a decade later and die about three years after that. We also know that HIV (called HTLV-III in 1985) is not necessarily confined to the "high-risk groups," such as gay men and injecting drug users, although in North America and Europe they are much more likely to become infected. It is not whether you are a member of a "high-risk group" that predicts whether you will get AIDS or not, but whether you engage in high-risk behaviors. While there is good evidence to suggest that men can infect women somewhat more easily than women can infect men, it is now clear that both men and women can readily infect each other through intercourse without using condoms.

In the relatively short span of three years, over 7,000 cases of ... [AIDS] have been diagnosed in the United States. ... With a mortality [rate] that two years from diagnosis exceeds 80%, this illness now ranks as one of the most serious epidemics confronting man in modern time. ...

It is hoped that only some people infected with HTLV-III will develop overt AIDS. . . . It is [also] hoped that prospective studies . . . will determine which factors are responsible for the host response to infection. . . .

Another major issue of AIDS is whether the disease will remain confined to . . . high-risk groups. . . . It is unknown whether heterosexual transmission will ever become important in the epidemiology of AIDS in the United States . . . [or whether women will be as] efficient as . . . men in transmitting the virus. . . . [However], the potential for extension of AIDS outside the present high-risk groups remains a real possibility.

Source: Thomas C. Quinn, "Editorial," *Journal of the American Medical Association* 253(2): 247–248 (January 11, 1985).

DOCUMENT 15: The "Coming Great Plague"

By the beginning of 1987, it was clear to public health officials that they were dealing with a global epidemic of massive proportions. Some of the projections for the future were very bleak, often not taking into account the success of prevention efforts or other potential factors that would slow the epidemic. Dr. Bowen estimates in this reading a global death toll in the tens of millions by 1997, and 50–100 million HIV-infected by 2007. Though the first estimate was too high, since only 6 or 7 million were dead of AIDS by 1997, his second estimate of 50–100 million HIV-infected by 2007 appears to be perhaps an underestimate.

A worldwide AIDS epidemic will become so serious that it will dwarf such earlier medical disasters as the Black Plague, smallpox and typhoid, the nation's top health official said today.

"You haven't heard or read anything yet," Dr. Otis R. Bowen, the Secretary of Health and Human Services told the National Press Club. "If we can't make progress, we face the dreadful prospect of a worldwide death toll in the tens of millions a decade from now." . . . Dr. Bowen said 50 million to 100 million people worldwide could become infected with the AIDS virus in the next two decades. . . .

Source: "AIDS May Dwarf the Plague," *The New York Times*, p. A24 (January 30, 1987).

DOCUMENT 16: The Changing Definition of AIDS

The Centers for Disease Control and Prevention (CDC) does not require mandatory HIV reporting from all states, only reporting of full-blown AIDS cases. The definition of exactly what constitutes an AIDS case has changed over time. It significantly changed in 1987 and again in 1993. The 1993 change was very substantial, since anyone testing positive for HIV and having a weakened immune system (with a count below 200 T4 cells) is now defined as a person with AIDS. Before 1993, many women (and some injecting drug users) with HIV and weakened immune systems were dying of invasive cervical cancer, recurrent pneumonia, or pulmonary tuberculosis but were not being counted as AIDS cases. Now they are being counted.

Since federal funding for AIDS is linked to the number of reported AIDS cases in a particular area, this revision in the definition allowed for a more accurate assessment of the true number of AIDS cases. Also, it was known that the change in definition would result in a sharp increase in cases and draw attention to the insufficient level of funding for AIDS by the Bush administration. It is believed by many that the decision to wait until after the 1992 election before implementing the change was a political decision.

The revised HIV classification system provides uniform and simple criteria for categorizing conditions among adolescents and adults with HIV infection and should [assist] efforts to evaluate current and future health-care and referral needs for persons with HIV infection. The addition of a measure of severe immunosuppression . . . will enable AIDS surveillance data to more accurately represent those who are recognized as being immunosuppressed, who are in greatest need of close medical follow-up, and who are at greatest risk for the full spectrum of severe HIV-related [diseases]. The addition of . . . pulmonary TB, recurrent pneumonia, and invasive cervical cancer to [the AIDS profile] reflects the documented or potential importance of these diseases in the HIV epidemic.

Source: Centers for Disease Control and Prevention, "1993 Revised Classification System for HIV Infection and Expanded Surveillance Case Definition for AIDS Among Adolescents and Adults," *Morbidity and Mortality Weekly Report* 41 (RR-17): 9–10 (1992).

THE SHAPING OF PUBLIC OPINION

Unlike the massive publicity that occurred when Legionnaires' disease broke out in the 1970s and toxic shock syndrome in 1980, the advent of AIDS in 1981 went virtually unnoticed by the national media for nearly two years. Until the mid-1980s, the national media rarely reported on gay-related issues and politics. On the other hand, the gay newspapers and magazines (which began to proliferate throughout the United States during the 1970s) had excellent coverage of the growing health crisis. By early 1983, the gay and lesbian community in the United States was increasingly aware of and concerned about the epidemic, while few nongay Americans (outside of the medical community) had even heard about AIDS. Gay Men's Health Crisis, the first and largest AIDS service organization, organized a major fund-raiser, filling an 18,000-seat auditorium with mostly gay men and lesbians, in New York City in April 1983. This event drew considerable publicity, and in May 1983, newspapers, magazines, and radio and television stations throughout the nation reported about AIDS as if it had just been discovered.

With this publicity came both concern and fear. Many people avoided going into predominantly gay neighborhoods to dine and shop, and many gay waiters and salesmen lost their jobs either for being openly gay or due to a lack of business. Haitian-Americans, who were similarly characterized as being at high risk for AIDS, also were often shunned and fired from their jobs. The growing anti-gay religious right in the United States used the AIDS issue to condemn homosexuality. Throughout the mid-1980s, there were concerted political efforts to confine all persons with HIV to quarantine camps for life. In 1986, for example, a ballot proposition was put before California voters that would have put tens of thousands of HIV-infected Californians behind barbed wire in quarantine camps. Fortunately for the growing number of HIV-infected persons in that state, the proposal did not pass.

During the early and mid-1980s, the federal government, most states, and most municipalities in the United States did little or nothing to support AIDS research, education, or services. Indeed, from a political perspective AIDS could not have occurred at a worse time. The year that AIDS was first noticed was the same year that Ronald Reagan took office as president. From the very beginning, there was no funding at the CDC and the NIH for AIDS research, and it was not until President Reagan's second term in office that he first uttered the word "AIDS" in public. While his conservative advisers, such as Gary Bauer and Pat Buchanan, were telling him that he should not do anything about

AIDS, Surgeon General C. Everett Koop was actively meeting with congressional members to support a massive AIDS education program.

In 1985, Rock Hudson was diagnosed with, and died of, AIDS. He was the first celebrity known to have AIDS, and the publicity about the disease was renewed. By the following year, evidence from HIV testing in Africa and inner-city America was making it clear that the virus was far more widespread than previously believed, that it was spreading very rapidly, and that it was affecting more heterosexuals in the world than homosexuals. Emergency meetings were held at the very highest levels of government in North America and Europe to attempt to cope with this emerging heterosexual plague. Now that it was no longer seen as "just" a homosexual or an injecting drug user disease, government planners throughout the developed world were taking this enormous health crisis very seriously. Some feared that it would lead to massive global depopulation similar to the great plagues of past centuries. In 1987, condom ads began to appear in the media.

In the late 1980s, AZT (zidovudine) became a drug widely used by AIDS patients in the developed nations, though it was initially very expensive and produced serious side effects in many people who took the large dosage recommended. During this period, AIDS activism grew in the larger cities of North America and Europe, where demonstrators demanded that governments take a more active role in funding AIDS research and programs. ACT-UP (AIDS Coalition To Unleash Power) demonstrators succeeded in getting the NIH to reduce the time it took to review AIDS research proposals by a few months, and in getting the Food and Drug Administration (FDA) to speed up the approval process for new experimental drugs to combat HIV.

Throughout the late 1980s and early 1990s, community-based AIDS service organizations grew in size as they provided education and psychosocial and other services for persons with AIDS (PWAs). Thousands of people volunteered to serve as buddies to PWAs, and to assist with food programs and a variety of other much-needed services. Large fund-raisers, including AIDS walks and gala parties, were organized to supplement the inadequate government funding available. In 1990, the Ryan White program, named after a teenager with hemophilia who died of AIDS after galvanizing the country with stories of both AIDS discrimination and then caring by the public, began to bring tens of millions of federal dollars into metropolitan areas hit hardest by the epidemic. By 1995, the funding levels of the Ryan White program grew larger, and it was funded for another five years. In 1991, the basketball player "Magic" Johnson announced to a stunned world that he had become infected with HIV through unprotected sex with a woman. Millions of heterosexual men and women in the United States began to take the threat of sex without a condom more seriously.

By 1993 and 1994, the situation seemed very bleak as word spread that AZT was proving to be largely ineffective when used without other drugs, and AIDS patients were developing resistance to the drug. Also, efforts to develop a vaccine were proving unsuccessful. However, by 1996 a new optimism began to prevail within the HIV community as studies showed that the new protease inhibitor drugs, when used with two of the older drugs (including AZT), dramatically reduced viral load levels and increased the immune levels in those who took them. People in developed nations, where these very expensive treatments could be afforded, began to talk for the first time of HIV/AIDS becoming a chronic but controlled disease, like diabetes.

Today, as AIDS continues to take a heavy toll, there is a growing realization that AIDS, even as a chronic illness, is here to stay for the foreseeable future. With still neither a cure nor a vaccine available, more people appear to be practicing safer sex. Clearly, AIDS is not an easy disease to get, providing a few simple precautions are taken, such as using condoms during penetrative sex, practicing forms of nonpenetrative sex, and not sharing needles if engaging in recreational drug use. There is certainly no need to panic over AIDS. We will, however, be facing new and challenging policy decisions on a societal level, and difficult and demanding decisions on a personal level. It is vital that everyone learn as much as possible about the issues surrounding AIDS, to be able to make informed and intelligent choices.

DOCUMENT 17: AIDS: A Moral and Political Time Bomb

From the very beginning of the AIDS epidemic, the political right in the United States and a few other countries has used AIDS as a tool to support its very conservative political agenda. In the same way that Adolf Hitler blamed the Jews for what was wrong with life in Germany during the 1930s and 1940s, the political right has been focusing upon gay men and lesbians as their scapegoat during the 1980s and 1990s. In this article, they blame gay men instead of the virus for the AIDS epidemic. Pat Buchanan, Jesse Helms, Gary Bauer, Pat Robertson, and many others have used AIDS to bolster their comments supporting anti-gay bigotry. AIDS has even been used to support anti-gay propositions on the ballot in a few states. In reading the following selection, try substituting your own or a friend's ethnic group for the word "homosexual."

AIDS is most frequently, in fact, primarily, spread by homosexual contact. The more promiscuous the homosexual, the greater his risk. The bloodier the homosexual act, the greater the risk. . . . Infants, children, surgical patients, and hemophiliacs are being struck down in ever greater numbers via contaminated blood transfusions. . . .

AIDS is deadly—that much is known. All 1979 and 1980 AIDS patients are dead. Of those suffering from AIDS for as long as two years, 82% no longer suffer—they too are dead! . . .

More precisely, AIDS knocks out a person's immune defenses and then allows some of the most horrible killer diseases known to man to ravage the victim's body. . . .

[T]he homosexual lobby is so powerful and the homosexual influence in the media so pervasive that an entire nation stands essentially defenseless before a malignant minority. . . .

[W]hy have federal health authorities not stipulated . . . that homosexuals:

(1) be forbidden from working in food handling businesses,

(2) be forbidden to donate blood—both on pain of legal penalty?

[H]omosexuals and their practices can threaten our lives, our children, can influence whether or not we have elective surgery, eat in a certain restaurant, visit a given city or take up a certain profession or career— all because a tiny minority flaunts its lifestyle and demands that an entire nation tolerate its diseases. . . .

Source: Ronald S. Goodwin, "AIDS: A Moral and Political Time Bomb," *Moral Majority Report*, pp. 2, 8 (July 1983).

DOCUMENT 18: Rock Hudson Dies of AIDS

In 1985, the popular actor Rock Hudson flew to Paris in a failed attempt to be treated for AIDS. He was the first household name known to have AIDS, and the massive publicity drew new attention to the spreading epidemic. Since few people knew that he was gay, and since the disease at that time was so closely identified with being gay, his publicist at first tried to claim that he had liver cancer instead. But when it was clear that the treatment in Paris was not effective, he disclosed that he was indeed suffering from AIDS. President Ronald Reagan had refused to discuss AIDS until then. After Hudson's death, he acknowledged his passing in sorrow, but did not utter the uncomfortable word "AIDS" for another two years. Below are two related readings.

A.

Rock Hudson is in a Paris hospital suffering from inoperable liver cancer, his publicist said here yesterday. The 59-year-old actor is appar-

ently being seen by physicians specializing in acquired immune deficiency syndrome.... [A spokesman said] that reports suggesting that
Hudson was suffering from AIDS were merely "speculation." AIDS destroys the body's immune system, leaving its victims vulnerable to disease. As of yesterday, Hudson was "being tested for everything" at
American Hospital in Paris.... Asked whether such testing included
AIDS, [the spokesman] repeated: "Everything."

Source: "Actor Reportedly Being Treated by AIDS Specialists," *San Francisco
Chronicle* (July 24, 1985), Newsbank 85 NIN 1:C10.

B.

Rock Hudson confirmed Thursday through a spokeswoman that he
has been battling AIDS for a year, and gay rights activists said his "cou-
rageous" disclosure may be the breakthrough they needed to publicize
the severity of the epidemic.... Hudson, the first American celebrity to
acknowledge having acquired immune deficiency syndrome, may also
be the first AIDS victim that President Reagan knows personally, activists said. "If a friend is a friend, you're going to be there for him or her
regardless of what they're dying of. We hope President Reagan is the
same," said [a spokesperson for] the San Francisco AIDS Foundation....
Hudson, who is under the care of Paris doctors, has also highlighted
"the fact that people with AIDS are being forced to flee the country to
seek treatment," said [the coordinator of] a San Francisco political lobbying group.

Source: Kathy Holub, "Rock Hudson Confirms He Has AIDS," *San Jose Mercury
News* (July 26, 1985); Newsbank 85 NIN 1:D1–1:D2.

DOCUMENT 19: California to Vote on AIDS Proposition

At the height of the AIDS hysteria in the mid-1980s, California voted
on a public referendum that would have quarantined thousands of persons with AIDS throughout the state for the remainder of their lives,
and would have forced thousands more with HIV to lose their jobs.
Fortunately for the persons with HIV/AIDS in that state, the measure
lost.

California is poised to be the first state in the nation to attempt to deal
with AIDS by public referendum.... Citizens will vote on a ... measure
that would legally declare AIDS an "infectious, contagious, and easily

communicable disease." Ballot Proposition 64 . . . could force public health officials to establish camps to quarantine AIDS patients, as well as anyone who carries the AIDS virus. The measure would also . . . ban persons infected by the virus from attending or teaching in public schools or holding jobs that involve food handling.

Sponsored by a Lyndon LaRouche organization called PANIC (the Prevent AIDS Now Initiative Committee), Proposition 64 embodies all of the deepest fears about AIDS in one cold legislative package. PANIC, based in Los Angeles, had no trouble getting 683,000 California voters to sign the petition that put [it] on the ballot. Opposition to the AIDS measure among health officials, physicians, and academics is strong and mounting. . . .

Source: Charles Petit, "California to Vote on AIDS Proposition," *Science* 234 (4774): 277–278 (October 17, 1986).

DOCUMENT 20: Magic Johnson: HIV Positive!

Magic Johnson, famed basketball player, stunned America in 1991 by announcing that he is HIV positive. A successful athlete, neither gay nor an injecting drug user, he apparently became infected from failing to use a condom during sex with a woman. Millions of American men who thought they were invulnerable to HIV began to think seriously about using condoms with their female sex partners for the first time. Two related readings follow.

A.

Nearly an hour before the news conference aired on the East Coast, the lights on the switchboard began to dance. The callers were mostly men, most of them heterosexual, all eager—some desperate—to know when they could be tested for the virus that can end in AIDS. Inquiries tumbled in at a breakneck speed. Late that evening when DC AIDS Information Line coordinator Ronald King took a break, he discovered they were up a staggering 500 percent. And while heterosexuals make up 49 percent of callers on a routine day, they made up 95 percent on Thursday. That was the day a brilliant star of the National Basketball Association . . . retired because he had tested HIV positive. . . . Earvin "Magic" Johnson made his astonishing announcement, and America began reassessing one of the most feared of the world's incurable diseases.

Source: Anne Reifenberg, "Magic Johnson Spurs New Look at AIDS Peril," *Dallas Morning News* (November 10, 1991): Newsbank 91 NIN 202:E6.

B.

Basketball superstar Earvin "Magic" Johnson abruptly announced Thursday that he would retire from the Los Angeles Lakers because he had tested positive for the AIDS virus. Mr. Johnson, whose charismatic style and personality revived interest in the National Basketball Association, was composed as he delivered the grim message. . . .

"I plan to go on living for a long time," Mr. Johnson said. "I'm going to miss playing. My life will change, no question about it. But I still intend to be a part of the game. And I will become a spokesman for the HIV virus. I want people to understand that safe sex is the way to go."

Source: David Moore, "Move Stuns Basketball World," *Dallas Morning News* (November 8, 1991); Newsbank 91 NIN 202:E9.

DOCUMENT 21: Anyone Can Get AIDS

Many people still do not believe that anyone can get AIDS. They assume, since most people in the United States with the disease are gay or bisexual men, injecting drug users or their sex partners, or the poor (migrant workers, crack users, and the homeless), they (white heterosexual middle-class men and women) cannot get it. Unfortunately, they are very wrong. While the risk in the developed nations remains quite low, many white heterosexual middle-class men and women have become infected with HIV and have died from AIDS. In the United States, through December 1995, a cumulative total of 2,924 white, non-Hispanic men and 6,474 white, non-Hispanic women had developed AIDS through heterosexual contact. Alison L. Gertz was one of them.

Alison L. Gertz, who contracted AIDS in a single encounter with a man at the age of 16 and drew international attention by telling her story as a warning to heterosexuals, women and teenagers, died yesterday at her family's summer home in Westhampton Beach [Long Island]. She was 26 years old and lived in Manhattan. Her parents, Jerrold and Carol Gertz, said she died of AIDS.

[Ms. Gertz did not fit the profile of high-risk categories that prevailed in 1989, when she publicly told her story. Her story was all the more dramatic because of the privilege she was born into, with artistic talent, affluence, private schools and social prominence.]

Ms. Gertz became a crusader, speaking at schools, colleges and public events. . . . "Unfortunately, a lot of people just flip by" AIDS reports about gay men and addicts, she said. "They think it doesn't apply to them. They can't turn the page on me. I could be one of them, or their daughter, and they have to deal with this."

Source: "Alison L. Gertz, Whose Infection Alerted Many to AIDS, Dies at 26" [Obituaries], *The New York Times*, August 9, 1992.

SUGGESTED READINGS

"AIDS: The Devastating March of a Killer, Through People's Eyes." *People Weekly* 41, pp. 259–261 (March 7–14, 1994).

"Arthur Ashe Says Magic Should Not Have Quit." *Jet* 83, p. 50 (January 11, 1993).

Brandt, Allan. *No Magic Bullet: A Social History of Venereal Disease in the U.S. Since 1880*. New York: Oxford University Press, 1987.

Brown, David. "Biology: Evolving Theories on Origin of AIDS." *The Washington Post*, p. A2 (April 17, 1995).

Cohen, J., and E. Marshall. "NIH-Pasteur: A Final Rapprochement." *Science* 265, p. 313 (July 15, 1994).

Curtis, T. " 'Origin of AIDS' Update." *Rolling Stone*, p. 39 (December 9, 1993).

Duesberg, Peter H., & Bryan J. Ellison. *Inventing the AIDS Epidemic: The Truth Behind the Biggest Medical Deception of Our Time*. New York: St. Martin's Press, 1994.

Ezzell, C. "New Evidence Supports a Cofactor in AIDS." *Science News* 139, p. 133 (March 2, 1991).

Fee, Elizabeth. *AIDS: The Making of a Chronic Disease*. Berkeley: University of California Press, 1992.

Garrett, Laurie. "Scientists Search for the Origins of the AIDS Virus." *Philadelphia Inquirer*, p. A4 (January 4, 1994).

Masood, Ehsan. "Anomaly Admitted in 'First' AIDS Case." *Nature* 375 (6526), p. 4 (May 4, 1995).

Piel, G. "AIDS and Population 'Control.' " *Scientific American* 270, p. 124 (February 1994).

Santiago, R. "Playing One on One." *Essence* 22, p. 126 (March 1992).

Thomas, C. A., et al. "What Causes AIDS? The Debate Continues." *Reason* 26, pp. 32–41 (December 1994).

Weiss, R. "How Does HIV Cause AIDS?" *Science* 260, pp. 1273–1279 (May 28, 1993).

2

The Impact of the Epidemic

The impact of the HIV/AIDS epidemic in the United States and through-out much of the world has been enormous. By the mid-1990s, over a third of a million Americans had died of AIDS, but the Centers for Disease Control and Prevention (CDC) had revised their estimate of living persons with HIV/AIDS downward from about a million to a more conservative estimate of 650,000 to 900,000 people. On the other hand, the World Health Organization (WHO) was continually increasing its estimate of persons living with HIV/AIDS throughout the world up to over 20 million and were expecting over 40 million in less than five years. By the end of 1997, the United Nations revised their estimate of persons with HIV upwards to 30.6 million.

In the United States, even with a cumulative total of about 1.1 million HIV/AIDS infections and AIDS deaths in a nation of some 260 million, the social fabric has been irrevocably altered in ways that we may never fully understand. With AIDS disproportionately taking the lives and affecting the health and thoughts of so many Americans in the arts (visual, theater, dance, photography, writing, film, television, and others), it is difficult to imagine how the various artistic fields would have evolved since 1981 without the profound influence of AIDS. How the world has been changed by the untimely deaths due to AIDS of Peter Allen, Howard Ashman, Michael Bennett, Brad Davis, Perry Ellis, Halston, Keith Haring, Robert Mapplethorpe, Freddie "Mercury" Bulsara, Vito Russo, Sylvester, and many others will never be truly known.

The readings in this chapter begin with a discussion of various topics relevant to the current situation in the United States: the increasing spread of HIV among African-Americans, Puerto Ricans, Mexican-Americans, minority women, and gay youth; the major development of protease inhibitor drugs that potentially promise to make AIDS and

HIV infection a manageable chronic illness like diabetes; the discovery that AZT taken during pregnancy will significantly reduce an HIV-positive pregnant woman's chances of having an HIV-infected infant; the pattern of many terminally ill persons with AIDS moving back to their parents in rural America, only to learn that the health professionals there are ill-equipped to treat their opportunistic infections or manage their illness; and the need for more HIV testing and counseling.

The chapter then broadly discusses the global crisis of HIV/AIDS, including the rapid spread of HIV/AIDS in India and Southeast Asia; the current alarmingly high rate of persons with HIV/AIDS in much of sub-Saharan Africa; the meager resources available to prevent HIV transmission and treat AIDS in the developing world; the existing pattern in which women are nearly as commonly infected with HIV in developing nations as are men; and the reality that other sexually transmitted diseases are quite prevalent throughout the world, indicating the frequency of unsafe sexual behaviors and posing an increased risk for HIV infection upon exposure and accelerating disease progression among those who are HIV-infected.

The chapter concludes with selections on how the epidemic has taken its toll, both economic and psychosocial, including the extraordinary costs involved in paying for the new protease inhibitor drugs and other medical expenses; the need for more effective HIV prevention programs, which have proved to be highly cost-effective; the high rate of AIDS-related suicides; the alarming increase of uninsured and underinsured persons with AIDS slipping through the "safety net"; the growth of the National AIDS Quilt to keep alive the memories of thousands who have died from AIDS; the rapid increase in the number of children, both HIV-positive and HIV-negative, who have been orphaned by the AIDS-related deaths of their mother or both parents; and the continuing stigma and prejudice against persons living with HIV/AIDS. Subsequent chapters will go into greater detail about issues touched upon in this chapter.

THE SITUATION IN THE UNITED STATES

DOCUMENT 22: Prognosis for the Next Century

This reading summarizes the status of the HIV epidemic in the United States and points to some areas of concern. One such area is the increasing number of AIDS cases among injecting drug users, women, blacks, and Hispanics. Although there is still no cure for AIDS, there are some extremely positive developments in treatment with new drugs and in the reduction of HIV transmission to newborns through pregnant women's treatment with AZT (the first federally approved medicine to work against AIDS). In an important study, only 8 percent of pregnant HIV-positive women who took AZT (also known as zidovudine) had an HIV-positive child, while 25 percent of pregnant HIV-positive women who did not take AZT had an HIV-positive child. And while there is not yet a vaccine that has proved to be effective for humans, much success has been achieved in animal studies, and dozens of preventive vaccine trials are ongoing. Amazingly, despite all the publicity about AIDS, more than half of all HIV-positive persons in the United States still do not know that they are infected.

The HIV epidemic is a multifaceted national and international problem. . . . Without treatment, about 50 percent of [all] people [with HIV] develop AIDS within ten years [after] becoming infected. . . . Groups at special risk have been identified and include: [injecting] drug abusers and their sex partners, people with large numbers of sex partners, men who have sex with men and their female partners, and people who exchange sex for money or drugs. . . . [T]he most rapid increases are occurring among [injecting] drug abusers, women, and babies born to women in high risk groups. An estimated 20 to 35 percent of infants of infected mothers develop HIV infection. Approximately 60 percent of AIDS patients are white, 25 percent are black, and 15 percent are Hispanic. . . . The development of a safe and effective HIV vaccine is a high priority for the coming decade. Other prevention and control strategies are vital to stopping the spread of HIV infection. Most HIV-infected people in the United States do not know they harbor the virus, and increased counseling, testing, and follow-up services are needed. Public education efforts on risks and precautions are essential to slowing the spread of the disease.

Source: *Healthy People 2000: National Health Promotion and Disease Prevention Objectives* (Washington, D.C.: U.S. Department of Health and Human Services, Public Health Service, n.d.), p. 74.

DOCUMENT 23: Why Everyone Should Care About AIDS

The Citizens Commission on AIDS for New York City and Northern New Jersey began its work in 1987, a time of widespread panic about AIDS. By the time it released its report three and a half years later, apathy about AIDS and hostility toward people living with AIDS had become a growing concern. In the following selection, the Citizens Commission discusses this problem and offers ten very compelling reasons why everyone should care deeply about AIDS.

The AIDS epidemic continues its relentless course, with no end in sight. But AIDS is fading from public concern. When the Citizens Commission on AIDS was created [a few] years ago, AIDS was an unpopular cause. It is now [1991] rapidly becoming a "post-popular" cause without ever having truly engaged widespread public support.

While [the statistics] are alarming in themselves, what is even more ominous is the apparent peak in public interest long before the [New York/New Jersey metropolitan area] feels the full onslaught of the epidemic. Political leadership appears to be following the public mood rather than taking bold initiatives. With a few exceptions, leadership at all levels has been lacking. The public mood that the Citizens Commission confronted at its inception was a mixture of hysteria and confusion. As the Commission ends its work, the prevailing mood is apathy and hostility. Outside the most devastated communities, the epidemic seems hidden, happening to someone else, somewhere else. An invisible wall seems to separate those who are suffering from everyone else.

Ten Reasons to Care about AIDS

Why should people who are not at risk themselves—or who believe they are not at risk—care about those who are? Because:

1. *They may be wrong about their own risk.* ... [A]ny sexually active person, or any person who uses injectable drugs or crack cocaine, may be at risk.

2. *They may be wrong about their children's risk.* AIDS threatens a generation of adolescents and pre-teenagers whose experimentation with sex or drugs can now lead to HIV infection and death.

3. *AIDS is an epidemic.* More precisely, HIV/AIDS is a series of still unfolding epidemics, with different peaks and valleys among different populations, each with no end in sight.

4. *HIV transmission can be prevented.* Consistent, ongoing, supportive, multicultural educational programs, linked to direct services, motivate and sustain safe behaviors.

5. *In the vast majority of cases, AIDS is ultimately fatal.* There is no cure or vaccine, and no way to reverse HIV infection.

6. *Early medical treatment can help people who are already HIV-infected.* Lives can be prolonged and improved through early medical and psychosocial intervention and appropriate counseling.

7. *AIDS is decimating a generation of otherwise healthy adults in their most productive years.*

8. *AIDS threatens to overwhelm an already strained health care and social welfare system.* Society needs a health care system available to all who need it, when they need it, and for whatever reasons they need it.

9. *Deferring costs now will increase burdens later.* Failing to provide drug treatment and HIV-related services in community-based settings will lead to greater acute-care costs as more and more people fall ill.

10. *AIDS tests our humanity, decency, and dignity.* If we turn our backs, we diminish ourselves and quite possibly jeopardize our futures.

Source: Ten Reasons to Care about AIDS (New York: Citizens Commission on AIDS for New York City and Northern New Jersey, February 1991), pp. 1–3.

DOCUMENT 24: Looking at the Growing Numbers

AIDS is a difficult disease for many young people to understand, since it takes a decade, on the average, for most persons infected with HIV to become sick. It is misleading to read the following selection and think that teenagers and young adults rarely get AIDS, since only 3 percent of all people who died of AIDS were under twenty-five years of age. Most of the people who die of AIDS in their late twenties were infected in their teens, and most of those who die in their early thirties were infected in their early twenties. Three out of every four persons who die of AIDS were probably infected before they were thirty-five years old. Like other sexually transmitted diseases, HIV hits teenagers and younger adults more than middle-aged and older persons.

In 1991, 29,850 U.S. residents died from HIV infection; of these, 3% were [under] 25 [years of age], 74% [were] 25–44 . . . and 23% [were 45 and older]. HIV infection was the ninth leading cause of death overall, accounting for 1% of all deaths, and the third leading cause of death among persons aged 25–44 years, accounting for 15% of deaths in this age group. . . . [F]or men and women aged 25–44 years, the death rate for HIV infection steadily increased. . . . The findings in this report underscore the role of HIV infection as a cause of death among men and women aged 25–44 years in the United States. . . . [These] deaths impose a disproportionately high impact on society because of the loss of productive years of life and the loss of parents from families with young children. The impact of HIV infection on death patterns is even greater in many large cities than in the total U.S. population. For example, for persons aged 25–44 years in 1990, HIV was the leading cause of death among men in 64 (37%) of 172 cities with populations of at least 100,000 and among women in nine (5%) such cities. . . .

Source: "Update: Mortality Attributable to HIV Infection/AIDS Among Persons Aged 25–44—United States, 1990–1991," *Morbidity and Mortality Weekly Report* 42(25): 481–485 (July 2, 1993).

DOCUMENT 25: AIDS Is Becoming a Rural Problem, Too: A Case Study from Iowa

Relatively few AIDS cases are reported from Iowa and the other rural states. Among the general population, HIV infection rates are lower in these areas. Therefore, when people with HIV disease move back to rural areas, medical and social services available elsewhere are often very difficult to find; patients may have to travel to the nearest major city for help. Along with the difficulties of living with a serious illness, they often experience a great deal of stress from the move itself, the loss of a job, and separation from friends.

Although many rural areas have a low number of reported AIDS cases, the "iceberg" phenomenon [the fact that many more people are infected with HIV than the reported AIDS statistics show] continues to leave most of the problem submerged. . . . [I]nterviews indicate that most people move back to Iowa for reasons of family support, often still grieving losses in significant relationships and support networks due to AIDS-related deaths. . . . When . . . [people] change residence with an HIV diagnosis, they may encounter family members who are unprepared to meet their needs. This problem may be compounded if there are no local services or if their physician is not prepared to care for them. . . .

Professionals need to prepare to provide support for patients who are grieving multiple losses, often having left behind a job, home, and friends in addition to the losses they may have experienced through deaths of friends and peers.

Source: Kristine A. Davis, Barbara Cameron, and Jack T. Stapleton, "The Impact of HIV Patient Migration to Rural Areas," *AIDS Patient Care* 6(5): 225–228 (October 1992).

DOCUMENT 26: The Second Wave of HIV Infection Among Gay Men

To prevent sexual transmission of HIV, safer sex practices must be consistent and maintained on a long-term basis. Reports that some gay men have gone back to high-risk sexual practices is alarming because rates of HIV infection in this population are already high. For example, in San Francisco 29 percent of a group of young gay men between the ages of twenty-seven and twenty-nine were recently found to be HIV-positive. This "second wave" of the HIV epidemic is alarming because it appears to be concentrated among young men in their twenties. There are several reasons for sexual risk-taking among young gay men. Drug and alcohol use is one factor. Another is underestimating and denying the actual risk of infection. For many young gay men, health concerns are not nearly as important as the acceptance of their friends and the affection of their partners or lovers.

Many gay men [in San Francisco], saying they are numb with loss, fatalistic about their own survival, unwilling to face a measure of sexual deprivation and eager for the attention showered on the sick and the dying, are again practicing unprotected anal intercourse. . . . The surveys indicate that one of every three gay men . . . is engaging . . . [in this behavior]. A man at a recent safe sex forum . . . [said] "It makes you feel like what's the point. . . . Eventually you're going to get it, so why resist? We're surrounded." . . .

One 46-year-old man who works in an AIDS clinic and is thus fully informed about the disease recently became infected. He explained himself to a friend by saying, "So I'll live to be 55 or 60. That's not what I had in mind, but it's better than another 30 years worrying about this and living without sexual intimacy."

Source: Jane Gross, "Second Wave of AIDS Feared by Officials in San Francisco," *The New York Times*, pp. 1, 8 (December 11, 1993).

DOCUMENT 27: A Turning Point in the Struggle Against AIDS

Perhaps the most significant turning point in the war against AIDS occurred in 1996 when the XI International Conference on AIDS, held in Vancouver, Canada, made it widely known that a combination of one of three new "protease inhibitor" drugs with two of the established anti-AIDS drugs dramatically reduced the level of HIV in patients (by decreasing their viral load count from tens or hundreds of thousands to below 500) and significantly strengthened their immune system (by increasing their T4 count substantially). Amazing but true stories were being told of some people with AIDS who were literally on their deathbeds, emaciated and suffering from unbearable pain, but after receiving the three-drug "cocktail" regained their full weight, were successfully treated for their opportunistic infections, and felt healthy and were prepared to return to work. The new three-drug "cocktail" did not help many in the final stages of AIDS, but was remarkably successful for patients in the earlier stages of HIV infection.

Combination therapy, including a protease inhibitor [a class of new drugs] and two drugs based on AZT, is showing promise for many AIDS patients, leading experts to the conclusion that AIDS may soon be seen as a long-term, manageable disease. After years of development and testing, scientists may have found the appropriate combination of drugs to control HIV. In a new approach that researchers hope may be a cure, scientists are targeting newly-infected patients, rather than those in the advanced stages of disease. Martin Markowitz of Aaron Diamond AIDS Research Center claims that the effort "will answer the question of whether HIV infection can be eradicated in man." Nearly 60,000 Americans and 10,000 more people in other countries have already received the new drugs, the first of which was approved in mid-December [1995]. The cost of the drugs and possible side effects are drawbacks to the therapy, but many in the AIDS community are optimistic about the recent advances.

Source: Michael Waldholz, "New Drug 'Cocktails' Mark Exciting Turn in the War on AIDS," *Wall Street Journal*, p. A1 (June 14, 1996), CDC National AIDS Clearinghouse (Bethesda Md.: Information, Inc., 1996).

DOCUMENT 28: The New Protease Inhibitors

Will AIDS become a manageable disease like diabetes? Thanks to the new protease inhibitor drugs, this seems to be quite likely. However, it is possible that HIV, which mutates about 1 percent each year, might develop defenses against the new drugs and become resistant. In the meantime, though, for those who are taking one of the three new drugs, in combination with two of the older available drugs, it feels like a new lease on life!

After battling the AIDS virus for three years, Sam Viet was ravaged last January by parasitic disease, ulcers and 105-degree fevers. Listed in critical condition, he told friends he might leave the hospital in "a body bag."

Today, Viet, 26, is healthy and strong—and thinks he'll stay that way.

... [He] and thousands of other AIDS patients ... across the country are reaping the benefits of new drugs known as protease inhibitors.

Thanks to the near-miraculous effects of these drugs, doctors believe they may be on their way to converting a fatal disease into a controllable condition like diabetes. So successful have protease inhibitors been in early tests that some physicians and AIDS activists have even begun to think the unthinkable: Might they have found a cure for the so-far invincible virus?

... In basic terms, protease inhibitors—Crixivan, Norvir and Invirase—block the action of protease, an enzyme that ... HIV ... needs to reproduce.... Only time will tell whether HIV is resilient enough to defeat protease inhibitors and whether the new drugs prove to have long-term toxic effects. In the meantime, the early results are stunning....

Source: Joe Nicholson, "Fighting AIDS: Wonder of Life After AIDS," *New York Daily News*, pp. 16–17 (August 25, 1996).

THE GLOBAL CRISIS

DOCUMENT 29: Implications of a Global Epidemic

The increase in new HIV infections is particularly rapid in India and Southeast Asia, where sexual transmission is an important factor. For example, in Thailand, the commercial sex industry has contributed to the very rapid spread of HIV. In other regions, such as Latin America and the Caribbean, HIV infection is also spreading quickly. Sub-Saharan Africa already has one of the highest rates of HIV infection and a large number of deaths from AIDS. Since as many women as men are infected in Africa, families have lost adults in the most productive period of their lives, children have been orphaned, and those remaining in the affected households have been impoverished. Unfortunately, resources in developing nations are often meager; consequently, the financing of prevention efforts and treatment programs is grossly inadequate and cannot begin to match those in wealthier countries. By the end of 1997, the United Nations estimated that 16,000 people become HIV-infected each day.

WHO [the World Health Organization] estimates [in 1992] that 10–12 million adults and children have been infected with HIV since the start of the pandemic, and projects that this cumulative figure will reach 30–40 million by the year 2000. As these infected people develop HIV-related illness and ultimately AIDS (a progression that takes on average 10 years from initial infection), . . . AIDS prevention and control [programs] will increasingly be judged by the quality of the care they offer.

Hospital, ambulatory and home care . . . must at [a] minimum include pain relief and treatment for common opportunistic infections. . . . In addition, infected individuals need understanding and compassion if they are to maximize their remaining health potential and refrain from infecting others. Families and friends, the prime support of infected persons, must in turn receive assistance in fulfilling this function. . . .

Because AIDS incapacitates people at ages when they are most needed for the support of the young and elderly, the impact on families with one or more HIV-infected members is enormous. . . . The global strategy calls for direct action, as well as research, to lessen this impact and in particular to reduce the burden on women, who often carry the primary responsibility for providing AIDS care. It stresses the need to plan immediately for the care of the 10–15 million children who will be orphaned by maternal AIDS by the year 2000.

The impact of AIDS on society at large is equally damaging. Among the direct and indirect economic costs are spiraling health care costs, decimation of the workforce, loss of investment in skilled [labor] and educated professionals, and loss of consumers and purchasing power. In the developing countries, the pandemic may well cause social disintegration and political turmoil.

Source: *Global Strategy for the Prevention and Control of AIDS: 1992 Update* (Geneva: World Health Organization—Global Programme on AIDS, 1992), pp. 1–19.

DOCUMENT 30: The Vulnerability of Women in the Developing World

Throughout most of the world, heterosexual HIV transmission is an increasing risk for women. For instance, in Africa there are about as many women as men who are infected with HIV. The role of women in society contributes to their vulnerability. Social inequality between the sexes and economic dependence of women upon men make it more difficult for women to assert themselves in their sexual relationships. Male sexual behavior, such as a reluctance to use condoms and not discussing their extramarital sexual relationships, places women at risk. In order to protect themselves properly, women need the strength and autonomy to negotiate their relationships with men and to make their own choices.

In the battle against AIDS, theirs is an "unheard scream" that must now break into the global consciousness. . . . The scream is that of girls and young women who, according to Dr. Elizabeth Reid of the United Nations Development Programme, are "excessively vulnerable" to AIDS infection.

Action, Reid says, must be taken to . . . address the factors . . . that contribute to HIV infection. . . . Practices that allow women's sexual bondage and early initiation into sexual relationships—such as incest, early marriage, and dowry—must be eliminated. Girls should be assisted in getting an education so they will not have to consent to sex to pay for their schooling.

Source: Estrella Miranda-Maniquis, "The Silence About Women," World Press Review 40(2): 26 (February 1993).

DOCUMENT 31: STDs Are a Good Indicator of Unsafe Sexual Behavior

With one-third of a billion new cases of sexually transmitted diseases (STDs) occurring in the world each year, it is clear that unsafe sexual behavior continues in spite of the AIDS epidemic. Diseases such as gonorrhea, syphilis, herpes, hepatitis, chlamydia, chanchroid, lymphogranuloma venereum, granuloma inguinale, scabies, pubic lice infestation, and many others are very common and cause considerable suffering around the world. A few countries have lower STD rates than in previous years, suggesting that fear of AIDS or HIV prevention campaigns are at least partially effective. Other countries, unfortunately, have increasing or constant STD rates. We also know that some STDs make it more likely for persons exposed to HIV to become infected, and those who are infected with both HIV and certain other STDs will tend to develop AIDS symptoms more rapidly.

The World Health Organization (WHO) said on Friday that many more people contract sexually transmitted diseases (STDs) [333 million new cases per year] than was previously believed. In addition, it seems that such infections "greatly increase the risk of contracting HIV," the Organization said. A new study . . . was conducted by WHO's Global Programme on AIDS and the Rockefeller Foundation. The results suggested that STDs are increasing in China and parts of the former Soviet Union, while decreasing in recent years in Norway, Sweden, Chile, Costa Rica, Thailand, and Zimbabwe because of safer sex. However, "There is strong evidence that these curable STDs, because they cause genital lesions or inflammation, greatly increase the risk of sexual transmission of HIV," the report said. Antonio Gerbase, the study's leading author at

WHO, added that "the huge number of sexual infections sets the stage for the amplification of HIV."

Source: Stephanie Nebehay, "333 Million New Cases of Sexual Disease a Year" (Reuters, August 25, 1995); CDC National AIDS Clearinghouse (Bethesda, Md.: Information, Inc., 1995).

THE EPIDEMIC TAKES ITS TOLL

DOCUMENT 32: Forecast of the Cost of Medical Care for People with HIV

Billions of dollars are spent each year to treat patients with HIV infection and AIDS. During the 1980s, costs came down as hospital stays for persons with AIDS were shortened. However, in the future, medical expenses for AIDS patients are expected to increase. In developed nations, new drugs and new combinations of drugs, specifically the protease inhibitors used with nucleoside analog drugs, are now becoming available. Survival time will increase, and access to care should improve. As AIDS continues to become more of a chronic disease with people living many years after being diagnosed with AIDS, it is likely that the lifetime costs of treating the malady will continue to rise.

It is estimated that the cumulative (i.e., national) cost of treating people with AIDS (PWA's) is about three times the cost of treating seropositives without AIDS [those infected with HIV but not diagnosed with AIDS], and that the cost of treating all people with HIV in 1991 will be $5.8 billion. . . .

Recent cost studies [estimate] that the lifetime medical care cost of treating a person with AIDS from the time of diagnosis is between $40,000 and $75,000. [My studies have calculated] that the [annual] cost of treatment is $32,000, and the lifetime cost of treating an individual with AIDS is $85,333. The chief reasons for the increased estimate of lifetime cost are longer survival times and the [widespread use] of costly outpatient drugs. . . . [I]t is assumed that the average cost of treating a seropositive [person] without AIDS [symptoms] will remain at $5,150 per year in 1990 dollars for the years 1991 through 1994.

These forecasts are based on numerous assumptions. . . . More information about a variety of issues is needed to improve forecasts of HIV-related costs. . . . More information on the cost of treatment for specific subpopulations such as women, children, [injecting] drug users, and [gay] and bisexual men would improve the sensitivity of forecasts to changes in the composition of people with HIV. . . . [Then] analysts could multiply projected numbers of PWA's in each subpopulation by their estimated cost of treatment.

Source: Fred J. Hellinger, "Forecasting the Medical Care Costs of the HIV Epidemic: 1991–1994," *Inquiry* 28(3): 213–225 (Fall 1991).

DOCUMENT 33: AIDS Is Expensive

Many AIDS patients are without private health insurance. Those who do have insurance run the risk of surpassing the total expenditures allowed. The result is that the public will carry the burden of the cost, through the Ryan White Program, Medicare, and Medicaid. Estimates of total future costs are difficult to make with great precision because there are so many unknown factors. However, it is likely that medical expenditures will substantially increase because of the availability of new treatments, as well as escalating medical costs.

Joe Luevanos, chief financial officer for Cedars-Sinai Medical Center, said the west Los Angeles facility is beginning to see a new phenomenon—AIDS patients with insurance who are beginning to reach the lifetime caps on their medical coverage. . . . [M]any insurance policies have lifetime caps of $100,000 or $250,000. Now that AIDS patients are living longer, "some of these AIDS patients are in here six or seven times." . . . There are new drugs and new therapies to prolong their lives. These drugs are expensive.

[The director of AIDS programs for Los Angeles County] said it is impossible to know how much AIDS will cost in the future because that depends on how fast the disease spreads. "The big impact, in terms of the spread of the virus among drug users to women and children, hasn't hit Los Angeles yet. . . . It's just beginning."

Source: Liz Mullen, "Taxpayers May Shoulder Increasing AIDS Outlays," *Los Angeles Business Journal* (August 17, 1992).

DOCUMENT 34: . . . And Now Getting Even More Expensive

The discovery in the mid-1990s that the protease inhibitor drugs, when combined with two of the other anti-AIDS drugs, will significantly lower the viral load counts and boost the immune systems of persons with HIV/AIDS has revolutionized treatment for persons with HIV in the developed world. However, the new drugs are so prohibitively expensive, the key question is: Who will pay for them? Intense political activism forced the price of AZT, the first FDA-approved anti-AIDS drug, down from an exorbitant $8,000 per year when it was first released to the public in the 1980s to about $1,800 per year at discount pharmacies in 1996. It will probably take similar political activism to bring down the price of the new protease inhibitor drugs.

To the pharmaceutical industry [the new protease inhibitor drugs] represent a financial bonanza, given the desperate need of millions of people [worldwide] for an anti-HIV drug that works. Today, the *least* expensive protease inhibitor, Crixivan (Indinavir), manufactured by Merck & Co., is sold to suppliers at $4,380 for a year's supply, compared with $6,500 for Abbott's drug [Norvir] and $5,700 for Hoffman-La Roche's Invirase— two to three times the cost of AZT. While cost-versus-sales figures are any company's best-kept secret, a look at Abbott's reported first-quarter earnings proves that its wonder drug is bringing home the bacon: Norvir garnered approximately $10 million in sales in the first three weeks of being on the market. . . .

Only people with money will be able to afford these drugs; everybody else will have to settle for AZT. . . .

Source: Anne-Christine D'Adesky, "Rich Man's Drug," *Out! Magazine*, pp. 62–65, 100, 102–103 (August 1996).

DOCUMENT 35: Good News/Bad News About the New Drugs

Larry Kramer, author and playwright, has been a longtime AIDS activist. In this selection, he discusses both the good news that the protease inhibitors are so far extremely effective in helping people with HIV/AIDS, and the bad news that the drugs may be out of reach to hundreds of thousands of HIV-infected people in the United States who do not have good private health insurance. It is ironic that when this milestone development in pharmaceutical technology comes along, so many cannot afford it.

There has been much recent excitement about protease inhibitors, a new class of drugs that promise to prolong markedly the lives of and in some cases possibly help cure those with HIV. But because of the cost, a great many who would benefit from such drugs will not have access to them.

For many people already infected, like myself, treatment with proteases might offer at least "two to three years of additional life—which is a lifetime, because new drugs are appearing so fast," says Dr. Steven A. Miles, director of the AIDS research center clinic at the University of California at Los Angeles. For those just infected, Miles says, proteases "quite possibly are a cure, if you get them into you quickly enough."

But drug companies are charging historically high prices for their new wares, insurers are finding ways to get out of reimbursing for them and what little Government help there was in past years is rapidly evaporating as the nation turns away from public support for the needy, a group that now includes a lot more people than it ever did before.

A *New York Times* article earlier this year estimated that drugs for someone with full-blown AIDS cost about $70,000 a year. . . . Indeed, the seriously sick can find their annual drug cost exceeding $150,000. . . .

Finally there are drugs that may allow people to live longer, but here's the punch line: Few can afford them. . . .

Source: Larry Kramer, "A Good News/Bad News AIDS Joke," *The New York Times Magazine*, pp. 26–29 (July 14, 1996).

DOCUMENT 36: Who Should Pay for AIDS Care?

The AIDS epidemic has proved to be costly. Not only is it expensive to care for patients with HIV, but the indirect costs are substantial. Many who die of AIDS are in their most productive years. The loss of their labor, their contributions, and their potential is difficult to replace. In this reading, the author refers to a distinction sometimes made by others between those who acquired HIV through behaviors that could have been avoided (unprotected sex and injecting drugs with infected needles and syringes) and those who acquire HIV through other means (such as through birth or a blood transfusion). However, this distinction between "guilty" and "innocent" sufferers is a faulty one. No one asks to be infected with the virus. Most of the persons who died from AIDS during the 1980s and early 1990s were infected at a time when little was known about how people should protect themselves from the virus. Safer sex practices reduce risk of infection but do not eliminate risk entirely. Blaming people for the diseases they get is mean-spirited and unproductive. The author argues that we should set aside our prejudices and moral judgments. What do you think? Why do you think that?

The economic burden of AIDS medical care will be shared between the public (federal, state, and local government[s]) and private (insurance industry, private corporations) sectors. Equity of distribution of this financial burden is the issue underlying policy decisions at all levels of government. . . . The numerous hospitalizations and extensive care AIDS generally requires means that the economic impact is great. Economic losses occur as a result of direct costs (health care expenditures) and indirect costs (work-years lost after diagnosis, loss of lifetime earnings due to premature death). . . .

The question of who should bear the financial burden of AIDS health care is being fought within both public and private sectors. What proportion . . . should be borne by the government, the insurance companies, hospitals, and the patients themselves? . . .

Several difficult issues regarding AIDS have been superimposed on . . . [the allocation of funds]. [One] issue involves social prejudice and moral judgment. It attaches a cost-of-care/benefit-of-life ratio to . . . [those who engage in] willful self-destructive behaviors while attaching the same cost/benefit ratio to children with AIDS engaging in innocent behaviors. . . .

[P]olicymakers and the public will respond to the AIDS crisis in direct proportion to their sense of vulnerability to AIDS. . . . AIDS is a crisis that has been imposed on an imperfect health care system . . . [whose] flaws are easy to recognize but difficult to treat. Difficult choices about who pays for the medical care for AIDS patients will be made by upper-class and upper middle-class policymakers who are influenced by their own sense of vulnerability. . . . Social prejudice and moral judgment must be set aside.

Source: Linda J. Kerley, "The Escalating Health Care Cost of AIDS: Who Will Pay?" *Nursing Forum* 25(1): 5–13 (1990).

DOCUMENT 37: HIV Prevention Is the Best Economic Solution

Preventing one case of AIDS saves many times the eventual cost to society. The direct costs of medical care and other patient care services, combined with indirect economic and social costs, are considerable. Yet prevention and public health efforts are not always given the funding and support they deserve. In the developing countries of Africa, Asia, and Latin America, AIDS has been allowed to worsen because of the lack of sufficient funds to develop effective prevention programs.

This has usually resulted in a situation where AIDS has cost the society more than it would have spent on prevention. Every person who is prevented from becoming infected with HIV saves society from a worsening economic and social burden.

The powerful negative impact of AIDS on households, productive enterprises, and countries stems partly from the high costs of treatment, which divert resources from productive investments, and mostly from the fact that AIDS primarily affects people during their economically productive adult years, when they are typically responsible for the support and care of others. . . . Since there is no vaccine or cure for AIDS, primary prevention is the only current method of fighting the epidemic. . . .

Studies in nine developing and seven high-income countries suggest that preventing one case of AIDS saves . . . about twice the GNP per capita in discounted lifetime costs of medical care. . . .

If [the world's] communities wait until they recognize significant illness from HIV before acting, the epidemic will most likely have penetrated deeply into the population, at which point HIV will be much more costly and difficult . . . to halt.

Source: Seth Berkley, Peter Piot, and Doris Schopper, "AIDS: Invest Now or Pay More Later," *Finance & Development*, pp. 40–43 (June 1994).

DOCUMENT 38: Increasing Costs and Scarce Funds

Outpatient treatment for HIV infection or AIDS is more cost-effective than inpatient hospital care. And yet AIDS clinics are being squeezed by greater demand for their services, increased costs, and decreased funding. Over time, there will be the danger of burnout or battle fatigue among private and public funding sources. During the mid-1990s, Ryan White funding from the United States government alleviated much of the lack of funding for AIDS-related outpatient programs. Fortunately, the Ryan White Care Act was renewed in 1996 for an additional five years. However, the enormous costs of the new protease inhibitor drugs threatened to bankrupt existing HIV funding resources.

Innovations in outpatient treatment for AIDS have helped patients live longer while improving their quality of life. . . . [However,] the rapid growth in ambulatory care for AIDS patients—supported in part by the development of new, expensive drug therapies—has contributed to a growing price tag for AIDS treatment. . . .

Institutions that operate AIDS clinics are being financially squeezed by rising costs, growing demand, inadequate reimbursement from Medicaid and other payers, and tougher competition for grants from foundations. . . .

One of the largest private funders of AIDS care, the Robert Wood Johnson Foundation, is winding down its $17.2 million, four-year initiative to fund new outpatient programs at nine sites. The Princeton, NJ-based foundation has no plans to provide additional seed money for a similar multi-site project. . . .

[A hospital spokesman said] there is "burnout among private foundations in giving money for AIDS" [and predicted] "very high competition among providers for grants from a small pool of donors."

Source: Howard J. Anderson, "Outpatient AIDS Care Squeezed by High Costs, Low Payments," *Hospitals*, pp. 40, 42 (May 5, 1991).

DOCUMENT 39: The Insured vs. the Uninsured and Underinsured

The AIDS Drug Assistance Program (ADAP) was designed to give anti-AIDS drugs to people with HIV who do not have insurance or do not have adequate insurance, and cannot afford the cost of these expensive medications. However, with the advent of the new protease inhibitor drugs, this program has rapidly become inundated with applicants and the available financial resources are not nearly sufficient to deal with the increased need.

Due to increased demand for new AIDS drugs, and the high cost of the treatments, government programs designed to provide the drugs free to needy patients are failing. The AIDS Drug Assistance Program was established by Congress to give states money to provide the drugs to uninsured or underinsured people. Recently, however, states have been forced to limit the drugs they provide, or make applicants wait for treatment. Nearly half of all states are limiting or expecting to limit access to the new protease inhibitors. A lobbying group for AIDS patients estimates that the $190 million appropriated for the program in the 1996 budget is less than half of what is needed.

Source: Gina Kolata, "AIDS Patients Slipping Through Safety Net," *New York Times*, p. 24 (September 15, 1996), CDC National AIDS Clearinghouse (Bethesda, Md.: Information, Inc., 1996).

DOCUMENT 40: Familiar Names, Sewn on a Quilt

The Names Project Foundation, which sponsors the AIDS quilt, has helped Americans remember the hundreds of thousands of people who have died of AIDS. Friends and family create a panel that is displayed with thousands of others throughout the country. By 1992, the AIDS quilt covered an area the size of twelve football fields; over 20,000 panels were displayed in Washington, D.C., on the grounds of the Washington Monument. In October 1996, it was exhibited again in its entirety on the lawn of the Great Mall in the nation's capital. By 1996, over one-third of a million Americans had died of AIDS. Below are a selection of some of the more familiar names.

Names You May Recognize: Peter Allen, entertainer; Arthur Ashe, tennis player; Howard Ashman, lyricist for "The Little Mermaid" and "Beauty and the Beast"; Michael Bennett, director/choreographer best noted for "A Chorus Line"; Amanda Blake, actress best known for "Gunsmoke"; Kimberly Bergalis, advocate for HIV testing of health care workers; Mel Boozer, black and gay rights activist; Arthur Bressan, Jr., filmmaker; Michael Callen, singer and AIDS activist; Tina Chow, fashion model and clothing designer; Roy Cohn, attorney and conservative political insider; Brad Davis, actor; Neal Dickerson, AIDS activist and television news producer; Perry Ellis, fashion designer; Wayland Flowers, comedian and puppeteer; Michel Foucault, postmodern French philosopher; Alison Gertz, AIDS activist; Elizabeth Glaser, AIDS activist; Miguel Godreau, lead dancer with Alvin Ailey American Dance Theater; Halston, fashion designer; Keith Haring, artist; Robert Hershman, television producer; Jon Hinson, U.S. Congressman (Mississippi); Rock Hudson, actor; Philip C. R. Jerry, choreographer and lead dancer with the Joffrey Ballet; James Kirkwood, writer; Stephen Kolzak, casting director for television show "Cheers"; Liberace, performer and pianist; Robert Mapplethorpe, innovative photographer; Kiki Mason, AIDS advocate and writer; Sgt. Leonard Matlovich, gay rights activist; Stewart McKinney, U.S. Congressman (Republican, Connecticut); Freddie "Mercury" Bulsara, lead singer of rock group Queen; Rudolf Nureyev, famous ballet dancer; Anthony Perkins, actor; Robert Reed, actor; Norman Rene, theatrical director; Max Robinson, ABC news anchor; Vito Russo, writer; Jerry Smith, Washington Redskin; Willi Smith, fashion designer; Stephen Stucker, actor; Sylvester, disco singer; Dan Turner, AIDS activist; Tom Villard, actor; Dr. Tom Waddell, Olympic athlete; Ryan White, teenage AIDS activist; Ricky Wilson, guitarist with the B-52's; David Wojnarowicz, painter, writer, and filmmaker; Pedro Zamora, AIDS educator, focusing on youth, and star of MTV's "The Real World."

Sources: The Names Project Foundation Factsheet; "A Decade of Loss," *Newsweek* 121(3): 22–23 (January 18, 1993); CDC National AIDS Clearinghouse (Bethesda, Md.: Information, Inc., 1994, 1995, 1996).

DOCUMENT 41: Orphans of the Epidemic

The HIV epidemic has left children and young people without parents or family to care for them. In the near future, there will be well over 100,000 orphaned in the United States as a result of the epidemic. Some of these children are themselves infected with HIV and are already ill, although most are not infected. Properly caring for these children is a major challenge for society.

By the year 2000, as many as 125,000 children and adolescents will be motherless because of a single disease. Their mothers, and in many cases their fathers too, will have died of AIDS. And the end of the epidemic is nowhere in sight.

The vast majority of these youngsters are not HIV-infected but are at high risk for a range of behavioral and developmental problems. At least 80 percent of them come from poor communities of color, which have already been devastated by society's neglect. The teenagers are at risk for engaging in sexual and drug-using behaviors associated with HIV transmission.

Along with their unique problems, the orphans of the HIV epidemic share some characteristics of children whose parents have died of other causes; all such children grieve the loss and need care. They also share some characteristics of children living in the same communities whose families are not directly affected by HIV; all such children need better education, improved living conditions and greater economic opportunities, as well as freedom from violence, discrimination, and the ravages of drugs and alcohol. [But] [t]he orphans of the HIV epidemic are of particular concern because [they have been affected by all of these problems].

The phenomenon of a very large group of orphans whose parents have died of a single disease appears to be unprecedented in American history. . . . The various categories of children and adolescents who are infected with or affected by HIV can be represented [by] an iceberg.

The tip of the iceberg represents the . . . pediatric AIDS cases in the United States reported to the CDC (including the small but growing number of reported adolescent cases. . . . [P]ediatric AIDS has received the most public and professional attention, since these fragile children and their families have urgent medical and social service needs. Just below the tip of the iceberg . . . are known cases of HIV-infected children and adolescents. There are many more HIV-infected newborns than known pediatric AIDS cases . . . which means that a large portion of this section of the iceberg is still hidden.

The second largest portion of the iceberg represents the uninfected siblings of the group with AIDS or HIV infection. These may be older brothers and sisters, born before their mother contracted HIV, or younger children who escaped maternal–fetal transmission. . . .

By far the largest and most hidden portion of the iceberg . . . includes uninfected children and adolescents whose parent or parents, another adult relative, or a committed caregiver unrelated by birth or marriage has either died of AIDS or is living with serious HIV disease. To carry the image one step further, the iceberg itself is situated in a stormy sea of violence, homelessness, drug and alcohol use, poverty, discrimination, and community disintegration.

Although in recent years the term "orphan" has been used most commonly to describe a child who has lost both parents, it has historically meant a child who has lost one or both parents. A definition that focuses on motherless youth was chosen . . . partly because [it] conforms to the realities of life as these families know it. For the vast majority of youth whose caregiving parent dies of HIV, that parent is the mother. There are, of course, families in which an HIV-infected father is the primary caregiver; however, these situations appear to be rare. There are also families in which the death of the father from AIDS, even when the mother is uninfected, is a traumatic event that results in a family breakup.

Source: *Orphans of the HIV Epidemic: Unmet Needs in Six U.S. Cities* (New York: The Orphan Project, 1994).

DOCUMENT 42: Catastrophic Loss in the Artistic and Creative World

Artists, musicians, actors, dancers, and writers are the visible symbols of the nation's creative and cultural life. The AIDS epidemic has greatly affected this community because so many of its members have been lost. The number of gay men who were talented in the visual, theatrical, musical, and literary arts and have succumbed to AIDS is enormous and has undoubtedly had a devastating impact upon the direction of these arts that we shall never fully know.

The cultural world is getting used to untimely deaths. Every week someone's friend, collaborator, colleague, or lover dies. . . . All lives are irreplaceable, but the death of an artist leaves a void that echoes beyond the circle of loved ones. There is the art work that will never be made. There are the lessons that can't be passed on to a new generation. . . .

[George Davidson, theatrical artistic director, remarked:] "The impact on the arts and culture is incalculable. . . . The problem, aside from the horror of the deaths, is that the system by which we encounter art is a system of passing things down, and when you break the circuit the way it is being broken by AIDS, the damage may be irreparable." . . .

The crisis . . . has not just struck the world of art, it is just that its ravages are more visible there—and have an impact on everyone whom culture touches.

Source: David Arsen, Donna Foote, Katrine Ames, Jack Kroll, Abigail Kuflik, and Pete Plagens, "A Lost Generation," *Newsweek* 121(3): 16–20 (January 18, 1993).

DOCUMENT 43: From the Depths of Despair

Suicide rates are much higher for people infected with HIV than for patients with other chronic diseases. The social stigma, emotional isolation, and personal problems that people experience can be overwhelming. Support groups and services provided by community-based organizations are invaluable in helping people to cope. By 1996, however, with new advances in treatments and the potential for greatly diminished viral load counts, increasing T-cell counts, and improving health, the cloak of despair is beginning to lift.

Among people with AIDS, it is an open secret. When the time comes . . . [many] are going to take control of their death. [Many of them] are going to enlist the help of friends, family, lovers and sympathetic doctors, and they are going to take an overdose of pills or put a plastic bag over their heads or add a little too much morphine to an intravenous drip, and they are going to kill themselves. . . .

Several studies . . . have consistently shown that people with AIDS kill themselves at a much higher rate than people with other chronic diseases and that the suicide rate among people with AIDS is from 10 to 20 times that of the general population.

"In the AIDS community it's widespread, it's ethical, it's noble," said Martin Delaney, the director of Project Inform, an advocacy group for people with AIDS. . . . [B]ecause the community tends to be closely knit, those contemplating suicide often seek the advice of others. . . . But even an advocate like Mr. Delaney cautioned that "this whole assisted-passage stuff isn't for everyone."

Source: "AIDS Patients Seek Solace in Suicide, but Many Find Uncertainty," *The New York Times*, p. B5 (June 24, 1994).

DOCUMENT 44: You Know Someone with HIV, Even If You Think You Don't!

Even if you think you do not know anyone with HIV or AIDS, there is no question that you do know several people with HIV infection whom you watch every week on television or in the movie theater. AIDS discrimination is unfortunately quite common in the entertainment industry, and it is the public's perception of AIDS as a stigmatizing syndrome that keeps it alive. If you learned that your favorite actor on television or in films was HIV-positive, would you remain a loyal fan? What if you learned that a popular leading man, or male "sex symbol," was HIV-positive as a result of unprotected homosexual behavior?

Many Hollywood celebrities, moved by personal losses from AIDS, have been leaders in speaking out about the disease and in urging compassion for AIDS patients. Actors with HIV and AIDS, however, have criticized the industry for shunning them from the business. In a job market where competition is intense, physical appearance and stamina are highly valued, and public perceptions about an individual's personal life are critical, HIV-positive actors often keep their infected status closely guarded. While insiders say that insurance claims for people working in Hollywood indicate that hundreds of actors are infected with HIV, most choose to keep their condition confidential. Some say the situation has improved and that producers would only consider an actor's HIV status a liability if he or she was to play in a long-running series. One HIV-positive television actor said that the real point of actors not disclosing their HIV status is to keep the audience in the dark.

Source: Rodger McFarlane, "Taking a Hit," *Advocate*, p. 91 (August 20, 1996), CDC National AIDS Clearinghouse (Bethesda, Md.: Information, Inc., 1996).

SUGGESTED READINGS

Alexander, S., and J. Rapaport. "The Real AIDS Numbers." *Mademoiselle* 98, p. 104 (March 1992).

———. "The No-Futures Market." *Harper's* 285, pp. 25–26 (November 1992).

Black, R. F., et al. "The Hidden Cost of AIDS." *U.S. News & World Report* 113, pp. 48–52ff. (July 27, 1992).

Brown, David. "AIDS's Economic Impact Contradictory, Complex." *Washington Post*, p. A3 (July 11, 1996).

Colacello, B. "The Last Days of Nureyev." *Vanity Fair* 56, pp. 182–189 (March 1993).

Dellamora, Richard. *Apocalyptic Overtures: Sexual Politics & the Sense of an Ending*. New Brunswick, N.J.: Rutgers University Press, 1994.

"The Economics of Disease. "*Investor's Business Daily*, p. B1 (November 3, 1995).

Elmer-Dewitt, P. "How Safe Is Sex." *Time* 138, pp. 72–74 (November 25, 1991).

Feldman, Douglas, and Thomas Johnson, eds. *The Social Dimensions of AIDS: Method and Theory*. Westport, Conn.: Praeger, 1986.

"Foreign Aid Cuts Threaten National and International Health, Experts Say." *Nation's Health* 25(7), p. 5 (August 1995).

Harris, W. "Art and AIDS: Urgent Images." *Art News* 92, pp. 120–123 (May 1993).

Katz, J. "AIDS and the Media: Shifting out of Neutral." *Rolling Stone*, pp. 31–32 (May 27, 1993).

Koop, C. Everett. "AIDS and American Values." *World Affairs Journal* 6, pp. 24–29 (Fall 1987).

Levine, A. Carol, ed. *Death in the Family: Orphans of the HIV Epidemic*. New York: United Hospital Fund, 1993.

Lovejoy, Margot. *The Book of Plagues*. Purchase, N.Y.: Center for Editions, Visual Arts Division, S.U.N.Y. Purchase, 1994.

Mandel, Michael J. "The Economics of AIDS." Business Week no. 3442, p. 34 (September 18, 1995).

Mann, J. M. "AIDS and the Next Pandemic." *Scientific American* 264, p. 126 (March 1991).

McCoy, F. "AIDS: We All Pay in Different Ways." *Black Enterprise* 23, p. 65 (February 1993).

"The Numbers Debate." *World Press Review* 41, p. 40 (January 1994).

Nunn, P., and A. Kochi. "A Deadly Duo—TB and AIDS." *World Health*, pp. 7–9 (July/August 1993).

Strauss, A. L., et al. "AIDS and Health Care Deficiencies." *Society* 28, pp. 63–73 (July/August 1991).

Swartz, M. "The Price of AIDS." *Texas Monthly* 22, pp. 88–89 (March 1994).

Ulak, Richard, and William F. Skinner, eds. *AIDS and the Social Sciences: Common Threads*. Lexington: University Press of Kentucky, 1991.

3

HIV/AIDS Within Communities and Populations

It is not *who* you are that will predict whether or not you will get AIDS, but *what* you do. Being a gay male does not give you AIDS. Having repeated anal sex with an HIV-positive male without using a condom is very likely to give you AIDS. If an HIV-negative gay man is in a permanent, completely monogamous relationship with another HIV-negative gay man, neither man can become HIV-infected even if they engage in anal sex without using a condom. Being an injecting drug user does not give you AIDS. Using a needle and syringe to shoot up drugs that were just used by an HIV-infected person is very likely to give you AIDS. An HIV-negative injecting drug user who always uses his or her own clean drug injection equipment cannot become HIV-infected from injecting drug use.

However, some communities and populations are particularly vulnerable to HIV infection, and some have been severely impacted by the epidemic. This chapter will focus primarily upon the situation in the United States, while the next chapter will take a more international view. By December 1996 (Centers for Disease Control and Prevention 1996), 581,429 Americans were reported to have or have had AIDS; 362,004 had died of AIDS and 219,425 were living with AIDS. It is very conservatively estimated by the CDC that an additional 450,000 to 700,000 persons were living with HIV infection but had not yet developed AIDS.

Of the 581,429 persons with AIDS, 7,629 were children under thirteen years old, 2,754 were teenagers (thirteen–nineteen years old), 21,097 were young adults (twenty–twenty-four years old), and 549,949 were adults twenty-five or over. The modal age category (with the greatest number) was the early thirties (thirty to thirty-four years old). Of the 581,429 persons, about half (49 percent) were men who had sex with men (gay, bisexual, and self-defined heterosexuals who had sex with other men but were not injecting drug users), 6 percent were men who had sex with men and were also injecting drug users, 25 percent were men and women who were injecting drug users, 1 percent were men, women, and children with hemophilia/coagulation disorder, 4 percent were men and women who had heterosexual sex with an injecting drug user, 4 percent were men and women who had heterosexual sex with an HIV-infected person but the risk was not specified, 1 percent were men, women, and children who received infected blood, blood components, or tissue, 1 percent were children of mothers with HIV infection or at risk for HIV infection, and 7 percent were men, women, and children who had another risk or whose risk was not reported or could not be identified.

Among the total number of reported AIDS cases, 85 percent were male and 15 percent were female; 46 percent were white (not Hispanic), 35 percent were black (not Hispanic), 18 percent were Hispanic, 1 percent were Asian/Pacific Islanders, and 0.3 percent were American Indians/Alaskan Natives. The states with the highest rates of new cases of reported AIDS during January 1996–December 1996 were New York, Florida, New Jersey, Maryland, and Delaware. The metropolitan areas with a population of over 500,000 having the highest rates of new cases of reported AIDS during that same period were New York City, Miami, Jersey City (New Jersey), San Francisco, and West Palm Beach (Florida).

This chapter will focus upon teenagers, women, children, injecting drug users, gay men, commercial sex workers (prostitutes), the homeless, prisoners, and persons with hemophilia. We will look at the vulnerability of each of these groups or communities and how each is responding, or failing to respond, to the AIDS crisis. It is important for us to understand the social context of how people live in order for us to develop successful programs that prevent HIV infection and to properly care for those who have already become infected.

Source: Centers for Disease Control and Prevention, *HIV/AIDS Surveillance Report* 8(2): 1–39 (1996).

TEENAGERS

DOCUMENT 45: Attitudes and Social Factors Contribute to AIDS Among the Young Urban Poor

---

Young people growing up in poor neighborhoods are particularly vulnerable to high-risk sexual encounters and drug use. In this environment, unprotected sex and the drug culture offer immediate rewards and satisfaction to young people. On the other hand, success through education or work opportunities seems unattainable, and hope for another kind of life, unrealistic.

Teenagers and young women [in poor, urban neighborhoods] who are particularly at risk for HIV infection do not have access to economic or educational institutions that reward postponed childbearing.... Sexual activity begins as young as age 11 or 12 for girls and a few years older for boys. The role of sex in these [preteens' and teenagers'] lives is neither an erotic expression nor a response to romantic love, but rather . . . a part of the "warm body syndrome" or search for comfort. For many urban poor there is neither privacy nor time for loving sexual encounters, and many of those which lead to pregnancy (and perhaps to HIV transmission) occur in hallways with both partners fully dressed. Sex in a drug culture tends to produce either money to buy drugs or the drugs themselves. Many of these young people live in unsupervised . . . settings. Because truancy from school is the norm rather than the exception, socializing and sex, rather than education, establish the basic structure of the day.... The expansion of the drug culture and the unprecedented economic power it has brought to the young people who become enmeshed in it have removed the possibility of planning for alternative futures.

Source: Carol Levine, "Uncertain Risks and Bitter Realities: The Reproductive Choices of HIV-Infected Women," *The Milbank Quarterly* 68(3): 123–142 (Fall 1990).

DOCUMENT 46: The Surgeon General Discusses Teenagers and AIDS

It is important that the problem of HIV infection among teenagers be recognized by national leaders. The danger is that HIV can spread quickly among the young because this is the age when experimentation with sex and drugs begins. Teenagers need guidance and support during this period of intense personal change and confusion. Dr. Antonia Novello gave this speech while she was the U.S. Surgeon General during the early 1990s.

In this, its second decade, AIDS is a disease that is increasingly female, increasingly heterosexual and increasingly young. . . . The need to address the issue of HIV infection among young people is immediate. The legal, ethical, social and medical challenges that you young people represent to our current legal and health care systems . . . [make] this a cumbersome process. AIDS in young people presents many more social issues than I ever would have imagined. . . . [A]dolescence is a period of profound physiological, psychological and social change. Many young people often feel alienated from the rest of society, and society, in turn, often finds it difficult to understand their emotions and behaviors. . . .

The behaviors that lead to HIV infection in adolescents are often deemed socially unacceptable, and there is a temptation to stigmatize most of the adolescent population as "high risk," or "hard to reach." It is crucial for us adults to understand that *most* young people find themselves at times in situations that are risky for acquiring HIV, even if these situations are encountered only infrequently, for only a few minutes, a few hours, or a few weeks. . . .

We must work to provide HIV prevention education immediately . . . as an integral element of a . . . health curriculum that also provides education about sexuality and drug abuse. A dialogue between young people and their parents is critical . . . and all views should be acknowledged and accommodated.

Source: Antonia C. Novello, "Health Priorities for the Nineties: The Quest for Prevention," *Vital Speeches of the Day* 58(21): 666–672 (August 15, 1992).

DOCUMENT 47: Assisting Runaway Youth with Behavioral Changes

Runaway youth are at greater risk for HIV infection than other young people their age because they are more likely to engage in unprotected sexual intercourse and to inject drugs. In this study, intensive counseling proved successful in changing runaways' sexual behavior. This is encouraging because it shows that given enough of the right kind of help, teenagers can change their behavior to protect themselves.

The high seroprevalence rates among runaways exist despite reports of relatively high knowledge about HIV and . . . AIDS and positive be-

liefs about safe acts, highlighting the importance of [intervention pro-
grams] for HIV/AIDS among runaways that emphasize behavior
change.... Runaways' sexual risk behaviors (oral, anal, and vaginal intercourse) and [injecting] drug use place them at risk for AIDS infection.
... [U]nprotected sexual intercourse appears to be the primary behavior
leading to HIV transmission among runaways.... The goal of [our]
study [was] to evaluate an intervention program targeting the reduction
of sexual risk behaviors of these runaways.... [Our] program differed
from earlier adolescent HIV/AIDS programs in intensity, with a minimum of 10 sessions considered to be necessary for changing behavior.
Because the program targeted runaways, a group experiencing many
stressful events and unstable living situations, access to ongoing health
and mental health care to maintain safe sexual behaviors was also included as part of the HIV/AIDS prevention program.... [W]e found
significant increases in consistent condom use and reductions in the percentage of youths reporting a high-risk pattern of sexual behavior following the intervention.... This study ... has potentially important
implications [because it showed that] adolescents do change their behaviors in response to an intensive intervention, even adolescents with multiple problem behaviors and unstable life situations, who have been
described as resistant to change.

Source: Mary Jane Rotheram-Borus, "Reducing HIV Sexual Risk Behaviors
Among Runaway Adolescents," *Journal of the American Medical Association* 266(9):
1237–1241 (September 4, 1991).

DOCUMENT 48: Youth HIV Prevention Projects

Some young people are at greater risk for HIV infection than others.
For example, those who inject drugs or who exchange sex for drugs or
money are much more vulnerable than those who do not. Recognizing this fact, the Centers for Disease Control and Prevention (CDC),
state departments of education, and other organizations are sponsoring
HIV prevention programs specifically designed to reach high-risk teenagers.

[Beginning in the mid-1980s] the CDC [began] a variety of programs
designed to prevent HIV infection among youth in high-risk situations.
These include runaway and homeless youth, ... migrant youth, youth
who barter or sell sex, drug injectors, juvenile offenders, youth with sexually transmitted diseases, and those who seek counseling and testing
for HIV infection. These young people are frequently difficult to reach
with school-based HIV prevention education.

Implementing programs that can effectively prevent HIV infection among this population is difficult because of the characteristics of these youth. . . . These young people often have no access to societal institutions that provide important social support and services. . . .

State and local departments of education receive technical and . . . [financial] support to help to implement HIV prevention education programs in schools and communities. . . . These activities often include HIV prevention programs for students in alternative schools, training staff of community-based agencies, and participating in community and state coalitions that address the needs of youth. . . .

Currently USCM [the U.S. Conference of Mayors] is funding eight projects targeting children at high risk, including both out-of-school and in-school youth. For example, Atlanta's The Bridge will develop and provide an AIDS curriculum to the 200-plus runaway and homeless youth participating in its alternative classroom and counseling programs. Houston's Covenant House will provide weekly AIDS presentations to 800 clients, [and] comprehensive health education (including STD/HIV education) to 1,500 clients. . . .

In 1987, [the CDC] began providing funding to seven national organizations that address the specific needs of runaway, incarcerated, migrant, and other youth in high-risk situations.

For example, the National Network of Runaway and Youth Services provides HIV prevention education . . . to runaway and homeless youth throughout the nation. The Network trains staff in these agencies to provide HIV prevention education through street outreach programs, shelters, telephone hotlines, foster care, and individual and family counseling. . . .

[The] CDC also provides direct . . . support to community-based organizations serving youth. These programs encourage organizations to design specific prevention programs that reflect and respect the [youths'] culture and language, identify places where youth congregate, and form networks with other community organizations that are already serving this population.

The Neon Street Center for Youth in Chicago, for example, provides services to homeless and runaway youth and incorporates HIV risk-reduction messages into activities provided by the center. CDC works closely with the project . . . to assess behavior changes in the youth served.

The Massachusetts Committee for Children and Youth is a CDC-funded organization that has served as an advocate for children since 1959. It develops progressive child welfare policies, researches and documents children's needs, and links groups and other agencies on legal issues and educational forums that increase public awareness of critical children's issues. Its HIV programs include educational sessions for children in emergency shelters and teen peer education. . . .

CDC also conducts seroprevalence surveys and behavioral research to study the individual and social factors that motivate and shape adolescent risk behaviors. These activities are designed to determine the prevalence of HIV infection among children in high-risk situations, describe youth populations at risk for HIV infection, examine predictors of behavior, and evaluate intervention activities.

Ongoing coordinated programs are essential to ensure that youth in high-risk situations receive effective education to prevent HIV infection ... [because] [t]he lives of our most vulnerable children depend on the success of these programs.

Source: "HIV Education for Youth in High-Risk Situations," *HIV/AIDS Prevention*, pp. 10–12 (July 1991).

DOCUMENT 49: Requiring Parental Consent

Ideally, HIV education and prevention programs for young people would not require parental consent. Teenagers could then act on their own behalf without anxiety or fear. However, this is not always realistic from a political point of view; nearly all programs have incorporated parental consent into their design. Federally funded research, with only the rarest exceptions, requires parental consent in all studies involving those under eighteen years of age. Indeed, the National Institutes of Health, a major federal research center that gives out research grants, requires parental consent in research conducted among teenagers under eighteen even when the study is conducted outside the United States in a country where parental consent is not required. It is interesting to note that if the function of parental consent is to take decision-making control out of the hands of the teenager and put it into the hands of the parents, a teenager who does not want to participate in an HIV risk reduction program can still avoid participation even when his or her parents want the child to participate in such a program.

Because of their unique needs and legal status, adolescents should be able to obtain access to prevention education, HIV testing and counseling, medical care, and psychosocial services on their own initiative, without requiring parental consent. While the assistance of a parent, guardian, or supportive adult should be encouraged, many adolescents whose behavior puts them at risk of acquiring HIV disease do not have a supportive family network. New York and New Jersey should develop comprehensive community-based HIV health and education programs for adolescents.

Source: AIDS: Is There a Will to Meet the Challenge? Report (New York: Citizens Commission on AIDS for New York City and Northern New Jersey, February 1991).

DOCUMENT 50: Local Control of Sex Education Curricula

Educational policy decisions differ from state to state and city to city. In states like Maine, local school boards have broad authority over curricula and programs within the framework of minimal state guidelines. As a result, the response to a health crisis like the AIDS epidemic is a product of local politics and culture. Areas where current rates of infection are low should begin their efforts before the situation becomes serious. Unfortunately, aggressive action is seldom taken beforehand.

"Guys don't like them," a shy girl says as she stares down at the table. She adds in a whisper that sometimes, "guys get violent" if she insists. . . .

[Teenagers'] lack of information combined with their reluctance to use condoms will probably kill some of these teens, many of whom ran away from abusive homes. According to state and family planning estimates, about one in every 100 teens in Maine may be already infected with HIV, the . . . AIDS virus. . . . State officials say they are doing the best they can considering their limited funds and the sanctity of local control over sexuality education in Maine. . . . "It's not worth having the state mandate AIDS education" [said a member of the Maine AIDS Alliance]. "The tradition of local control in Maine is strong. People elect their school board members and those boards need to hear . . . from people who are in favor of [sex education]."

Source: Christine Kukka, "Unsafe Sex," Maine Times (January 4, 1991); Newsbank, 1991: HEA 1:G1–G4.

DOCUMENT 51: Gay Male Teens Have Special Emotional and Informational Needs

Male teenagers who are gay or bisexual face an unusual situation because of the AIDS epidemic. During this critical period of their development, lack of knowledge can place them at very high risk for HIV infection. They may believe that if someone looks healthy, he must be healthy. This is a common misunderstanding. Sexually active gay or bisexual male teens are at considerably higher risk for HIV infection (perhaps as much as a hundred times greater!) when engaging in un-protected sex with another male, especially if the male partner is an older adult, than are sexually active heterosexual teens or lesbian teens who engage in risky sex. What they need to know is where to find information on "safer sex" and support for avoiding high-risk behavior. The following selection from a book chapter written in the late 1980s briefly discusses these issues.

[As the AIDS epidemic escalates, gay and bisexual] male teenagers . . . today [in the late 1980s] face considerable adversity during their "coming-out" process. Not since the mid-1960's have so many obstacles been placed in the path of gay youth during the formation of their gay identity and self-esteem. It appears that as a result of the AIDS epidemic, many gay male adolescents are delaying the development of their gay identities and postponing homosexual relationships. Denial of same-sex orientation is often easier for gay youth to cope with than the hostility, stigma, and possible terminal illness facing gay men. . . .

Gay and bisexual adolescents often may not have other gay or bisexual friends, read gay publications, or have access to the same kinds of formal and informal social networks and informational [sources] that adult gay men usually have. Gay bars and bathhouses, places where gay men can learn about AIDS and safe-sex techniques, are usually closed to gay and bisexual teenagers.

[A] common myth held by many gay and bisexual teenagers is that if the sex partner is healthy, or appears healthy, then it is all right to have sex with the individual. . . . It is . . . likely that this lack of adequate in-formation translates into unsafe sexual practices . . . [and] it is not clear if gay and bisexual teenagers are also using condoms in any significant numbers.

It would certainly be psychologically damaging to the gay individual if the fear of AIDS prevents him from normal homosexual development during his teenage years. On the other hand, the message that sex be-tween males should be practiced safely with condoms and spermicidal lubricants urgently needs to reach all gay and bisexual teenagers. It has become a matter of wellness or ill-health, of life or death.

Source: Douglas A. Feldman, "Gay Youth and AIDS," in G. Herdt, ed., *Gay & Lesbian Youth* (New York: Harrington Park Press, 1989), pp. 185–193.

DOCUMENT 52: Targeting Young Gay Men for Behavioral Research and HIV Prevention

Like other teenagers, young gay men may deny their susceptibility to HIV infection. They believe they are invulnerable and feel "immortal." This is a dangerous illusion, considering the high rates of HIV infection among gay or bisexual men in cities such as New York and San Francisco. Rates as high as 18 percent have been found among sexually active gay men aged eighteen–twenty-nine in San Francisco.

A number of factors militate against [young people] taking the risk of AIDS seriously, including the illusion of immortality characteristic of the young and the knowledge that there are few people in their age range diagnosed with AIDS. But the fact is that infection is taking place during the teen years even though diagnosis does not occur until later in the twenties, due to the long latency period between infection and the appearance of symptoms.

In addition, there is a danger to gay youths who, when they come to terms with their sexual orientation and come out, are not sufficiently knowledgeable about risk reduction techniques to protect themselves. Should their first sexual encounters take place with high-risk individuals, perhaps older men, they place themselves in danger, in part also because of their inexperience. . . .

We need to learn how to reach gay youths early with adequate information and motivational programs. Given the difficulties that the experimental programs in counseling of gay students in high schools have faced, it is extremely problematic to deal with this pressing issue. Likewise, gay college students must be reached. We need basic information about the lives of gay students at all levels.

Source: Ralph Bolton, quoted in *Meeting the Challenges of AIDS: Recommendations for the University of California* (Sacramento, Calif.: Assembly Subcommittee on Higher Education, 1989), pp. 1–44.

DOCUMENT 53: Knowledge Is Only Step Number One

As the following summary of a study of sexually active teenagers in San Francisco demonstrates, knowledge alone does not change behavior. These young people knew that condoms protect against sexually transmitted diseases, yet this knowledge did not lead to their planning to use them more frequently. Nor did they limit the number of their sexual partners. Knowing something abstractly is different from feeling personally vulnerable and then deciding to do something about it. Since changing behavior is complex, knowledge of potential health risks is just the beginning of that process.

Sexually active adolescents [in our study] report placing high value and importance on using a contraceptive that protects against STDs, and [they] know that condoms prevent STDs; yet, the females [did not plan] to have their partners use condoms, and the males' intentions to use condoms decreased. Although the study was conducted in a city with a high prevalence of AIDS, and where media and school coverage of the epidemic was increasing over the time studied, sexually active adolescents continued to have multiple sex partners and did not substantially increase their use of condoms, thus continuing to place themselves and their partners at possible risk for STDs, including HIV infection. . . .

Solely providing information to adolescents that condoms reduce the risk of contracting STDs may be insufficient to cause an increase in condom use. One problem may be that even if adolescents understand in abstract terms that condoms protect against STDs, . . . they may not feel personally vulnerable to contracting diseases from their sex partners.

Source: Susan M. Kegeles, Nancy E. Adler, and Charles E. Irwin, Jr., "Sexually Active Adolescents and Condoms: Changes over One Year in Knowledge, Attitudes and Use," *American Journal of Public Health* 78(4): 460–461 (April 1988).

DOCUMENT 54: How Do You Get Teenagers to Practice Healthy Sex When Health Is Not a Major Concern?

Efforts to prevent transmission of HIV among teenagers should take into account that the vast majority are sexually active by the end of their teenage years, before they reach their twentieth birthday. A great many sexually active teenagers have unprotected sex. Even when condoms are used, the pattern may be inconsistent. Teaching young people a realistic concern for their own health is not sufficient to significantly change their behavior. Understanding the reasons for their willingness to take risks, the reasons for their sexual choices, is necessary for developing effective intervention strategies.

The estimated one million pregnancies occurring among adolescents each year represent the apparent high rates of unprotected sexual intercourse (unprotected for either pregnancy [or] STD infection). Two-thirds of sexually active female adolescents, ages 15-19, use nonbarrier method contraceptives or nothing at all.

A common pattern occurs with respect to changes in teens' use of condoms and oral contraceptives. Condoms and withdrawal are the most commonly used contraceptives at first intercourse. Both are relatively effective at preventing male to female HIV transmission since in neither case is semen left in the female, although it is assumed that withdrawal is not as effective as condoms at preventing HIV transmission. As sexual experience increases, the use of oral contraceptives increases, and the use of condoms decreases.... These teens are not ... adopting a behavior that will protect them from contracting HIV and other STDs....

[Prevention-related] research regarding adolescents should be developed from the perspective of the teenager rather than ... the adult. It is important to remember that health considerations are not always the primary concern for adolescents and sexual activity represents a small part of their lives. Adolescents engage in sexual intercourse for many reasons, therefore, ... the role that sexual intercourse and sexuality play in their lives must be carefully considered.

Source: Cherrie B. Boyer and Susan M. Kegeles, "AIDS Risk and Prevention Among Adolescents," *Social Science & Medicine* 33(1): 11–23 (July 1, 1991).

DOCUMENT 55: Why Many Young People Don't Routinely Use Condoms

At a large Midwestern university 272 students were surveyed for their attitudes and behavior with regard to sexual transmission of HIV. A majority reported an episode of unsafe sex, and a significant number admitted to unprotected sex with a partner "they did not know well." Failure to use condoms or to use them consistently can be attributed to a variety of factors. One of these is the belief that safe partners can be recognized and identified by looking at them or by speaking with them for a while, and therefore protection is not needed. However, since the virus takes an average of ten years from infection until AIDS-related symptoms occur, most HIV-infected and potentially infectious persons look perfectly healthy most of the time. These erroneous assumptions and unsafe sexual practices put young people at considerable risk.

Over 25% of [survey respondents] who had some experience with condoms reported [in our study (of 272 university students)] difficulties with use, including inadequate lubrication, breakage, and poor fit. Persons who had not used condoms expected more problems than were actually encountered. . . . [T]he expectation of problems may . . . make them hesitant to try condoms, and they may be more apt to engage in [risky] behavior.

When comfort levels with a variety of safer-sex behaviors are examined, a troubling picture emerges. Participants reported significant discomfort with most of the protective strategies listed on the questionnaire. . . . [This] combination of problems with condom use and discomfort with safer-sex practices should lead to risk-taking. Thus, it is not surprising that the majority of respondents reported an episode of unsafe sex. [In addition,] 24% of participants who were in an ongoing relationship reported having intercourse outside the relationship . . . [and] [f]or 17% of [the] respondents, the last episode of unprotected intercourse involved a partner they did not know well. Given the risks involved, this is a frighteningly high percentage. Despite their stated perception that there are no obvious signs of HIV infection, participants appeared to believe they could identify whether or not a partner was infected. . . . [T]heir reason for unprotected intercourse was that they "just knew it was safe" or "just assumed that [their] partner was not infected."

Source: Mary L. Keller, "Why Don't Young Adults Protect Themselves Against Sexual Transmission of HIV? Possible Answers to a Complex Question," *AIDS Education and Prevention* 5(3): 220–233 (Fall 1993).

DOCUMENT 56: Increasing Teen Drug Use and Higher HIV Rates

From 1992 to 1996, the rate of drug use among teens rose dramatically, after declining during the late 1980s. During the 1980s, injecting heroin among youth declined in North America, in part because of fear of HIV infection by exchanging infected needles and syringes. But by the mid-1990s, heroin use was making a comeback, even among young, successful Hollywood actors and rock musicians. While most marijuana users do not go on to use more dangerous drugs, very few users of dangerous drugs fail to begin by using marijuana.

Pointing to an increase in teen drug use, the Dole campaign [for president in 1996] criticized the Clinton administration for not making the war against drugs a priority. Government studies found that the use of marijuana, cocaine, heroin, hallucinogens and other drugs by teens has increased 78 percent since 1992, and 33 percent [in 1995]. Moreover, data from the Department of Health and Human Services show that many youths are using drugs at an even earlier age than before—16.3 years—while another study indicates that 12-year-olds who use marijuana are nearly 80 times more likely to start using cocaine than others their age who do not use marijuana. Tom Hedrick, vice chairman of the Partnership for a Drug-Free America, warned that addiction, drug-related crime, and drug-related AIDS cases would increase if the rise in drug use is not stopped.

Source: Matthew Robinson, "Teen Drug Use: Issue of Epidemic?" *Investor's Business Daily*, p. A1 (September 3, 1996); CDC National AIDS Clearinghouse (Bethesda, Md.: Information, Inc., 1996).

WOMEN

DOCUMENT 57: Increasing Recognition of the Prevalence of AIDS Among Women

Compared with men with AIDS, women are often more seriously ill when they are first diagnosed. There are several reasons for this. First of all, their symptoms may be different when compared with the symptoms of men. Second, if they contract HIV as the result of heterosexual sex, physicians and other health care workers are not always alert to the possibility of HIV infection. As a result of late diagnosis and treatment, women with AIDS have not lived as long as men with AIDS. Today, there is growing recognition that all women in the United States, and not just women who have been seen as "high-risk," can—and sometimes do—get AIDS.

More women show up at hospitals suffering from what seems like advanced pneumonia when the real culprit is undiagnosed AIDS, researchers say. . . . "The lack of awareness is reflected in the fact that clinicians do not think of this diagnosis, and women are dying needlessly because of this," said Dr. Paula Schuman of Wayne State University's School of Medicine. Schuman and other doctors hope a five-year study on how AIDS affects women will help doctors . . . spot and treat the disease in . . . women. . . .

Part of the problem may be that many infected women don't fit the typical AIDS stereotypes as [commercial sex workers (prostitutes)] or [injecting] drug users, researchers say. "Unless you come in looking like a prostitute or you come with needle tracks all over your arms [doctors] are not considering that your chronic pneumonia may be [AIDS-related] *Pneumocystis*" [Dr. Schuman said].

Source: "New Study Will Track Women with AIDS," *AIDS Monthly* (Research Edition), p. 9 (April 1992).

DOCUMENT 58: In Developed Nations, Women Are at Greater Risk Than Men to Heterosexual HIV Transmission

Heterosexual transmission of HIV has become an increasingly important risk for women. Women whose male sexual partners are injecting drug users, bisexuals, from particular developing countries, blood transfusion recipients (who received blood before the mid-1980s), or persons with hemophilia are especially vulnerable. Usually HIV is more efficiently transmitted from male to female, rather than the reverse, in developed nations. During unprotected sex, a woman is more likely to be infected by a male partner than a man by a female partner, although both routes are quite possible. If a woman is unaware of her sexual partner's HIV status and becomes infected, she may not know she is HIV-positive until she becomes symptomatic. Because of the long latency period, women can remain asymptomatic for a dozen years or more, and miss the benefits of early diagnosis and treatment.

As is the case with several other sexually transmitted diseases, women are more susceptible to acquiring HIV from an infected male partner than the other way around. Their biological vulnerability is compounded by their frequent lack of awareness of their partner's HIV status, which often leads to a misperception of their personal risk. Women are, therefore, less likely than men to know they are infected until they manifest symptoms. And even when they do show symptoms, physicians are often slow to diagnose HIV infection.

Source: Kenneth H. Mayer, "Women and AIDS," *Scientific American* 266(3): 118 (March 1992).

DOCUMENT 59: Women and Bisexual Men

For women, heterosexual contact is an increasingly important risk factor for HIV transmission. Among reported heterosexual cases in the United States, most HIV-infected women become infected from sex with a male injecting drug user, though wives or sexual partners of bisexual men may be underreported. Women who have unprotected sex may be unaware of their partner's bisexuality and the risk that poses.

Among 3,555 women with AIDS who acquired HIV infection through heterosexual contact (excluding women born in African or Caribbean countries), 11% (. . . 405) reported sexual contact with a bisexual man and no other risk factors for AIDS. Another 114 women with AIDS [3%] reported sexual contact with a bisexual man and [sex with a heterosexual man at higher risk, such as an injecting] . . . drug user, . . . a transfusion recipient or [a] person with hemophilia. . . .

Nearly one quarter of bisexual men with AIDS who died were married at the time of death. Because many women may not be aware of their partners' behavior, the number of women with AIDS who have a bisexual partner is probably higher than reported. Thirteen percent of women with heterosexually acquired AIDS did not report the risk of their partner and 7% of all women with AIDS are reported without an established risk factor; some of these cases may have resulted from sexual contact with bisexual men.

Source: Susan Y. Chu, Thomas A. Peterman, Lynda S. Doll, James W. Buehler, and James W. Curran, "AIDS in Bisexual Men in the United States: Epidemiology and Transmission to Women," *American Journal of Public Health* 82(2): 220–224 (February 1992).

DOCUMENT 60: The Female Condom

The first female condom, Reality, was marketed in 1993. The advantage of this protective device is that it allows women to take control of their health and reproductive choices, rather than being dependent upon their partners. Many men refuse to use a condom when having sex with their female partners. The woman inserts the female condom inside her vagina just before the male partner has sexual intercourse with her. It clings to the inside of the woman's vagina instead of around the outside of the man's penis. While it is available in drugstores and appears to be gaining in popularity among women, the fact that it is much more expensive than a male condom may prevent its widespread use.

The importance in practice of the female condom will depend greatly on our ability as public health educators, teachers, and caregivers to achieve for this new method a prominent place in our prevention [options]. . . .

[However, there are other issues involved.] For example, feminists would not want the availability of the female condom for AIDS prevention to lessen efforts to address the consequences of gender imbalances in sexual relationships, and health educators would not want to reduce the responsibility in men for protecting themselves and their partners.

Besides conferring control on the woman, the new device has certain other advantages. . . . It can be inserted before intercourse without interrupting the sexual sequence—its placement does not require an erect penis. . . . [It] can also be in place before [sexual intercourse] to protect against potential HIV infection from pre-ejaculate seminal fluid ["precum" in the male].

Source: Erica L. Gollub and Zena A. Stein, "Commentary: The New Female Condom—Item One on a Women's AIDS Prevention Agenda," American Journal of Public Health 83(4): 498–500 (April 1993).

DOCUMENT 61: Pregnant Women and AZT

Current studies indicate that the probability of a baby being infected if the mother is HIV-positive is about 25 percent. With AZT, an antiretroviral drug, for mother and infant this risk can be decreased substantially, to about 8 percent in newborn infants of HIV-positive mothers. Quality counseling should provide the most up-to-date information and then support the mother's decision. Research has shown that nearly all women who are counseled about the benefits and potential risks of AZT decide to take AZT to try to protect their fetus (the unborn young from the end of the eighth week until the moment of birth). It is believed that future studies will show that HIV risk for infants can be lowered even further by giving HIV-positive mothers a combination of AZT, another similar drug such as ddI, and one of the new protease inhibitor drugs.

The Centers for Disease Control and Prevention (CDC) has published guidelines that call upon medical professionals to provide HIV counseling and voluntary testing for all pregnant women. In 1993 . . . , an estimated 7,000 HIV-infected women gave birth in the United States. The prevalence of HIV infection in women giving birth was about 1.6 per 1,000, or about 1 in every 625. Assuming an HIV transmission rate from mother to infant of about 15%–30%, about 1,000–2,000 HIV-infected infants were born in the United States in 1993.

For HIV-infected women and their infants to benefit optimally from AZT [a drug taken in pill form] and other medical treatment, it is important for women to know if they are HIV-infected before or early in pregnancy. CDC guidelines promote early HIV counseling and voluntary testing to help women learn if they are infected. This will enable women to seek and receive the care they need for themselves and for reducing the chances of transmitting HIV to their infants. If women do not receive prenatal [existing or occurring before birth] care, or if for any reason their HIV status is unknown, the guidelines recommend that HIV testing be offered to the mothers or their babies at or shortly after labor and delivery.

In February 1994, the results of the National Institutes of Health (NIH) AIDS Clinical Trials Group Protocol were announced, indicating that . . . AZT could reduce perinatal [occurring near the time of birth] HIV transmission by as much as two-thirds in some infected women and their babies. . . . In August [1994], the Food and Drug Administration approved AZT use for pregnant women and the U.S. Public Health Service issued guidelines on using AZT during pregnancy. . . .

The finding of a 67.5% reduction in HIV transmission is promising, and there were no serious short-term side effects observed in the study. But several questions remain unanswered. The trial included a select group of women in the early stages of disease, who had not previously taken AZT long-term, and who had access to prenatal care. The therapy may differ in effectiveness in women who differ from these characteristics. Since researchers do not know exactly how the therapy prevented transmission, they also don't know the effect of any therapy variations—such as using AZT only during labor or later in the pregnancy, or using it for a shorter time during pregnancy. Moreover, scientists don't know about the long-term effects of AZT on both mothers and infants. Researchers continue to seek answers to these questions. NIH is continuing to monitor the mothers and babies in the trial.

The combined strategy of HIV counseling for all pregnant women and voluntary HIV testing is already proving effective in several communities. Voluntary testing means that after a woman receives appropriate counseling from her health care provider, she is able to make an informed decision about having a test for HIV. Studies show that when her health care provider talks with a pregnant woman about the test and what it means for her and her baby, most women choose to be tested and then to be treated as their doctor recommends. For example, in one inner-city hospital in Atlanta, Georgia, 96% of women chose to be tested after being provided HIV counseling and offered voluntary HIV testing as part of prenatal care. . . .

. . . The dramatic reduction in HIV transmission in the trial dictates that every HIV-infected pregnant woman should certainly be offered

AZT therapy to reduce the risk of transmitting the virus to her baby. Because of the uncertainties, a woman should make a personal decision about taking AZT only after she discusses the benefits and potential risks for herself and her child with her health care provider.

Source: U.S. Public Health Service, *PHS Guidelines for HIV Counseling and Voluntary Testing for Pregnant Women* (Washington, D.C.: U.S. Public Health Service, July 1995).

DOCUMENT 62: Poverty Among Women with AIDS

This passage is testimony to frustrations that poor women with HIV/ AIDS feel. They are very dependent upon the health care system and the social services available in their communities. Often the working poor, who often do not have health insurance and are not eligible for Medicaid because they are working, have the poorest access to medical care and social services. The Ryan White Program has assisted many such women in major metropolitan areas, but there are many areas of the United States where these services are not available or are still inadequate. The speaker in this selection briefly discusses this within the framework of a much broader context.

Too often we are denied services or cannot find services that adequately address the real needs in our lives because of gender issues, economic issues, politics, racism, sexism, and because we do not yet have a single strong voice of advocacy. We are so preoccupied with meeting the needs of others that there is never enough attention focused on our own needs. Many of us are poor and must improvise and compromise ourselves or simply do without much needed support, basic services, love and attention, and all the simple things in life which help people develop whole and wholesome attitudes about themselves.

Source: Janice Jireau, person with AIDS, quoted in *America Living with AIDS*, Report of the National Commission on Acquired Immune Deficiency Syndrome, p. 116 (Washington, D.C.: Superintendent of Documents, 1991).

DOCUMENT 63: Condoms Versus Other Birth Control Methods

Birth control pills and devices, unlike condoms, female condoms, and spermicidal lubricants, will not prevent HIV or other sexually transmitted diseases. It is alarming how many women erroneously believe that birth control pills and devices will somehow protect them from these diseases. Or it may be that many do not really care about it, since many women who are not practicing birth control have their male partners use a condom, not in order to protect them from HIV or other STDs but to protect them from pregnancy.

Many women who use birth control pills, Norplant [a birth control device surgically implanted in a woman's arm], and surgical sterilization wrongly believe that these contraception methods provide some protection against HIV and other sexually transmitted diseases, [government] researchers reported. A study conducted by researchers at the Centers for Disease Control and Prevention found that more than half the women surveyed who had steady partners and one-third of those who engaged in casual sex had not used condoms the last time they had intercourse. Women who had been surgically sterilized were about four times less likely to use condoms than women who used condoms for contraception. Women using hormonal contraception were twice as likely to not use condoms.

Source: Mara Bovsun, "UPI Science News: Birth Control Pills Without Condoms Put Women at Higher Risk for HIV Infection" (United Press International, September 26, 1996), CDC National AIDS Clearinghouse (Bethesda, Md.: Information, Inc., 1996).

CHILDREN

DOCUMENT 64: AIDS in Children Becomes a Concern as the Epidemic Begins Its Second Decade

The publicity on AIDS and HIV infection in children has been excellent for focusing attention on the disease itself. Most of the children were infected by their HIV-infected mother during birth, by infected blood, or by infected blood products. By the early 1990s, half of all AIDS funding for research was targeted to children with AIDS, who comprised less than 2 percent of the total population living with AIDS. It is much easier to raise private funds or allocate government funds for children with AIDS than for adults with AIDS.

Introduction of Resolution to Designate June 10–16, 1991, Pediatrics Awareness Week

While the nation's attention is turned toward the Persian Gulf fiasco, we must not forget that we have another kind of war right here in our own backyard. That war is called AIDS. A war that is killing hundreds of people in the prime of life, and even worse, those who may never have a chance—our children. It is vital that the United States adopt a domestic policy to rescue our children from all destructive forces. This resolution is designed to focus more attention on one of this country's most explosive health problems.

AIDS has become the number one killer in America. It is a national health emergency affecting individuals, their families and the health care system in all 50 states. . . . Conservative estimates suggest that the numbers [of those diagnosed with AIDS] in America will more than double in the next two years. Sadly more than half those diagnosed include children and these numbers are expected to increase at an alarming rate.

[P]ediatric AIDS refers to patients under the age of 13 at the time of diagnosis with . . . [HIV]. . . . For every child born or diagnosed with the disease, there is another who is also infected, and a father, who too carries the disease. Certain groups of women are especially vulnerable to contracting AIDS, solely as a result of their relations with men who are intravenous drug users, or with men who engage in . . . relations with other men. . . . [O]ne of the fastest growing components of the epidemic [is] women. . . .

One successful course of action available is an effective public education campaign aimed at providing information to all persons and especially to high risk groups about the consequences of the disease. . . . Educational tools sensitive to the different ethnic and high-risk groups, and especially children, must be devised and deployed in our cities to further help curtail the spread of this fatal disease. . . .

I urge my colleagues to join me . . . and cosponsor this measure which designates the week June 10 through 16 as "Pediatric AIDS Awareness Week."

Source: Remarks by the Honorable Jose E. Serrano of New York in the House of Representatives, *Congressional Record*, pp. E294–295 (January 24, 1991).

DOCUMENT 65: AIDS in Children Presents New Implications

HIV infection in children is usually the result of transmission from mother to child during pregnancy or the birth process. Most of the mothers were infected because of injecting drugs or heterosexual contact with a male injecting drug user. As a consequence of this, the increase in the number (but not the proportion) of pediatric cases puts pressure on the health care system and social services to provide specially designed programs for these families.

While [injecting drug use] is still the primary means of maternal infection in the United States (42%), infection through heterosexual contact [usually with a male partner who is an injecting drug user] has been increasing at a more rapid rate. [A recent study showed that] 29% of children with ... AIDS were born to mothers infected through heterosexual contact. ...

As the number of cases of pediatric AIDS increases, and the number of perinatally transmitted cases increases and is documented, all communities must face the reality that HIV-infected children will be attending their schools and living and playing in their communities. The medical and social service systems must *anticipate* the needs of these children and their parents. Unlike other chronic and terminal diseases affecting children, ... HIV-infected children will be living in an environment where at least one parent either has died of HIV infection or is currently infected and possibly ill and dying.

Source: Harold M. Ginsburg, Jennifer Trainor, and Eric Reis, "A Review of Epidemiologic Trends in HIV Infection of Women and Children,"*Pediatric AIDS and HIV Infection: Fetus to Adolescent* 1(1): 11–13 (1990).

DOCUMENT 66: Caring for the HIV-Infected and Orphaned Children

Care of HIV-infected children poses a unique challenge to society. With regard to medical treatment, the availability and effectiveness of new drugs for infants and children is critical. For example, as discussed in a previous reading, zidovudine (ZDV/AZT) has been found to decrease the rate of HIV transmission from mother to infant dramatically. Once an infant or child is infected, support services for families are needed. Parents as well as children may be infected, and at some point children from these families may become orphaned.

Children, who have historically been under-represented in clinical trials, should have access to promising drugs. Access to trials should be ensured after Phase I/II studies have demonstrated safety ... in adults. An exception to this principle are seropositive but asymptomatic babies under 15 months in whom a positive HIV test may reflect the presence of maternal antibodies, not true infection. Perinatal transmission rates are now believed to [average about 25 percent]; therefore, most HIV positive infants are not infected. Drug trials may offer [a] benefit, but also [a] risk; since non-infected children can obtain no benefit and may be harmed by participating in HIV drug studies, they are generally not appropriate trial participants. Furthermore, to ensure the ethical acceptability of the informed consent process . . . children not in the custody of their parents, and therefore especially vulnerable, should be provided advocates to make appropriate decisions for them.

[We] must be prepared to assist the tens of thousands of children who have been and will be orphaned because of the loss of their parents to HIV disease. Some of these children may themselves be infected with HIV and already symptomatic; others may be infected but asymptomatic; and still others—[certainly] the majority—are uninfected. The vast majority of these children come from impoverished families. . . . Solutions must be developed soon to help these very vulnerable, at-risk children.

Source: AIDS: Is There a Will to Meet the Challenge? Report, Citizens Commission on AIDS for New York City and Northern New Jersey (New York: The Commission, February 1991).

DOCUMENT 67: What Do You Tell Your Child with HIV?

This a mother's poignant account of her young son's struggle to live with HIV infection. It is a reminder that clinical research can change the lives of patients. New drugs and treatments can relieve suffering, prolong life, and provide hope. Five years after this testimony was given, remarkable progress was beginning to be made in this area.

I have a son who is infected with HIV. . . . He was doing very well, up until a couple of months ago. He had to have his tonsils removed. And since then, he's been very tired and just worn out. And he's just tired of fighting this whole thing. But he'll hear little things from people, from school, from the media. "I heard about a miracle cure." He came home saying, "Mom, I heard about this cure. You know, can we check on it? Can we go somewhere in France or something. It comes from some snake's head or something—you know." And he gets his hopes up so much.

. . . Just today when I called to see how he was, he said, "Did you testify yet? Did you tell them? . . . Did you tell them to hurry up and find a cure?" What do I tell him? What do I tell him now? I mean, he knows ddI is helping him, but now what do I tell him when he hears there's something going on in France that is definitely a cure? "It's a real cure, Mom. It is. That's what they're saying."

How do I explain to him that maybe it's not? What do I tell him? What happens after ddI? I don't know. I don't have the answers. I know what I need to tell him, but I don't. I can't. He wants to have hope. I want to have hope, but I don't see any hope on the horizon as far as a vaccine goes. He was so excited about a vaccine and I said, well, that wouldn't really help you. It would help other people like us—like your brothers and myself who aren't infected. And he said, "So it wouldn't do a damn thing for me, huh?"

I mean, he deals with it very, very well. But he's starting to see the injustice and the prejudices and I know it's got to hurt. It's got to hurt, but he handles it so well. I don't know, I don't know how he does it. I just think he's a remarkable child.

Source: Sheila Swain, mother of an HIV-infected child, quoted in *America Living with AIDS*, Report of the National Commission on Acquired Immune Deficiency Syndrome (Washington, D.C.: Superintendent of Documents, 1991), p. 92.

DOCUMENT 68: Trends Among Children with AIDS in the United States

The information presented in this reading strongly suggests that the shift to using AZT among pregnant women who have HIV has been effective in reducing the number of children born with HIV/AIDS. On a global level, AZT is too expensive to be used in most African and Asian countries. But shorter and more simplified courses of AZT treatment are being evaluated in these countries to see if they would also be effective.

As of September 30, 1996, a total of 566,002 . . . AIDS cases, including 7,472 cases among children [under] 13 years [old] . . . , had been reported to [the] CDC. . . . Most children reported with AIDS acquired . . . HIV infection perinatally [around the time of their birth] from their mothers. During 1988–1993, an estimated 6,000–7,000 children were born each year to HIV-infected women; an estimated 1,000–2,000 of these children were infected annually. In 1994, results of clinical trials demonstrating effective therapy for reducing perinatal HIV transmission indicated a two-thirds decrease in such transmission associated with [AZT] therapy for HIV-infected pregnant women and their newborns. The Public Health Service (PHS) issued recommendations in 1994 for [AZT] treatment to reduce perinatal HIV transmission, and in 1995 for routine HIV counseling and voluntary testing for all pregnant women in the United States.

Risk exposures for HIV infection among the mothers of the 6,750 children with perinatally acquired AIDS included injecting drug use (41%), sexual contact with a partner with or at risk for HIV/AIDS (34%), and receipt of contaminated blood or blood products (2%); for 13%, no risk was specified.

The estimated number of children with perinatally acquired AIDS peaked at 905 during 1992, followed by a decline in incidence.... From 1992 through 1995, the estimated annual number of perinatally acquired AIDS cases declined 27%, from 905 to 663. During this time, the estimated annual number of cases declined 39% among non-Hispanic white, 26% among non-Hispanic black, and 25% among Hispanic children. The proportionate decrease in the number of children with perinatally acquired AIDS from the six areas reporting the highest number of cases was greater than the decrease for all remaining areas and for all areas combined.

Through September 1996, [the 28 states that require confidential reporting of children with HIV infection and with AIDS] reported 29% (2,155) of all children with AIDS and 1,447 children with HIV infection [but not AIDS]. During 1995, these states reported 228 AIDS cases among children and 302 children with documented HIV infection who had not developed AIDS.... During [that year], these states received 1,464 additional reports of children who were born to HIV-infected mothers but who require follow-up with providers to determine their HIV infection status.

... Because the number of HIV-infected women who gave birth each year was stable during 1989–1994, [the] decline [of children with AIDS] suggests that the decrease in perinatal HIV transmission rates probably reflected the effect of perinatal [AZT] therapy. Increasing proportions of women may be accepting voluntary prenatal HIV testing and using [AZT] to prevent perinatal transmission.

... The [AZT] regimen recommended in the United States is not an affordable prevention strategy in many countries where HIV prevalence rates among women are highest. Worldwide, an estimated 8.8 million women and 800,000 children have HIV/AIDS; most of these persons reside in sub-Saharan Africa where resources for health services ... are limited.... [The] CDC and other organizations are collaborating with ministries of health in Africa and Asia to evaluate the effectiveness of shorter and simplified [AZT] regimens, other [similar] medications, and other interventions for reducing perinatal HIV transmission. However, because [AZT] treatment or other potential interventions are not universally effective in preventing perinatal transmission, primary prevention of HIV infection among children will continue to require preventing new HIV infections among women in the United States and other countries.

Source: "AIDS Among Children—United States, 1996," *Morbidity and Mortality Weekly Report* 45(46): 1005–1010 (November 22, 1996).

INJECTING DRUG USERS

DOCUMENT 69: The Need for Treatment Programs for Injecting Drug Users

The HIV epidemic is closely linked to the epidemic of recreational drug use. Transferring (or sharing) contaminated needles and syringes is the cause of the spread of HIV among drug users. The infected blood from the needle or syringe directly enters their blood stream upon injecting heroin or cocaine. There is a potential ripple effect: sex partners of injecting drug users can become infected through vaginal and anal sex, and their children become infected through the birth process. Chronic crack users frequently develop bleeding gums, and can become infected or be infectious while performing oral sex. What can be done about this situation? Innovative prevention strategies, such as needle exchange programs and street outreach programs, have proven very effective. Programs have combined drug treatment with HIV counseling and testing. However, the general conditions that affect drug use are more difficult to address because they are chronic and systemwide, and it is unclear whether there is a sufficient commitment within our society to work on social problems such as poverty, medical care, and housing.

The failure of the Federal government to recognize and confront the twin epidemics of substance use and HIV infection has become glaringly apparent to the [National AIDS] Commission throughout its nearly two years of hearings and site visits. The Federal government's strategy of interdiction and increased prison sentences has done nothing to change the stark statistics:

- Approximately 32 percent of all adult/adolescent AIDS cases are related to [injecting] drug use.
- Of the pediatric AIDS cases related to a mother with [HIV infection or] at risk for HIV infection, 70 percent are directly related to maternal exposure to HIV through [injecting] drug use or sex with an [injecting] drug user.

- [Seventy-one] percent of all female AIDS cases are linked directly or indirectly to [injecting] drug use.
- [Nineteen] percent of AIDS cases among men are directly linked to [injecting] drug use, and an additional 7 percent of AIDS cases among men are linked to both homosexual/bisexual contact and [injecting] drug use.
- African-American and Hispanic communities are being extremely hard hit by the twin epidemics. While African-Americans make up 28 percent of all diagnosed AIDS cases and Hispanics make up 16 percent; of the cases attributed to [injecting] drug use, African-Americans account for 45 percent of cases and Hispanics for 26 percent.
- The City of New York has an estimated 200,000 [injecting] drug users (who are 50 percent HIV positive) with only 38,000 publicly funded treatment slots.
- The National Institute on Drug Abuse (NIDA) recently estimated . . . that approximately 107,000 persons are currently on waiting lists for drug treatment.

These twin epidemics transcend all economic, geographic and racial boundaries; everyone is affected. Substance use enhances the spread of HIV infection through the [transferring] of needles and the practice of unsafe sex related to crack (the smokeable form of cocaine), alcohol, and other substances. Despite this insidious and indisputable link between substance use and HIV infection, the Office of National Drug Control Policy continues to virtually ignore it, and neglect the real public health and treatment measures which could and must be taken to halt its spread.

Repeatedly, medical and treatment experts have come before the Commission and stressed the absolute importance of treatment on demand. Increasing treatment slots is a stated goal of the Federal drug control policy, yet, as Dr. Robert Newman told the Commission, ". . . There seems to be nothing . . . to indicate that any government agency either at the Federal or at any of the 50 state levels is indeed pursuing the objective of expansion on a massive scale to make treatment for addicts who want it readily available." Providing quality treatment and treatment on demand may be an expensive proposition, but so is the unchecked spread of HIV infection. . . .

We must also take immediate steps to curb the current spread of HIV infection among those who cannot get treatment or who cannot stop taking drugs. Outreach programs which operate needle exchanges and distribute bleach not only help to control the spread of HIV, but also refer many individuals to treatment programs. Legal sanctions on injection equipment do not reduce illicit drug use, but they do increase the [transferring] of injection equipment and hence the spread of HIV infection. . . .

Finally, all levels of government and the private sector must work together to attack the deep-rooted social and economic problems which promote and sustain substance use. The poor of this nation, especially in communities of color, have been inordinately hard hit by the twin epidemics of HIV and substance use. In order to combat these epidemics which affect the entire nation, we must provide basic needs such as housing, medical care and food. HIV education and drug treatment often seem like luxuries to individuals who do not know where they will sleep at night or where their next meal will come from. To reach the point where our nation's drug epidemic is really a thing of the past, we must create communities and neighborhoods which promote health and hope, not addiction and despair.

Source: *National Commission on Acquired Immune Deficiency Syndrome, The Twin Epidemics of Substance Use and HIV* (Washington, D.C.: National Commission on AIDS, July 1991).

DOCUMENT 70: The Social Context of HIV Transmission Among IDUs

The epidemic of HIV infection is closely connected to the epidemic of injecting drug use and addiction. Sharing contaminated needles and syringes spreads the virus from one drug user to another, who may then infect his or her sexual partners. Breaking into this chain of events is difficult because of the nature of addiction and the unstable lives of injecting drug users. One way to reach this population is to integrate HIV prevention into existing drug treatment programs.

AIDS is not the primary disease; drug abuse is. If you start talking about AIDS intervention and education and you don't tie it up with treatment you are going to lose the addict. . . . I have addicts who are infected and are becoming reinfected over and over again [possibly with different strains of the virus]. . . . The addict and the disease of addiction [go] from periods of surviving to periods of [increased drug] use. And when the person is using [drugs], it doesn't matter how much they know about AIDS intervention and education. They're not going to use safe sexual techniques; they are also not going to clean their syringes.

If you tell an [injecting] drug user who is a male, and you have his wife tell him, about safe sex and he doesn't know about it, she gets hit. . . . That point was driven home in San Francisco in an AIDS Train the Trainer program . . . when one of the trainers went out and told Latina women to go out and tell their husbands to [practice safe sex] and demand that they use a condom: One of the women was killed and two of the women were hospitalized for severe battery. What I'm trying to get

across is [that] people keep on looking at AIDS as the problem. AIDS is
one of many of the problems. . . .

Source: Testimony of Dr. German Maisonet, medical director of Van Ness Recovery House, before the Assembly Subcommittee on Higher Education, in *Meeting
the Challenge of AIDS: Recommendations for the University of California* (Sacramento:
Assembly Subcommittee on Higher Education, May 1989), pp. 11–12.

DOCUMENT 71: Changing Behavior Among IDUs

In states such as New York and New Jersey, drug use and HIV infection
have combined to produce a large number of people with HIV disease.
While research shows that drug users are capable of changing their
behavior, the situation calls for aggressive action. Injecting drug users
are more likely to practice safe injection techniques than safer sex techniques. A comprehensive strategy would include counseling and testing, needle exchange programs, legalization of the purchase and
possession of needles, safer sex programs, and increased availability of
drug treatment programs.

Drug-related HIV infection . . . represents the fastest growing source of
transmission in New York and New Jersey; yet programs developed to
tackle drug use are dwarfed by the magnitude of the problem. The tragedy of this poorly addressed problem is not only the numbers of infected
and ill drug users but also its impact on the sexual partners of drug
users, including women who do not themselves use drugs, and on . . .
infants born to HIV-infected mothers. As a result of the link between
drug use and HIV infection, the bi-state region has the nation's highest
rates of HIV disease among women and children.

The [Citizens] Commission [on AIDS] stressed the importance of available treatment both as a compassionate measure to treat those who wish
to be free of drugs and to prevent further HIV transmission among drug
users, their sexual partners, and their children. The diverse treatment
[methods] were examined, as was research demonstrating that while
drug users and their sexual partners are difficult to educate, they should
not be considered unreachable. . . . [A] large number of drug users (in
many studies, the majority) report changes in their drug-using behavior
to reduce their risk of contracting HIV. . . . However, more drug users
reported changes in drug injection behavior than changes in sexual behavior. . . .

The Commission [in 1991] also considered the ongoing controversies
regarding risk reduction and concluded that distribution of bleach

should be supported within the context of a comprehensive approach that primarily emphasizes drug treatment, education, and counseling, and that needle exchange programs should be evaluated.

Source: AIDS: Is There a Will to Meet the Challenge? Report, Citizens Commission on AIDS for New York City and New Jersey (New York: The Commission, February 1991).

DOCUMENT 72: HIV Prevention Education Among IDUs

The term "sharing needles" among injecting drug users (IDUs) is rather misleading, since in "shooting galleries" or "get-off houses" where IDUs go to rent "works" (drug injection paraphernalia), IDUs do not engage in good-natured sharing. The social interaction in a shooting gallery is usually not anything like friends passing around a six-pack of beer or a marijuana joint. Instead, the IDU frequently rents the works because he or she cannot gain access to clean needles and syringes, and shooting galleries are a good way to avoid carrying the equipment if stopped by the police. A better term might be "transferring" needles and syringes. In this brief selection, we learn more about the social behavior of IDUs in Denver, Colorado.

Besides drug sharing, many injecting drug users have other drug-related risk behaviors for HIV infection, researchers at the University of Colorado report. [Dr.] Stephen Koester [an anthropologist] and colleagues found that the sharing of drug injection paraphernalia, including water, drug-mixing containers, and drug filters was twice as prevalent as sharing of syringes. They also discerned that heroin injectors were at the greatest risk of contracting HIV through risky injection practices. Individuals who received some community HIV prevention education reported a lower rate of injection-related risk behaviors.

Source: "Many Injection Drug Users Uninformed About HIV Transmission Risks" (Reuters, June 13, 1996); CDC National AIDS Clearinghouse (Bethesda, Md.: Information, Inc., 1996).

DOCUMENT 73: Heroin Use Again on the Rise

Drug use patterns change over time. In the late 1960s and early 1970s, hallucinogenic drugs like LSD became very popular. In the late 1980s, crack cocaine became increasingly available and used. Recently, after years of a declining trend, heroin use is again increasing in popularity. While it is now possible to snort or smoke heroin, chronic heroin users are frequently injecting it into their veins. This may have serious implications for a new wave of HIV infections for injection drug users.

Heroin use is on the rise in the United States since changes in the drug industry have resulted in a more powerful, cheaper, and safer product. In the 1980s, the average $10 bag of heroin was only 2 percent to 8 percent pure. In 1994, however, average purity was 63 percent, pure enough to snort or smoke—and avoid the risk of HIV infection linked to injecting. The price also fell, due to a doubling in production over the last decade. Many new users begin using heroin by snorting, but eventually progress to injecting. About 50 percent of users who sought treatment last year were using needles, and up to 75 percent are now. Injecting is a concern for two reasons: injection drug users now have the highest rates of new HIV infection, and fluctuations in purity increase the risk of overdose. Many people working to prevent and treat drug use say support for such programs is inadequate to deal with the growing heroin problem.

Source: John Leland, Peter Keitel, and Mary Hager, "The Fear of Heroin Is Shooting Up," *Newsweek* 128(9): 55 (August 26, 1996), CDC National AIDS Clearinghouse (Bethesda, Md.: Information, Inc., 1996).

THE GAY COMMUNITY

DOCUMENT 74: The Remarkable Achievements of the Gay Community

During the first years of the epidemic in the United States, gay men were the most affected. Men who have sex with men are still the largest number of AIDS cases, by "exposure category," diagnosed each year among adults and teenagers. In response to the crisis, the gay community pulled together in several important ways. They raised the awareness within the gay community and the general public, lobbied Washington for funds, campaigned for changes in drug development and distribution, and organized community-based support networks. These remarkable achievements are models of political activism that benefit the larger society as well as the gay community.

[Gay people have] carried the stigma of [AIDS since the early 1980s] and have buried [many] of their friends. At the same time, they have educated themselves and have organized extraordinary support systems that now serve as examples to other cities and other countries.

If there is ever a vaccine for AIDS, it will ... be the result of their strength and their efforts. For more than half a decade they have been isolated by most communities, have allowed doctors to experiment with them, suffered incredible side effects from experimental drugs, ... and participated in anything that promised a cure. In the end, they have succeeded in forcing people to see that AIDS is not just a "gay disease," but affects everyone.

Source: Elisabeth Kübler-Ross, *AIDS: The Ultimate Challenge* (New York: Macmillan, 1987).

DOCUMENT 75: Gay Community Recognized Need for Behavioral Changes Early in Epidemic

For gay men, the 1970s were a time when sexual freedom and political power were closely identified. But toward the end of the early 1980s, it became clear to those within the gay community that there is no escaping the grim reality that high-risk sexual behavior can lead to a life-threatening illness. After a diagnosis of AIDS, there were few long-term survivors at that time. Radical changes in sexual behavior were clearly called for.

The nightmare rumors that swirled through the homosexual communities of New York, San Francisco and Los Angeles [about two] years ago have become cruel fact. ... Suddenly everyone seems to know a [person with AIDS]. ... If it had not developed first among homosexuals, it could well have struck some other risk group. But clearly, urban gay life-style has put many homosexual males at risk. ... More than 300 gay men have already died [in 1983], and the fear of further contagion has led to a slowing down of life in the fast lane. ... [M]any ... say tentatively that they have moved beyond shock and fear and anger to a feeling of relief that they finally have a medical reason to slow down their lives.

Source: Vincent Coppola, Richard West, and Janet Huck, "The Change in Gay Life-Style," *Newsweek*, p. 80 (April 18, 1983).

DOCUMENT 76: Gay Persons Mourning the Deaths of Lovers Have Special Needs

The loss of a lover or partner is one of life's most traumatic experiences. For gay men who have lost a lover to AIDS, the grief is often compounded by the stigma associated with the disease and with being gay. The isolation and pain of such a loss can be intensified by disapproving family members, friends, and associates.

Gay lovers of AIDS patients probably experience triple stigma. The first is a change in attitude that takes place in society when a person dies.... [T]his type of stigma may ... be insignificant in gay bereaved people if the relationship was not acknowledged, accepted, or known to others.

The second ... stigma is directly related to sexual orientation.... [T]he stigma of homosexuality may prolong ... the grieving process by denying gay bereaved people the support they need while they mourn their loss. Third, the person who has lost a lover through AIDS has to deal with the stigma of this particular disease.... The deceased is often the survivor's only real family,... [and] [t]he family and heterosexual friends may be resentful and unable to support the survivor.

Source: Hildur Helgadottir, "Grieving Alone," *Nursing Times* 86(37): 28, 31–32 (September 12, 1990).

DOCUMENT 77: Stress and HIV Among Gay Men

Coping with a serious illness is very stressful. Gay men with HIV infection have this and many other reasons for seeking emotional support and counsel. In this selection that summarizes a study conducted among gay men, it was found that peers, or one's friends, were the most helpful in lessening anxiety and depression.

The AIDS epidemic confronts the gay community with a wide range of profound stressors. Gay men may be coping with the stress of their own illness, witnessing the sickness and death of friends and acquaintances, attempting to modify their life-style to protect their health, deciding whether or not to take the AIDS antibody test, or confronting the increasing violence and threats of discrimination directed at the gay community.... [R]esearch has demonstrated that an individual's social network can buffer the impact of a wide variety of stressful life experiences, including those related to physical illness.... However, very little is known about the extent to which gay men use social network resources and how effective these sources are in coping with AIDS-related concerns....

The gay men in [the study sample] ... reported both high psychological distress and a high degree of help-seeking from their social networks. The high levels of anxiety and depression ... are testimony to the profound psychological needs within gay communities ravaged by the AIDS epidemic.... High percentages of men diagnosed with AIDS sought help from all categories of sources (peers, professionals, and family), [while] seropositive, seronegative and untested men were more likely to seek help from [their] peers. Regardless of the men's HIV status, peers were perceived to be the most helpful ... [and] the most effective source of support for gay men, with the perceived helpfulness of one's peers associated with less anxiety and depression.

Source: Robert B. Hays, Joseph A. Catania, Leon McKusick, and Thomas J. Coates, "Help-Seeking for AIDS-Related Concerns: A Comparison of Gay Men with Various HIV Diagnoses," *American Journal of Community Psychology* 18(5): 743–755 (October 1990).

DOCUMENT 78: The Demographics of Men Who Have Sex with Men

Recent studies of sexual behavior in the United States estimate the number of self-identified gay men to be about 3 percent of the adult male population, and self-identified bisexual men and self-identified heterosexual men who also have sex with other men collectively comprise an additional 3 percent of the adult male population. This accounts for at least 6 million Americans. About 200,000 gay, bisexual, and other men who had had sex with men had reportedly died of AIDS in the United States by mid-1996. An estimated additional 380,000 gay, bisexual, and other men who had had sex with men were living with HIV in the United States by mid 1996, if we calculate from CDC's perhaps conservative figures. It is interesting to note that many men who have sex with men, even exclusively, do not define or think of themselves as "gay" or even "bisexual." They separate their sexual behavior from their sexual identity. Prevention strategies need to be designed differently for each group of men. Lesbians (women who have sex with women), by the way, very rarely get AIDS, and then only if they are infected by an HIV-positive bisexual woman or an HIV-positive woman who is an injecting drug user.

Since the first reports of AIDS were published, homosexual and bisexual men have been and will continue to be of major importance for the epidemic of HIV infection in this country. . . . The total number of men who have sex with men has not been well established but appears to be considerable. . . . For this large and diverse group of men, there are several important public health challenges concerning the HIV epidemic. . . . Prevention efforts need to be [ongoing and appropriate to their intended audiences]. . . . Strategies for men who are gay-identified may be less relevant for men who [have sex with men but think of themselves] as bisexual or heterosexual. . . . [R]ecent reports of "relapse" to unsafe sexual practices among some of these men indicate the importance of continuing prevention programs to reinforce risk reduction practices. . . . Educational messages for bisexual men should also stress prevention of heterosexual transmission.

Source: Alan R. Lifson, "Men Who Have Sex with Men: Continued Challenges for Preventing HIV Infection and AIDS," *American Journal of Public Health* 82(2): 166–168 (February 1992).

DOCUMENT 79: Should the Baths Be Closed?

Gay baths, where sex between men often occurs, have a unique opportunity to educate their gay and bisexual male clients on prevention of HIV and other sexually transmitted diseases. Some would argue that they are likely to increase the risk of infection by increasing the number of anonymous partners. However, in the following selection, the authors learn from a study conducted at two gay bathhouses in Brussels, Belgium, and among other gay and bisexual men who do not go to the bathhouses, that condoms are used more by the bathhouse clients than by those who are not bathhouse clients.

In the United States, the debate on the gay baths has political as well as public health aspects. With the support of some members of the gay community, New York City's public health officials closed the St. Mark's Baths and eventually nine of thirteen other gay baths in 1986 because they felt that the risks outweighed any other considerations. In 1984, the San Francisco Health Department closed gay baths and other gay commercial establishments. These actions were challenged in court. New York City's action to close the St. Mark's Baths and the other bathhouses was upheld. San Francisco's right to regulate sexual behavior in the baths was upheld, but it could not legally close the baths. The effect, nevertheless, was to close the baths. However, by the early 1990s private gay sex clubs began to open in major North American and European cities.

The most popular [gay] baths in Brussels [Belgium] cater to a large clientele. . . . The two most popular [gay] baths in Brussels operate in large multistory buildings in the center of the city. One is particularly elegant with spacious lounges (with televisions and reading materials), a bar and a restaurant in addition to the usual steamroom, dry sauna, showers, tanning booths, private rooms, orgy room, and Jacuzzi. It is elegantly decorated with art and elaborate floral arrangements. Patrons may walk around in towels or they may rent white terrycloth robes. . . .

Comparing sauna clients [gay men who go to the gay bathhouses] and non-clients [gay men who do not go to the gay bathhouses] on the highest risk behavior, anal intercourse, we note that it is the sauna clients who use protection [condoms] more than do the non-clients; non-clients practice more unprotected anal sex [without a condom], both insertive [performing anal sex] and receptive [receiving anal sex], while clients practice more protected anal sex, insertive and receptive.

Sauna clients are more likely than non-clients to practice safer sex. This finding suggests that saunas may be safer [places] for [sex to occur] . . . than the alternatives. Therefore, closing or restricting sauna operations may actually increase HIV transmission, an effect just the opposite of the one anticipated by the advocates of restrictions.

Source: Ralph Bolton, John Vincke, and Rudolf Mak, "Gay Baths Revisited: An Empirical Analysis," *GLQ: A Journal of Lesbian & Gay Studies* 1, pp. 255–273 (1994).

DOCUMENT 80: "Closets" Are No Longer Necessary in the Age of AIDS

For gay men, AIDS activism has been a positive focus for personal action. Local organizations channel energy into changing state and local policies. On a national level, organizations have used different strategies to keep the public's attention and to push for change. ACT-UP (the AIDS Coalition To Unleash Power), for example, combines aspects of guerrilla theater with protest demonstrations to shake up complacent attitudes and to change policy. On the other hand, the Human Rights Campaign and the Lambda Legal Defense and Education Fund lobby in traditional ways for protection of human rights and provide legal services for people with AIDS. Both approaches have proven very effective in their own ways. The gay community in the late 1980s and early 1990s became very galvanized by the reality that staying in the "closet" is no longer necessary when you have only a few years left to live.

Gene Harrington has stopped flossing his teeth. Instead, he organizes meetings and protests. He writes press releases to the editor. Like dozens of other gay activists, Harrington, 51, is dying of AIDS. Acknowledging he probably has less than five years to live, he says it really doesn't matter if he flosses. His remaining days must be devoted to the meat of life.

"I don't have the luxury of giving up," said Harrington, a Texas Southern University law professor. "The disease is there whether I like it or not. . . . I am determined that I will fight this until my last breath."

AIDS has rocked the foundation of gay political power in Houston as nothing else has. It energizes but divides. It moves the infected to action—even while destroying them. . . . "Whether you are going to live or die is a pretty strong motive for political action," said Harrington. "There is a great irony here: Through our deaths, we have become re-energized."

Source: R. A. Dyer, "AIDS Fear Lends Sense of Urgency to Gay Activism," *Houston Chronicle* (December 16, 1990); Newsbank 1990 HEA: 130: G3–G6.

DOCUMENT 81: Gay Men and the Take-No-Prisoners Politics of Prescription Drugs

AIDS activist groups, such as ACT-UP, have helped change the Food and Drug Administration's (FDA's) policies with regard to the procedures for drug testing. New drugs can now be put on a "fast track" for approval, and compassionate use has been expanded so that patients have greater access to new drugs. The high price of important drugs, such as zidovudine (ZDV/AZT), was criticized and subsequently lowered. AZT can in the mid-1990s be purchased for about one-fourth of its original price a decade earlier. Activist organizations have been successful in getting drug companies to focus on patient issues.

A few years ago, AIDS activists were at war and pharmaceutical companies were the enemies. Activists marched, picketed and protested to be heard. And pharmaceutical companies, puzzled by an aggressive, questioning, highly motivated patient group, retreated behind corporate walls. . . .

Today, demonstrations still occur, but more sporadically. Now, the board room has taken precedence as the forum for working out differences. Clearly, activists and pharmaceutical companies have come full circle. Companies are more open; activists are more business-like in their approach. As a result, cooperative productive relationships have taken root and, in some instances, flourished. . . .

A company entering Phase II clinical trials [which help to determine whether the drug is effective] should be in touch with activists. Protocol design is a particularly volatile issue . . . [and] [a]ctivists can provide helpful information during . . . [this] phase that can save companies time and dollars in testing a drug for AIDS. . . .

Source: Ann Moravick, "AIDS Activists and Pharmaceuticals: The Struggle for Common Ground," *Public Relations Quarterly* 83(1): 31–32 (Spring 1993).

DOCUMENT 82: Caution: Being in the "Closet" May Be Hazardous to Your Health

Gay culture in the United States has changed dramatically since the beginning of the AIDS epidemic in the early 1980s. By the mid-1990s, gay men and lesbians have become more open and visible in the media and other social institutions. The gay community has come a long way from the 1977 Save Our Children campaign of Anita Bryant, who fostered a climate of hate and fear against gays for allegedly trying to "recruit" children into a "homosexual lifestyle," and the overt discrimination of 1983 when gay waiters had to pretend to be heterosexual in order not to frighten away restaurant customers who were afraid that "AIDS carriers" might touch and infect the food. By 1996, such issues as a national employment nondiscrimination act to protect the workplace rights of gay men and lesbians, and even gay marriage as an accepted and legal social institution, were being openly and seriously discussed. It is likely that AIDS played a major role in speeding up social change both within and outside the gay community.

Gay men with HIV who keep their sexuality hidden from the public develop AIDS and die more quickly than those who are open about being gay, a new study found. Steve W. Cole, psychologist at the University of California at Los Angeles, says there is no clear explanation for the effect, but suggests that men who conceal their homosexuality may suffer decreased immune function. The study, which followed 80 homosexual men for nine years, was published in the May–June issue of *Psychosomatic Medicine.* It found that men who were the most determined to conceal their homosexuality experienced serious losses of immune cells and developed AIDS 1.5 to 2 years sooner than men who were more openly gay. A related study by Cole found that infectious diseases and all types of cancers occurred more often in men as efforts to conceal their homosexuality intensified. Cole warns, however, that men who conceal their sexuality would probably not improve their health by coming out, since the reason for their concealing—an inhibited temperament—is ingrained in one's personality.

Source: B. Bower, "HIV Accelerates in 'Closeted' Homosexuals," *Science News* 149(25): 391 (June 22, 1996); CDC National AIDS Clearinghouse (Bethesda, Md.: Information, Inc., 1996).

COMMERCIAL SEX WORKERS

DOCUMENT 83: AIDS and the Rights of Commercial Sex Workers

Founded in 1973 by Margo St. James, COYOTE (Call Off Your Old Tired Ethics) is an advocacy group for female commercial sex workers, often referred to as "prostitutes." From these women's point of view, they are professionals who have chosen their work and are not simply victims; they believe their activities should be decriminalized. Nevertheless, except for Nevada, where prostitution is legal, their work is not considered a legitimate economic activity in the United States. Female sex workers are often at great risk for HIV infection because of unprotected sex or injection drug use. Because of these risks, intervention programs are important; peer educators and outreach programs have had some success in promoting safer sex among these women. The author of this reading, who is a member of COYOTE, writes from the perspective of a commercial sex worker.

Feminist debates within and among prostitutes' groups center on whether prostitution should be considered a forced or chosen profession. . . . COYOTE (Call Off Your Old Tired Ethics) emphasizes the range of prostitutes' experiences, and works actively for prostitutes' rights. . . . Especially in the midst of the AIDS epidemic, we must fight to protect everyone's right to engage in consensual sex. And we must fight against all those who would use this crisis as an excuse to legislate or otherwise limit sexuality....

[In the mid-1980s] a law took effect in California making it a crime to *agree* to take money for providing sexual services. Before, prostitutes were arrested—theoretically—only for solicitation, for initiating the sexual contract. This new law legalizes entrapment, in obvious violation of our civil rights. The situation is worse for poor women, especially blacks and Hispanics, who are forced to work on the street because escort services and massage parlors almost exclusively employ whites and Asians.

Since the onset of the AIDS epidemic, many prostitutes have been eager to assume roles as safe sex educators. CAL-PEP (California Prostitutes Education Project), a COYOTE offshoot, was recently awarded a ... grant by the California State Department of Health for the purpose of educating street prostitutes about safe sex and IV hygiene. In city- and state-funded programs ... prostitutes and ex-prostitutes in drug treatment centers and halfway houses assume key roles as social workers providing much needed outreach to street communities. Prostitutes' rights organizations in some cities have organized support groups to discuss a range of personal issues, including safe sex, [injecting drug use] hygiene, and HIV testing.

AIDS is not a crime. We must defeat all legislation that violates the rights of all those with AIDS ..., those testing HIV antibody positive, and those stigmatized as belonging to "high risk" categories....

Source: Carol Leigh, "Further Violations of Our Rights," in D. Crimp, ed., *AIDS: Cultural Analysis, Cultural Activism* (Cambridge, Mass.: MIT Press, 1989), pp. 177–181.

DOCUMENT 84: The Risk of HIV Infection Among Commercial Sex Workers and Their Clients

According to a Centers for Disease Control and Prevention (CDC) study of female commercial sex workers, rates of infection ranged from 0 percent to 47.5 percent in eight areas of the United States. The highest infection rate was for women in northern New Jersey, while the lowest was for women in southern Nevada, where prostitution is legal and regulated. The most important risk factor for these women is a history of injecting drugs. Infection rates were higher among women who injected drugs and who had a larger number of nonpaying sexual partners. Condom use was erratic with paying clients, but much more frequent than with nonpaying partners. Heterosexual transmission is a risk for men who have unprotected sex with an HIV-infected female partner, especially if she also has a sexually transmitted disease like herpes or syphilis. But it is more likely that a woman in the same situation will be HIV-infected than a man, since the virus is more efficiently transmitted from male to female in developed nations.

Data from the [CDC] study indicate that rates of HIV infection among female prostitutes vary greatly [from city to city] . . . and reflect two important factors. First, rates of HIV infection are much higher among sex workers who report a history of [injecting] drug use than among those who show no evidence of drugs. . . . Second, among women who do not report [injecting] drug use, HIV infection is associated with a larger number of personal (i.e., nonpaying) sexual partners. The [pattern] of [injecting] drug use among female prostitutes is not clearly understood, but it appears to be skewed toward streetwalkers and ethnic minority sex workers. . . .

The other major risk factor for female prostitutes is multiple nonpaying sexual partners. The available evidence indicates that prostitutes engage in unprotected intercourse more frequently with nonpaying partners than with their clients. [A CDC study of sex workers in seven large cities] found that only 16 percent of female prostitutes used condoms with non-paying partners (e.g., husbands, boyfriends), compared with 78 percent who used condoms at least occasionally with clients.

Yet, even with clients, some prostitutes report only sporadic use of condoms, perhaps because of the client unwillingness to [use them] and the pressure this reluctance exerts on women whose livelihood depends on fulfilling clients' demands. Thus far, the number of cases of AIDS ascribed to contact with female sex workers has been small, and the available data . . . suggest that there is little danger that female prostitutes will be a "bridge" of infection to the general population. . . . [On the contrary] it appears that female prostitutes are more at risk of *acquiring* HIV than they are of transmitting it. . . .

Various types of AIDS prevention programs for female prostitutes have been implemented, including street outreach to teach safer drug use and safer sex techniques. . . . Many of the outreach programs involve peer-led interventions delivered by ex-prostitutes or current sex workers.

Source: H. G. Miller, C. F. Turner, and L. E. Moses, eds., *AIDS: The Second Decade*, Summary Report (Washington, D.C.: National Academy Press, 1990).

DOCUMENT 85: The Plight of the Male Commercial Sex Worker

Male commercial sex workers (known as "hustlers" if working on the streets or in gay bars, and as "call boys" if working through an "escort service") have behaviors that place them at considerable risk for HIV infection. As is the case for female commercial sex workers, injecting drugs and unprotected sex are important risk factors for these young men. In particular, unprotected anal intercourse has been found to be the strongest predictor of HIV infection. Therefore, condom use is extremely important. Male commercial sex workers often do not use condoms with nonpaying sexual partners; with clients (or johns), condoms are used more often, but inconsistently. In one study of male street hustlers in Miami, conducted during the early 1990s, 62 percent were HIV-positive. In Miami, as is true for numerous other cities, many runaway youth and "throwaway" youth (teens who are thrown out of their home or abandoned by their parents or guardians) exchange sex for money or drugs. The authors of the following reading report on the results of another study.

Male prostitutes engage in several identified high-risk behaviors for sexually transmitted disease and HIV.... [T]hey have multiple paying and nonpaying sex partners whom they have little opportunity to screen, they engage in sexual behaviors that place them at high risk for HIV, they have high rates of sexually transmitted diseases, and they are often [injecting] drug users. They and their paying partners, who are almost invariably male, do not necessarily [think of themselves] as bisexual or [gay]; a substantial number view themselves as heterosexual [straight] and report having female sex partners....

The findings ... [of our study indicate] that in terms of HIV risks, the number of a person's sexual partners is less relevant than is the type of sexual acts in which the person engages. The strongest predictor ... was receptive anal intercourse [receiving anal sex] with nonpaying partners. Male as well as female prostitutes tend to be more at risk through sexual activities with their nonpaying partners than ... with their paying partners ... because they seldom, if ever, use a condom with their nonpaying partners whereas they frequently, but inconsistently, use condoms with paying partners.... The HIV rates were significantly higher among the homosexually- and bisexually-oriented prostitute, who were also more likely to engage in receptive anal intercourse than were their heterosexually-oriented peers. Intervention specifically targeted at male prostitutes is necessary to reduce the risk to them and their partners for HIV.

Source: Kirk W. Elifson, Jacqueline Boles, and Mike Sweat, "Risk Factors Associated with HIV Infection Among Male Prostitutes," *American Journal of Public Health* 93(1): 79–83 (January 1993).

DOCUMENT 86: Global Sex Tourism

In very poor farming villages in northern and northeastern Thailand (in Southeast Asia), it is customary and accepted that the parents of a teenage girl will enter into a contract to have their daughter work for two or three years in a brothel in a major Thai city. The daughter is often happy to help her parents in their struggle to bring much-needed income into the household. Neither she nor her parents are aware of the level of exploitation by the brothel owners and managers that awaits her. The teenagers are treated very badly in most of these brothels. When they return to their villages, many are HIV-positive. The following selection briefly discusses global sex tourism and its impact not only on teenagers and young adults, but on preteenagers, as well.

Sex tourism is spreading from Thailand and India to Latin America and Asia, said Christian Aid [a British charity]. Although it is not known how many children are bought for sex, . . . the child prostitution industry is growing at a significant rate. Sex tourists do not usually use condoms, which exposes children to the risk of AIDS. They also look for younger children in the belief that they will not have sexually transmitted diseases. "It is believed some 200,000 Nepali girls have been sold into sexual slavery in Indian brothels. It is [also] a serious problem in Brazil. Probably 60,000 children work as prostitutes in the Philippine sex industry, and perhaps as many as 200,000 in Thailand," Christian Aid said. [They] urged the British government to pass legislation under which people who commit abuses abroad could be prosecuted in British courts.

Source: Lyndsay Griffiths, "Charity Chronicles Spread of Sex Tourism" (Reuters, May 16, 1995); CDC National AIDS Clearinghouse (Bethesda, Md.: Information, Inc., 1995).

THE HOMELESS

DOCUMENT 87: A National Commission Addresses the Dual Problems of AIDS and the Lack of Housing

---

The housing crisis in America preceded the AIDS epidemic. Good, affordable housing for low-income people has been in short supply. In this situation, a crisis within a crisis quickly developed. People with HIV disease who once had homes were without shelter because of unemployment, discriminatory housing practices, or problems with their family. Their numbers were suddenly added to the existing homeless population. Local community-based organizations have worked hard to provide housing, but often do not have enough resources of their own to meet the demand. Federal, state, and city governments have helped create residences such as the Bailey House for persons living with AIDS in New York City, the Broward House in Fort Lauderdale, Florida, and the Chicago House apartments for families in northwest Chicago to meet the special medical and housing needs of people with HIV disease. Programs like these are not available in every part of the country.

The lack of affordable and appropriate housing is an acute crisis for people living with . . . (HIV) within the larger crisis of HIV/AIDS. Health and medical aspects of the epidemic have overshadowed the frequently desperate need for safe shelter that provides not only protection and comfort, but also a base in which, and from which, to receive services, care, and support.

Housing problems for people with HIV disease arise in a variety of ways. Many individuals are evicted when their HIV status becomes known; most of them are not even aware that this type of discrimination violates federal fair housing law and many state laws. For others, loss of income as a result of illness and inability to work creates an inability to pay the rent or mortgage. Some who are hospitalized find that when they are able to leave the hospital their already unstable living arrangements have fallen apart. Some had no homes before becoming HIV-infected and lived on the street; then, too ill to continue to fend for themselves, they shuttle back and forth between shelters and acute-care hospitals. Some children with HIV have spent their entire lives in hospitals because of the lack of adequate housing for them and their parents. Women with children are often excluded from the few residential programs that do exist. The scope of these problems is vast and solutions are difficult, but there is increasing awareness that the homeless of tomorrow are being created by the failure to provide housing options for thousands of people living with HIV disease today. . . .

Despite the best efforts of AIDS housing providers, there is an acute shortage of resources available for the development of housing for people with HIV disease. Community-based AIDS service organizations have attempted to meet growing housing needs by providing small-scale community-based group homes and rental assistance programs patched together with the few available local resources. Across the country, communities have sponsored projects ranging from bake sales to "Walks for Life" to raise money to supplement the few government programs that have been available to create AIDS housing. In the meantime, efforts to increase federal participation have met with limited success. . . .

Therefore the Commission recommends:

1. That HUD [the Department of Housing and Urban Development] make HIV/AIDS a top priority. The Federal government must help support AIDS housing. The failure to do so contributes significantly to unnecessary human suffering and is costing the nation millions of dollars.

2. That Congress mandate that HUD recognize HIV/AIDS as a disability and not continue to deny people with HIV/AIDS access to housing funds targeted toward the disabled.

3. That people with HIV/AIDS be granted access to traditional housing programs. By the same token, Congress and HUD must adapt program requirements to meet the specific housing needs of people with HIV/AIDS. . . .

4. That Congress make clear that HIV/AIDS-specific housing under Shelter Plus Care [a housing program designated for people with HIV/AIDS] and other Federal programs is both permitted and essential.

5. That Congress continue to play a leadership role in developing new funds to address the HIV/AIDS housing crisis.

6. That . . . the President of the United States name a lead official or agency to be responsible for a national plan to combat HIV/AIDS with cabinet level, interagency coordination.

7. [T]hat at the local level, a continuum of housing options be made available for people living with HIV disease that includes a range of alternatives from hospice care, and intermediate or supportive housing, to rental subsidies which could allow people to reside independently until . . . they need additional care.

Source: Housing and the HIV/AIDS Epidemic: Recommendations for Action (Washington, D.C.: National Commission on AIDS, 1992), pp. 2–14.

DOCUMENT 88: Profile of a Residence for the Homeless with AIDS

Bailey House in New York City is a model group residence for homeless people with AIDS. The largest such residence, it provides housing,
nursing services, counseling, and emotional support to residents. It is
an example of a humane and dignified place for people with AIDS at
the end of their lives.

What you don't expect at Bailey House are the odd moments of affir-
mation—irony . . . [and] laughter. There are children's voices. Sex forges
on. There's a basket of condoms on the front desk. . . . The Bailey House
administrator wants to start a softball team called The Dead. . . . [T]he
institutional memory teems with comic fictions, misadventures, tributes
to . . . pettiness, bravery, suffering, and grace. . . .

A home with a bed is the one thing anyone wants when they're sick,
but by the early Eighties it was apparent that many people with AIDS
had no place to live. Whether homelessness was a byproduct of AIDS
. . . or part of the pattern of a disenfranchised life, . . . lives were being
abridged because of it. Having no home . . . meant having no place to
die, apart from subway tunnels or city sidewalks.

Bailey House is still the nation's largest group residence for homeless
people with AIDS. In the five years since it opened, it has served as a
model of supportive AIDS housing for more than one hundred community organizations around the country working to develop smaller . . .
facilities. . . . [A]side from Bailey House, some 400 city-funded individual
apartments, and a handful of city-sponsored single-room occupancy ho-
tels, there isn't any place for homeless people with AIDS to go.

Bailey House . . . promised a safe, secure environment where homeless
people with AIDS would have their own keys and could come and go
as they pleased. With [city, state, federal, and private funding] Bailey
House began to offer a program of nursing support, counseling, even
recreation. . . . If homeless people with AIDS could not be redeemed in
the eyes of a society that reacted to them with fear and abhorrence,
perhaps at Bailey House they might be redeemed in their own.

Source: Chip Brown, "A Last Good Place to Live," *Harper's Magazine* 284(1701):
48–55 (February 1992).

DOCUMENT 89: The Measure of Greatness

The problem of homelessness for people with HIV disease is a pressing one in large cities like Boston and in smaller ones like Salt Lake City. The percentage of homeless people who also have HIV disease is high. A downward spiral of events can lead to homelessness in a short period of time: unemployment, loss of health insurance, housing discrimination, and lack of support from family or friends are all contributing factors. Shelters, as a place of last resort, are not equipped to provide adequate medical services or support for people struggling with a chronic and debilitating illness. This short reading and the three that follow it will give you different perspectives on the plight of the homeless with HIV.

Mayor Flynn [of Boston], flanked by nearly two dozen activists from organizations fighting AIDS, yesterday announced a housing initiative for homeless people with the disease, and pledged to appoint someone with AIDS to help lead a housing task force. . . . "I have always believed that the greatness of Boston must be measured by how it cares for those most in need," Flynn said. "We take pride in our city as a community which will never, ever look the other way."

Source: Michael Rezendes, "City's Goal: To House Homeless Who Have AIDS," *Boston Globe* (December 22, 1990); Newsbank, 1990 HEA 130:E10.

DOCUMENT 90: Why So Many Homeless Are HIV-Positive

It has been said that most Americans are three paychecks away from poverty and homelessness. Some gay men with AIDS become homeless when they are no longer able to work because they, like most Americans, have not been able to accumulate substantial savings and are no longer able to pay the rent or mortgage on their home, condo, or apartment. Many active injecting drug users with AIDS were homeless even before they became ill.

[In Boston] . . . AIDS activists estimate nearly half of the city's homeless are infected with the deadly virus and some 2,000 persons with the disease need housing . . . for a variety of reasons [according to a report to the governor-elect]. "They may be thrown into poverty when they lose their jobs and health insurance. Many persons with AIDS contracted the virus while living in shelters, doubled up with friends or relatives or living in housing of marginal quality."

[Said one homeless person with HIV:] "When you have HIV, you think about it all the time. You can't get it out of your head. It's scary. Being homeless just adds to the stress. If I had a place to live, it would be . . . one less thing to worry about."

Source: Joe Sciacca, "Homelessness Adds Hopelessness for AIDS Victims," *Boston Herald* (December 16, 1990); Newsbank, 1990 HEA 130: E11–E12.

DOCUMENT 91: Warning: Homeless Shelters Can Be Hazardous to Your Health If You Have AIDS

A homeless shelter is perhaps the last place that a person with a weakened immune system (immunosuppressed) would want to stay. He or she is susceptible to violence, theft, severe stress, lack of privacy, and a host of pathogens that a person who is immunosuppressed may find very deadly. Tuberculosis, pneumonia, and other opportunistic infections often spread rapidly in homeless shelters. A private apartment, even a small studio with a kitchenette, is far preferable.

AIDS patients are "downwardly mobile," losing first their health, then jobs, insurance and finally their homes. . . . Some stay for a time with friends or relatives, but many end up in homeless shelters. "People who carry the virus are in danger in homeless shelters, . . ." [said Patrick Poulin, director of the organization that manages Salt Lake City's largest shelters]. . . . "Someone who's HIV positive or with AIDS is going to be put at a much higher risk to catch other diseases. . . . It makes me angry. . . . [W]e've seen the problem coming for the last four or five years but [have] not done anything about it."

Source: Lois M. Collins, "Housing Crisis Adds to Woes Facing People with HIV, AIDS," *Salt Lake City Deseret News* (July 26, 1992); Newsbank 1992 HEA 86:E10.

DOCUMENT 92: Reaching Out to the Homeless with AIDS

While the homeless are among the most at risk for HIV infection, they ironically are often among the last to get tested for HIV, receive education about AIDS, or participate in risk reduction programs for HIV prevention. Homelessness and AIDS constitute a nationwide problem from Maine to California.

Unless Maine makes aggressive efforts to protect its homeless population from AIDS, the state's street people will be assaulted with an epidemic of the fatal virus.... The risk of AIDS among a homeless population living with poverty, disease, and certain at-risk behaviors such as unsafe sex and drug abuse is on the rise.... Sometimes it is recently released prisoners who show up . . . in Portland with AIDS, little money and no place to go.... Other times, it's someone who has tested HIV positive and has been evicted from an apartment when the landlord found out.... The homeless tend not to be tested for HIV, or to receive educational and preventive services.... Information about AIDS may not reach people in the streets....

Source: Karlene K. Hale, "Maine's Homeless at Risk of AIDS," *Kennebec Journal* (July 25, 1992); Newsbank 1992 HEA 86:E9.

DOCUMENT 93: Housing for Homeless PWAs Is Cost-Effective

It costs at least ten times more for a homeless person with AIDS to stay in a public hospital than to live in public housing. Housing is, of course, not the complete answer to homelessness. It must be combined with a variety of job skills, health, mental health, and other services on or near the premises. There remains considerable apathy about the plight of homeless people with AIDS. Housing Opportunities for People With AIDS (HOPWA), a Federal program that provides resources to local communities for the housing needs of people with AIDS, was nearly eliminated in 1995. Fortunately, it was restored through an intensive effort by AIDS political advocates.

This month [March 1995], the House Appropriations Committee decided to cut rental assistance in this year's budget for the disabled homeless and to eliminate federal housing assistance for homeless people with AIDS. Although this is not Congress' last word on how to care for "the poorest Americans," it sends a bleak signal.... The bottom line is that it costs considerably more not to house these people than to house them. The House panel cut $186 million from a program that would have helped fund 35,000 housing units for people with AIDS. Unless these people have a stable place to live and access to primary care, they are likely to live on the streets and in hospitals. The average cost of a hospital bed is $1,085 a day, while supportive housing costs $40 to $100 a day. If the cutbacks mean that even 1,000 AIDS patients are inappropriately housed in hospitals, the extra cost to taxpayers will be $360 million a year. The proven answer to homelessness for the majority of homeless people is supportive housing—combining permanent housing with services such as health care, job counseling, and therapy. . . .

Source: Julie Sandorf, "Building Homelessness, Not Housing," *The New York Times*, p. A19 (March 13, 1995); CDC National AIDS Clearinghouse (Bethesda, Md.: Information, Inc., 1995).

CORRECTIONAL FACILITIES

DOCUMENT 94: Managing the AIDS Crisis in Prisons and Jails

Prison and jail populations have large numbers of people with HIV disease. That is because many inmates have a history of injecting drugs. In addition, they may have engaged in high-risk sexual behavior, such as exchanging sex for money or drugs. Since people in the correctional system are, of course, captive populations, the policies of these institutions directly affect their health. For those already infected with HIV, the quality of medical care influences the course of their illness. For those who are not infected, prevention is critically important to their remaining uninfected. Prevention and control strategies include mandatory testing and segregation, education and counseling, and condom distribution. States vary in their policies. For example, with regard to testing, some states test all inmates; some test higher-risk inmates like injecting drug users; and others test only when symptoms occur. Controversial programs, such as condom distribution or clean needle distribution, have seldom been instituted. On the other hand, there is a consensus that educational programs are necessary, and nearly every correctional system had one in place by the early 1990s, although by the mid-1990s budget problems were forcing many prisons and jails to end or cut back on their programs.

. . . [I]ntravenous [injecting into a vein] drug use was always the most prevalent risk factor for incarcerated [imprisoned] victims. . . . Inmate populations are drawn heavily from the intravenous drug-using population outside prison. Up to 50% of criminal offenses leading to incarceration are drug-related. . . . Among incarcerated populations, women have shown higher rates [of testing HIV-positive]. . . . Although the reasons for these higher rates among incarcerated female populations are still unknown, higher rates of prostitution and intravenous drug use may be the explanation. . . .

Control efforts in correctional facilities include mandatory testing, segregation, infection control, education/training, condom distribution, and access to clean needles. . . . Mandatory testing/segregation policy options separate corrections from the remainder of the public health policy arena. . . . Although the American Medical Association advocated mandatory testing for inmates, the World Health Organization recommended against it. . . . The public health community has recommended that correctional authorities make prison life safer by distributing clean needles and condoms to inmates. . . . Unfortunately, very few correctional systems distribute either condoms or clean needles to inmates. Correctional officials are loath to encourage further disregard for the law by supporting intravenous drug use and sexual activity in prison. . . .

Correctional officials and public health authorities agree that education is the key management tool. . . . Nearly all United States [prison] systems provide AIDS-specific education programs. . . . Key elements of education programs include regular updates, planned curricula, treatment of issues specific to the correctional environment, and mandatory training for both inmates and staff.

Source: T. Ford Brewer and Janice Derrickson, "AIDS in Prison: A Review of Epidemiology and Preventive Policy," *AIDS* 6(7): 623–628 (1992).

DOCUMENT 95: Health Care, Human Rights, and HIV Education in Correctional Facilities

The inadequacies of AIDS health care, the frequency of HIV-related discrimination, and the weaknesses of HIV education and prevention programs that exist in the larger society are magnified in our nation's prisons and jails. This reading details the harsh findings of the National Commission on AIDS when it observed the status of HIV/AIDS in our correctional facilities.

[At the beginning of the 1990s] the National Commission on Acquired Immune Deficiency Syndrome . . . conducted a site visit and hearing to identify and understand the issues which face the nation and its Federal, state and local correctional facilities, in their management of detainees and prisoners living with . . . HIV disease, the continuum of conditions which begins with seroconversion and ends with AIDS. The findings were sobering and troubling. . . .

The commission's study . . . reveals that too many correctional facilities subject inmates to a series of unnecessary, arbitrary indignities which fundamentally affect their basic human rights. . . . The addition of HIV disease to the already difficult world of prison life has created special problems in three major areas: health care, human rights, and education. Lack of adequate health care and often overcrowded conditions subject inmates living with HIV disease to the dangers of tuberculosis and other opportunistic diseases. Lack of education and understanding among officials and other inmates create violations of rights for the inmate living with HIV disease regarding confidentiality and access to prison programs.

Health Care:

Inmates with HIV disease face many of the same difficulties in obtaining adequate health care as do people with HIV disease in the general community. However, due to the lack of mobility and choice which define the life of prisoners, they also face unique problems, . . . [which] include:

- A . . . study by the Correctional Association of New York suggests that prisoners with AIDS may be dying at twice the rate of non-prisoners with AIDS.

- Doctors and dentists often refuse to treat inmates who have tested positive for HIV and inmates speak often of the difficulty of receiving "hands-on" care for both HIV and non-HIV-related problems.

- Prisoners with HIV infection have much higher rates of tuberculosis and are at increased risk from the resurgent tuberculosis epidemic in the nation's prisons. Immunosuppression [weakening of the immune system] fosters progression of dormant [inactive] tuberculosis to active disease.

- Due, in part, to the confusion regarding regulations governing clinical research involving prisoners, inmates are often denied access to clinical research programs which could provide opportunities for new HIV treatments available in the general community.

- Inmates living with HIV disease are often denied access to specialists outside the correctional facility who could significantly improve their medical conditions.

- T-cell counts, essential for monitoring the progression of HIV disease, are often administered erratically. . . . Medications are not always available or distributed in a consistent, timely manner.

- Special diets or housing appropriate for those with HIV disease are often lacking.

- Access to *voluntary* testing with appropriate counseling is in very short supply. Prisoners are often tested without their knowledge and consent, and then informed of their seropositive status with inaccurate projections of life spans, treatments, etc.

• Health care, testing and counseling specific to the needs of women and adolescents is virtually non-existent.

Human Rights and Confidentiality:

The ignorance and prejudice which cause so many to mistreat people with HIV disease have, inside prisons, resulted in a loss of human rights for individuals living with HIV disease and lives of isolation and despair. The following are examples of the policies which help create these injustices:

• Prisoners with HIV disease are often segregated from the rest of the prison community despite the fact that there is absolutely no legitimate public health basis for the practice.

• Segregated inmates often lose access to religious services, work programs, visitation rights, libraries, including law libraries, educational and recreational programs, and drug and alcohol treatment.

• Prisoners with HIV disease are being denied access to early release programs.

• In small prisons, isolation because of HIV positive status can . . . become a sentence of solitary confinement. In larger prisons, inmates with HIV disease are often grouped together indiscriminately.

• Segregation [based on AIDS or HIV status eliminates the confidentiality of the] prisoners' health [condition] . . . to the rest of the community of inmates and officials.

• In . . . facilities where segregation is not practiced, confidentiality is often violated due to the lack of privacy when meeting with medical personnel and during the distribution of medication.

• Inmates with AIDS are dying inside prisons and hospitals without release, or the support of family, friends or counselors despite the fact that they are not a threat to society.

Education and Prevention:

Education and prevention programs are in many ways the key to solving some of the most dangerous problems confronting all members of the prison community. . . . These dangers include the risk of continuing to practice behaviors which may lead to HIV infection and the physical danger to inmates with HIV disease. . . . [E]xplicit, culturally appropriate education programs for all members of the prison community [will help solve the following persisting problems]:

• Fear and discrimination towards individuals with HIV disease and unjust policies, such as segregation of inmates with HIV disease, will continue without education programs for both inmates and correctional staff.

• Inmates' informed participation in their own medical care, including the decision about whether to seek HIV testing, is not possible without comprehensive HIV education programs.

• Inmates and staff will remain at risk of HIV infection until they are taught how to reduce or eliminate that risk. Without specific education geared towards correctional personnel, they will continue to impede their own and inmates' progress toward minimizing risk behaviors.

• Segregation programs are creating a false sense of security about HIV disease among the non-segregated prison community and wrongly suggest that by isolating those individuals who are infected, everyone else is now "safe."

• The means to prevent HIV transmission through the distribution of condoms has been adopted by only a handful of prisons despite the fact that distribution of condoms has resulted in no adverse security incidents thus far.

• Former prisoners are re-entering their communities with little or no added knowledge about HIV disease and how to prevent it.

Source: Report, *HIV Disease in Correctional Facilities* (Washington, D.C.: National Commission on AIDS, March 1991).

DOCUMENT 96: Sickness and Death Among Inmates in New York City

When the AIDS epidemic began to affect New York City's drug users, it also affected the city's inmate population. Injecting drug users in New York City are known to have high rates of HIV infection. Therefore, the New York City Department of Health's reasonable estimate back in the late 1980s that 20 to 25 percent of inmates are HIV-infected is not surprising. Of those who are infected, many become ill and die in jail. AIDS rapidly became the leading cause of death among New York City inmates.

The correctional system has experienced a dramatic growth in the number of inmates affected by the AIDS epidemic. . . . Given the extent of intravenous drug use among inmates prior to incarceration, the Department of Health estimates that between 20% and 25% of the total inmate population is HIV positive. . . .

The number of inmates suffering and dying from AIDS has been increasing. . . . Inmates showing symptoms of HIV-related conditions are cared for on an outpatient basis in prison clinics, [in] the Riker's Island Infirmary AIDS unit, [in] the infirmary isolation ward (for TB [tuberculosis] cases), in general infirmary beds, or in [New York City Health & Hospital Corporation] facilities. AIDS is presently the leading cause of death among males and females in the inmate population. At least half of the ... deaths ... among people in [Department of Corrections] custody can be directly attributed to HIV-related illness, and that proportion may in fact be considerably higher.

Source: "Social Services and Clinical Care," in *New York City Strategic Plan for AIDS* (New York: Interagency Task Force on AIDS May 1988), section D.5, pp. 1–25

DOCUMENT 97: The Special Needs of Women with AIDS in Prisons and Jails

The majority of women in state prisons and municipal jails are there because of drug-related problems. In fact, most are former injecting drug users or sexual partners of injecting drug users. As a result, HIV infection rates are high in this population. These women have special medical and psychological problems. Since some of the women are pregnant, prisons and jails need to counsel them on their pregnancy and to offer them appropriate treatment.

Incarcerated women [confined in prisons or jails] have been, and continue to be, a forgotten population. This can be attributed, in part, to the historically small number of women [compared with men] incarcerated in prisons and jails in the United States. In 1980, there were approximately 13,000 women in federal and state prisons. By the end of 1989, that number had more than tripled, to almost 41,000. In 1989 alone, the female prison population grew by 25%, compared with a 13% growth in the male prison population. . . .

According to the Federal Bureau of Prisons, about 60% of women in federal custody are serving sentences for drug offenses. A large number of women in prison have alcohol and drug dependency problems. . . . The estimates now range between 70% and 80%. . . .

The behavior profile of women in prison to a great extent mirrors the profile of those most at-risk of contracting HIV infection. The overwhelming majority of female prisoners have multiple drug problems. Many of them are [injecting] drug users. Even though women comprise only nine percent of AIDS cases, they are the fastest growing population to be affected by HIV disease. Among prison entrants, the HIV prevalence rates are generally [slightly] higher for women than for men. In New York State, the seroprevalence rate for female entrants is 18.8% compared to a seroprevalence rate of 17.4% among male entrants. . . . Additionally, preliminary results of [a similar study] indicate that among persons less than 25 years of age, female entrants to correctional facilities had significantly higher rates of HIV infection than male entrants.

Eighty percent of female prisoners have children, and of those, 70% are single parents. Prior to their incarceration, 85% of female prisoners, compared to 47% of male prisoners had custody of their children. These women are primarily young, between the ages of 20 and 34 years old. Further, a significant number of women give birth to children shortly before they begin to serve prison sentences, or are pregnant and give birth during their incarceration. The Bureau of Justice Statistics reports that about 25 percent of women in correctional institutions are pregnant or postpartum [the period shortly after childbirth]. In New York City, approximately 8% of female inmates are pregnant at the time of their incarceration.

Urgent attention must be given to the special needs of females. . . . In addition to the services available to their male counterparts, women in prison are in desperate need of HIV education regarding perinatal [around the time of birth] transmission and pediatric [childhood] AIDS, frequent Pap smears [to test for cancer or to evaluate a woman's hormonal condition] and other services sensitive to gender and the distinct history of female inmates regarding the conditions of their confinement. In addition, pregnant inmates are in need of prenatal [before birth] services where HIV testing is offered upon request. Special care to provide education and counseling in a context of freely available reproductive choice is essential.

Source: Report, *HIV Disease in Correctional Facilities* (Washington, D.C.: National Commission on AIDS, March 1991).

DOCUMENT 98: Understanding the Social Context

In this excerpt, the HIV/AIDS epidemic and its relationship to the criminal justice system are viewed from a broader perspective. The social and economic conditions that have an impact on illegal drug use and high-risk sexual behavior are deep-rooted and long-standing. The cost of failure to change these conditions is high both in financial and in human terms. Ironically, the cost of a year in prison is about the same as the cost of a year of college!

All too often the disadvantaged child lives in a neighborhood where there are no neighbors who demonstrate that education matters, . . . that steady work is a viable alternative to welfare and crime, and that a stable family is normal. The vacuum is filled by drug pushers, pimps and prostitutes. They're often the only successful people the kids see. It's no wonder, then, that [they] become hooked on intravenous drugs and harmful sexual behavior and become a part of . . . social dislocations, from robbery to personal violence, and in the process become incarcerated and perhaps infected with HIV. . . .

[In prisons] HIV infection . . . [appears as many symptoms, each of which requires treatment on several levels], driving up the medical costs. . . . The greatest increased cost will be the expense of providing a sophisticated range of care, drawing from medicine, nursing, psychology, social service, health education, and religion. . . .

. . . [P]overty, ignorance, neglect, and hopelessness . . . are major contributors to a child's progression to a life of crime. . . . Enlightened realism tells us that money for new jails and prisons must be matched by money for prevention. . . . And . . . we adults must live as examples for kids to emulate. Otherwise, the days ahead will be worse than anything we can now imagine.

Source: E. T. Chandler, "A Piece of a North Carolina Doctor's Mind: The High Cost of Failure," *North Carolina Medical Journal* 52(6): 255–258 (June 1991).

DOCUMENT 99: Where Should State Prison Systems Put Their Seriously Ill AIDS Patients?

In 1993, Florida announced plans for a special prison for patients with advanced HIV disease. The facility would provide medical care to as many as 150 inmates. The state believes its plan is more cost-effective in the long run than a decentralized system. The head physician argues convincingly that it would allow him to treat all AIDS patients more easily. However, civil liberties groups question segregation of inmates as potentially discriminatory if it is expanded to include HIV-infected inmates, and not just those who are seriously ill.

Florida's prison system will become the first in the nation to house together inmates in the final stages of AIDS. Plans are under way to move as many as 150 prisoners to an "AIDS-care" prison under construction. . . .

Some civil libertarians call it a throwback to the days of leper colonies, an attempt to warehouse those with the deadly condition. But prison administrators say the idea is to provide the best care possible in the most cost-effective way. They say the prison will be only for those who are seriously ill, not for all prisoners who have AIDS [or are HIV positive]. . . .

Attorneys for the American Civil Liberties Union . . . argue that savings are not reason enough. Segregating the inmates could confer second-class status on a group. . . .

But Dr. Charles Matthews, the prison system's top doctor, said the central setting is best because AIDS . . . requires special expertise and special drugs. "I'm responsible for the treatment of these people, and I need to have them where I can treat them best."

Source: David Kidwell, "Prison for AIDS Inmates Readied," *The Miami Herald*, pp. 1A, 5A (August 23, 1993).

DOCUMENT 100: The Need for HIV Intervention Programs in Our Nation's Prisons, Jails, and Youth Confinement Facilities

During the first four years of the 1990s, the proportion of correctional facilities that provided any form of instructor-led HIV/AIDS education dropped significantly. Programs that not only educate inmates, correctional officers, and administrators about HIV/AIDS, but also develop the self-esteem of the inmates, encourage their ability to successfully make changes in their lives, and give them verbal skills for practicing safer sex. Condom distribution is a difficult issue, since sex is not permitted in any correctional facility in the United States but frequently occurs anyway. Only two state prison systems and four city jails distribute condoms. If you do not give out condoms to inmates who have sex with other inmates, you might be jeopardizing the lives of some inmates. But if you do give out condoms, you may be indicating that the prohibition against inmates having sex is not to be taken seriously. If you were the warden, what would you do?

Prison and jail systems for adults participating in [a] 1994 survey reported 5,279 cases of AIDS among current inmates, representing 5.2 AIDS cases per 1,000 adult inmates—a rate almost six times that of the total U.S. adult . . . population. . . . Based on reports from all 51 state and federal systems, the percentage of systems providing instructor-led HIV/AIDS education in at least one of their facilities decreased from 96% in 1990 to 75% in 1994. . . .

Two state prison systems (Vermont and Mississippi) and four city/county jail systems (New York City; Philadelphia; San Francisco; and Washington, DC) reported making condoms available to inmates in their facilities. . . . Of 456 confinement facilities in the 40 state systems responding to the question, 31 (7%) were operating peer-led HIV/AIDS education, 258 (57%) were providing instructor-led education, 246 (54%) were using audio-visual materials, and 270 (59%) were using written materials. . . .

To assist in reducing the transmission of HIV in the United States, comprehensive and credible programs of interactive education, counseling, testing, partner notification, and practical risk-reduction techniques (e.g., safer sex and safer drug injection) should be implemented for adult inmates in prisons and jails and for juveniles in confinement facilities.

Source: "HIV/AIDS Education and Prevention Programs for Adults in Prisons and Jails and Juveniles in Confinement Facilities—United States, 1994," *Morbidity and Mortality Weekly Report* 45(13) (April 5, 1996).

PERSONS WITH HEMOPHILIA

DOCUMENT 101: The Death of Ricky Ray

Clotting medication for people with hemophilia is produced from the blood of thousands of donors. Prior to 1985, when screening for HIV began, 50 to 80 percent of people with hemophilia who received contaminated blood products were infected with HIV. Drug companies claim that they had no prior knowledge and that they acted responsibly by screening blood as soon as an HIV test was available. However, prior to that time, it was known that hepatitis was transmitted in these products, and that heating would destroy the hepatitis virus. This procedure was costly and was not done. Today, clotting products are routinely heat-treated. Families like that of Ricky Ray, a young person with hemophilia who died of AIDS, have received substantial out-of-court settlements from drug companies. The Ray family had their house burned down and were forced to move from Arcadia, Florida, because of fear, hate, and discrimination by some of the people in that town against persons with AIDS.

[I]n growing numbers, [people with hemophilia] are revealing [that they have] the virus that causes AIDS . . . [and Ricky Ray's recent death] from AIDS at age 15 will inspire even more to speak up. . . . Last month, persons with hemophilia took their first major stand. At a National Hemophilia Foundation meeting . . . many pushed for a congressional investigation into whether the federal government and pharmaceutical companies that make blood products knew before 1985 that supplies were tainted. . . . The pharmaceutical companies say they did nothing wrong. The Hemophilia Foundation says it knows of no successful court verdict against the companies. Many families, though, such as the Ray [family], settled out of court with the makers of the blood products. The Ray [household] received $1 million.

Source: John Donnelley, "Hemophilia, Ricky, AIDS: 'It Didn't Need To Happen,'" *The Miami Herald* (December 15, 1992); Newsbank 1992 NIN 12:B3, 12:B4.

DOCUMENT 102: Ryan White in Kokomo

Ryan White, a teenager with hemophilia, died of AIDS in 1990, at the age of eighteen. He contracted HIV from contaminated blood products. The publicity surrounding his expulsion because of his illness from the Kokomo, Indiana, public school system caused a furor. In court, Ryan White won the right to attend school in Kokomo. But at the invitation of Cicero, Indiana, he and his family moved to Cicero instead. He became a symbol of courage in the face of fear and discrimination. In his honor, funding of HIV/AIDS health and social services for the states and sixteen cities was named after him: the Ryan White Comprehensive AIDS Resources Emergency Act of 1990. The five-year program was renewed and expanded by Congress in 1995 for an additional five years.

Ryan White had that bright, youthful Huck Finn [look] . . . [a] Midwestern kid to the core. He was from Kokomo, Ind., a blue-collar town of 50,000 that would treat him and his illness with a mean-spirited fearfulness, as though he were a freakish monster. . . .

For a country that sometimes seemed unwilling to confront AIDS head-on, Ryan was an anomaly who demanded immediate attention. He suffered from hemophilia, a congenital disease in which the blood does not clot normally. A [person with hemophilia] bleeds excessively when injured and often becomes crippled from repeated bleeding into joints. [Ryan] needed blood products to treat his hemophilia, and some of what he received was contaminated. . . .

[Ryan] was banned from . . . school in Kokomo when school officials contended his presence would create a health risk to him and to other students. His ouster precipitated a legal battle and an inordinate amount of national and international attention. . . .

[Amid continuing acts of discrimination] the family moved to Cicero, Indiana, [where] the school . . . embraced the boy, who by that point had achieved great fame. . . . [Upon his death in April 1990] the people of Kokomo expressed remorse about their callous treatment years earlier. Indiana Governor Evan Bayh ordered flags at the Statehouse flown at half-staff . . . in Ryan's honor. He said, "Had the world not known Ryan White, our understanding, treatment and concern for people with AIDS would be harsher and more judgmental."

Source: Gary Pomerantz, "Hemophiliac's Life Became American Symbol of the '80's," Atlanta Journal (April 9, 1990); Newsbank 1990 NIN 136:B12–B14.

DOCUMENT 103: Who Was Responsible for HIV Among Persons with Hemophilia?

By June 1996, 4,508 persons with hemophilia/coagulation disorder were reported with AIDS. This includes 228 children under thirteen years old, 688 teenagers (thirteen–nineteen years old), and 580 young adults (twenty–twenty-four years old). Since the vast majority of persons with hemophilia are male, nearly all of the persons diagnosed with AIDS have been male. Who was responsible for the explosion of HIV infections in persons with hemophilia who used lifesaving, but unheated, Factor VIII back in the early 1980s? Was it the drug companies, the CDC, or the National Hemophilia Foundation? Or was it the federal government's apathy at that time in failing to control an epidemic that mostly targeted disliked gay men? Although this reading refers to testimony in Canada, it describes an event that occurred in the United States.

. . . [Dr.] Donald Francis, a retired epidemiologist with the U.S. Centers for Disease Control and Prevention (CDC), testified in Canada before the Commission of Inquiry on the Blood System. One of the first scientists to study AIDS, [Dr.] Francis testified that the CDC made a mistake in not being more forceful in the early days of AIDS. He admitted that the exact cause of AIDS had not been identified in the early years of the epidemic. He noted, however, that lack of public knowledge had not prevented public health officials from taking strong measures to block other threats, such as Legionnaires' disease and toxic shock syndrome. [Dr.] Francis also said that there was little hesitation among government officials to issue early, written warnings to health-care workers about tainted blood. That effort began in November 1982, long before HIV was identified. The warnings came just four months after the National Hemophilia Foundation first informed its members that the CDC had found three HIV-infected [persons with hemophilia]. [Dr.] Francis said that he and [Dr.] Bruce Evatt, the Foundation's main contact at the CDC, were shocked to see that the Foundation's newsletter urged people to continue using Factor VIII [a product developed to prevent excessive and life-threatening bleeding among persons with hemophilia]. The newsletter said that although a virus might be causing the disease, there was little risk and that the "CDC is not recommending any change in blood product use." [Dr.] Francis claimed that he and [Dr.] Evatt never said any such thing.

Source: Donna Shaw, "Learning from the Tragedy of AIDS," *Philadelphia Inquirer*, p. A4 (March 10, 1995); CDC National AIDS Clearinghouse (Bethesda, Md.: Information, Inc., 1995).

SUGGESTED READINGS

"AIDS & Nutrition." *Prevention* 45, pp. 28–29 (October 1993).

"Baltimore Plans to Use Old Mailboxes to Collect Needles from Drug Addicts." *Washington Times*, p. C3 (June 12, 1996).

"Beta-Carotene and AIDS." *Prevention* 44, pp. 30–31 (October 1992).

Brown, C. "Dying Young: AIDS Among Teens." *Mademoiselle* 99, pp. 74–76 (February 1993).

"Charting the Spread of AIDS." *Science News* 144, p. 68 (July 3, 1993).

Des Jarlais, D., and S. R. Friedman. "AIDS and the Use of Injected Drugs." *Scientific American* 270, pp. 82–88 (February 1994).

Goldsmith, B. "Women on the Edge." *The New Yorker* 69, pp. 64–72 (April 26, 1993).

Gorman, C. "Are Some People Immune to AIDS?" *Time* 141, pp. 49–51 (March 22, 1993).

———. "Moms, Kids and AIDS." *Time* 144, pp. 60–61 (July 4, 1994).

Henry, W. A. "An Identity Forged in Flames." *Time* 140, pp. 35–37 (August 3, 1992).

Lee, Felicia R. "Cuts Set Off Debate on Helping Homeless with AIDS." *The New York Times*, p. B1 (March 21, 1995).

Masters, Troy. "For Gay Men, a Cultural Change?" *The New York Times*, p. A16 (July 30, 1996).

O'Brien, Thomas R., William A. Blattner, David Waters, et al. "Serum HIV-1 Levels and Time to Development of AIDS in the Multicenter Hemophilia Cohort Study." *Journal of the American Medical Association* 276(2), p. 105 (July 10, 1996).

Price, Joyce. "Hormone May Raise HIV Risk in Women." *Washington Times*, p. A9 (October 1, 1996).

"Prostitutes Spread AIDS in China." *American Medical News* 39(2), p. 24 (January 8, 1996).

Reynolds, R. "AIDS and Young Adults." *Black Enterprise* 23, p. 47 (April 1993).

Sabatier, Renee. *Blaming Others: Prejudice, Race and Worldwide AIDS*. Washington, D.C.: Panos Institute, 1988.

"Saving Children from Sex." *Economist* 340(7981), p. 17 (August 31, 1996).

Sherr, Lorraine, ed. *AIDS and the Heterosexual Population*. New York: Harwood Academic Publishers, 1993.

"Study Finds AIDS Growing but Not Rampant Among US Prisoners." *AIDS Alert* 9(4), p. 57 (April 1994).

Weinberg, Martin S. *Dual Attraction: Bisexuality in the Age of AIDS*. New York: Oxford University Press, 1994.

"Women, AIDS, Condoms and Confidence." *Glamour* 92, p. 180 (May 1994).

Woodman, S. "The Push to Test Babies for HIV." *Ms.* 5, pp. 90–92 (September/October 1994).

Worth, Dooley. "Latina Women and AIDS." *Radical America* 20(6), pp. 63–67 (November/December 1986).

4

AIDS in the Developing World

The vast majority of persons with HIV and AIDS do not live in the United States—about only one in twenty-two persons did in 1996. They live mostly in sub-Saharan Africa and Asia. Many also live in Latin America, the Caribbean, the Pacific region, the Middle East, North Africa, Europe, and Canada. While the great majority of persons with HIV/AIDS live in the developing world, only about 1 percent of the world's economic resources that go to combat AIDS and support HIV prevention programs are spent there. By 1996, 5.8 million people, including 1.3 million children, died of AIDS in the world. By the end of 1997, the United Nations estimated that only one in ten of the 30.6 million people infected with HIV knew that they were infected.

This chapter will give the reader an overview of some of the key issues in the social and public health dimensions of HIV/AIDS in sub-Saharan Africa, Asia, Latin America, and the Caribbean. In Africa, HIV/AIDS is only one of many major concerns facing that continent today. For example, while Rwandans have very high rates of HIV seropositivity, the immediacy of that problem paled by comparison when in the mid-1990s about 800,000 Tutsis, Twa (pygmies), and moderate Hutus were massacred by their Hutu neighbors. The major tribes of Rwanda and Burundi are the Hutu, Tutsi, and Twa. Millions of African men, women, and children die each year from diseases for which vaccines are readily available in North America and Europe. Countless African children die each year from drinking polluted water, because no safe water supply is available.

In Africa, the subordinate role of women and the sexual attitudes of men (the beliefs that women need to be sexually dominated, that if women use a condom they must be promiscuous, and that only men may make the decision to use a condom) have hindered safer sex campaigns and condom use. Innovative approaches to safer sex messages, however, have proven successful in getting the information out to non-literate populations, such as the theatrical presentations in rural Mali (West Africa) described in one of the reading selections. Peer education in South Africa has also proven effective in getting HIV information across in the workplace.

In the developing world, millions of children who are HIV-negative have been orphaned by the death of their parents. While most are taken in by their grandparents or other relatives, in some cities many children have to fend for themselves, and become homeless street children with no familial supervision or care.

In parts of the developing world where Western medical care is extremely inadequate, and often available only for the wealthy, the traditional healer (curer or shaman, occasionally pejoratively called a "witch doctor") is respected by the people in the community, and has learned how to use local herbs (plants) to effectively treat or cure many health problems. He or she often treats AIDS patients with traditional herbal medicines, and sometimes a little magic, to alleviate symptoms and treat some of the opportunistic infections brought on by AIDS. The traditional healer has been an often overlooked resource for HIV education and AIDS-related treatments, especially in rural areas.

One of our readings on AIDS in Africa discusses the dilemma of a rising population growth rate and the resulting stress on scarce resources, but a declining life expectancy rate that results in a lessened quality of life. Another reading discusses new information which shows that breast-feeding is more dangerous to young children in the developing world than was previously thought, and may require us to rethink our current policy.

HIV is currently spreading at a faster rate in Asia than in Africa, and the number of people with HIV in Asia should soon outnumber those with HIV in Africa. The social conditions in India, where male truckers have unprotected sex (without condoms) with female commercial sex workers for about 28 cents, are similar to those of central and eastern Africa, where the virus has spread rapidly through the population. While governments have expressed dismay over the coming of AIDS, with few exceptions (such as Thailand, which initiated a major and well-funded campaign against AIDS), relatively little has been invested by the nations to stop the spread of HIV.

In South America, Mexico, Central America, and the Caribbean, HIV/AIDS has also been spreading rapidly. Religious factors, such as resistance to condom use by the Roman Catholic Church, have adversely affected HIV prevention messages in some Latin American countries. Also, in the reading about sexually active Brazilian female university students who know a lot about HIV and AIDS but do not consistently use condoms when having sex, we are reminded that knowledge does not necessarily lead to behavioral change. Last, in Cuba the forced quarantine for life, in place until very recently, of all persons who tested positive for HIV, raises important questions about how much we are willing to sacrifice basic human rights and liberties in an attempt to control the spread of a disease. If you were positive for HIV, would you want to spend the rest of your life in a quarantine camp to ensure that you could not spread the virus to anyone outside of the camp?

THE AFRICAN PANDEMIC

DOCUMENT 104: AIDS Joins Spectrum of Adverse Conditions Taking a Heavy Toll on the People of Africa

The AIDS epidemic in Africa is different, in certain respects, from the AIDS epidemic in the United States. In Africa, there are about as many male cases as there are female cases; in the United States, most cases are male. Heterosexual contact is slowly increasing in the United States; in Africa, it is the most important mode of HIV transmission. An entire family, including the children, is usually affected and often infected. As devastating as this disease can be to an African family, AIDS is but one of many severe economic and health problems facing Africans today.

The overall pattern of HIV transmission in central and East Africa is very different from the pattern . . . in North America and Europe. In central and East Africa, most HIV transmission . . . occurs through heterosexual penile-vaginal intercourse. . . .

The problems of malnutrition, poverty, diarrheal disease (especially in children), and diseases for which cures exist but are simply not available, far outweigh the impact of AIDS at this time. When we consider the spectrum of social and health ills that many Africans face constantly (unemployment, illiteracy, warfare, and the general scarcity of resources), AIDS [to most Africans in 1991] is a relatively minor concern. . . .

In Africa, the typical [male] with AIDS is in his most productive years and is usually financially supporting or caring for a growing family. Children are left fatherless, motherless, or entirely orphaned. The family of the person with AIDS must endure not only the economic deprivation of the loss of a breadwinner or caretaker but also the psychological impact of caring for a chronically ill patient who is physically deteriorating before his loved ones. . . .

In Uganda, . . . if the wife develops AIDS-related symptoms before her husband does, even if she became infected from him and has been completely faithful to . . . him, the husband assumes that she has been unfaithful and casts her out of the household. . . . But when the husband . . . develops AIDS before the wife, it is her responsibility to take care of him. Often he is not able to continue working, and the family faces severe economic hardship. If the children become ill, further pressure is placed upon the burdened family. And if the wife falls ill to AIDS, she must take care of herself. When both parents die from AIDS, the orphaned children move in with the paternal grandparents [their father's parents]. . . . The grandparents . . . are finding themselves straining to cope with this crisis.

Source: Douglas A. Feldman, "The Sociocultural Impacts of AIDS in Central and East Africa," in R. Ulack and W. F. Skinner, eds., *AIDS and the Social Sciences: Common Threads* (Lexington: University Press of Kentucky, 1991), pp. 124–133.

DOCUMENT 105: Societal Attitudes Contribute to AIDS Epidemic in Africa

There are social and cultural conditions in Africa that contribute to the spread of HIV. The subordinate role of women, combined with the sexual attitudes of men, makes it difficult to introduce sexual practices that decrease risk, such as the use of condoms. Women who do not have an independent means of making a living are likely to go along with men's wishes with regard to sex, even if doing so endangers their health.

In many developing countries condoms are prohibitively expensive. Even if they are available and affordable, religious beliefs or lack of information means many men have deep-set prejudices against their use. They are usually associated with disease and loose morals; some people . . . believe rumors that manufacturers intentionally contaminate condoms with the virus. . . . The low socioeconomic status of women in many traditional African societies perpetuates their sexual exploitation. Women are . . . excluded from many professions and income-generating activities. . . . Their worth is measured in the domestic sphere, where they are expected to rear children, as well as [keep house] and entertain menfolk—in addition to day-long labor in the fields, office, or marketplace. This attitude promotes the assumption that women should serve men in all respects, including providing sexual favors. Educators who hope to empower women to seek cooperation from . . . men for safer sex will [fail] unless they also address the factors which determine the sexual attitudes of men.

Source: Fred Mhalu, "Point of View: Can Men Change?" *WorldAIDS* no. 18, p. 2 (November 1991).

DOCUMENT 106: The Power of Traditional Theater

In societies that do not discuss sexual matters publicly, health education is a challenge. Innovative approaches, such as adapting traditional theater to prevention messages, are needed. In rural Africa, most men and women do not know how to read or write their spoken language. By watching a theatrical presentation, they can learn how to protect themselves from the risk of HIV infection.

In Mali, an original experiment called the "useful theatre" has succeeded in making the population aware of the problem of AIDS while entertaining them at the same time. Philippe Dauchez, a French state director and teacher of dramatic art at the Institut National des Arts in Bamako, drew his inspiration from a popular theatre tradition, the *koteba*, and created the "useful theatre," whose aim is to make messages about health acceptable by presenting them in an amusing way.

Five companies of actors, all former pupils of INA, regularly visit the most far flung villages to present plays on hygiene and especially on AIDS. The AIDS question is treated here with humour, though gradually the comedy turns to tragedy as one by one, towards the end of the play, the characters learn that they have contracted AIDS. The actors mime their convulsions and suffering and die on stage, despite the efforts of the healer and the doctor, who remain powerless. The aim is to show how the disease is transmitted and how to protect oneself by using a condom. After each performance a discussion is organized to make sure that the message has truly been understood, and condoms are distributed to the audience.

Source: "Playing AIDS: An Experiment in Popular Theatre in Mali," *Sociétés d'Afrique & Sida: Understanding and Action* no. 3, p. 8 (January 1994).

DOCUMENT 107: Peer Education in the African Workplace

The economic impact of AIDS in Africa is substantial. When skilled workers are affected, their labor may be difficult to replace. The loss of a farm worker strains family resources and decreases productivity. As described in this selection, peer education in the workplace in southern Africa can be effective in distributing HIV prevention information. ("Aids," "behaviour," and "programmes" are British spellings.)

[In Zimbabwe] . . . [s]ome companies are . . . noticing sharp increases in sick leave, . . . higher mortality rates among their employees, . . . [and] ever-increasing numbers of people [who] take days off from work to attend funerals or to nurse sick relatives.

[W]orkplace Aids education programmes in Zimbabwe are now helping to curb the spread of HIV and Aids through changes in sexual attitudes and behaviour. . . .

[T]he most crucial factor in these successful programmes is the role played by "peer educators." These are members of the work force who volunteer to carry out Aids education with their colleagues and sometimes even within the wider community. . . .

Nixon Mutote, . . . is a general worker at a tea factory. "People come to me at work with questions about Aids. I also keep condoms in my locker and distribute them during breaks or after work."

Source: "Workplace Education Schemes in Zimbabwe Help Curb the Spread of Aids," *African Business*, p. 11 (January 1994).

DOCUMENT 108: Millions of AIDS Orphans

In Africa, people depend upon their extended family (which includes not just the father, mother, and children, but also grandparents, aunts, uncles, in-laws, and close cousins) when they cannot take care of themselves. When people are very ill, or children are orphaned, extended family members step in. When both parents have died of AIDS, the grandmother frequently takes care of the children. In some parts of Africa, the oldest child may assume the role of family head. If the family cannot care for them, the children may become part of the growing number of homeless street children. In the United States, these functions have largely been replaced by the health care system, charities, and government agencies. Most children of HIV-positive mothers are themselves HIV-negative.

By the year 2000, there may be as many as 2 million [African] children without one or both parents as a result of the disease. . . . In Zambia [by the early 1990s], at least 80,000 children have lost one or both parents and officials expect that another 30,000 new orphans will join them in each coming year of this epidemic.

One reason these numbers will skyrocket is that few HIV-infected women take precautions against further pregnancies . . . because the mother may have seen one child, already born infected, sicken and die, and so she chooses to have another to survive her. Such a gamble is risky: Nearly one of every three of these newborns will be infected. The majority, however, are uninfected and eventually survive their parents as orphans.

To date . . . [t]he burden of care has been left with the extended family. . . . Elderly women so regularly assume the role of caregivers—tending their dying son or daughter, possibly his or her spouse, and then the children left behind—that AIDS is now known as "The Grandmother's Disease."

Abandoned children are becoming more common. . . . The newest phenomenon emerging in southern Africa is child-headed households, in which the eldest orphan becomes the parent because no relative can or will.

Source: B. J. Kelso, "Orphans of the Storm," *Africa Report* 39(1): 50–55 (January/ February 1994).

DOCUMENT 109: The Important Role of Traditional Healers

Traditional healers in much of the developing world, including South Africa, provide a number of essential services. Some treat diseases with herbs and other medicinal preparations; some use Christian religious rituals in their work; and others use traditional religious and magical practices. In most poor countries, outside the urban areas, doctors and nurses are very rare, and the traditional healer (or shaman) is often the only person available and trusted to help if a family member becomes sick. We also now know that many of the traditional medicines given by traditional healers are effective in treating illness. Rather than re-place traditional healers with Western health care professionals, planners need to expand the role of traditional healers to include vital functions, such as HIV education and prevention.

[I]n remote areas and in urban "townships" many people turn to traditional healers in times of sickness, and for them primary health care may be synonymous with traditional medicine. For the foreseeable future ... it would seem that traditional healers will continue to offer greater accessibility. "Culture" is a further reason for developing the role of traditional healers. . . . [C]olonial rule has systematically eroded [the] African life style to the detriment of the African people. Not only [has] people's land been appropriated [with] Africans impoverished through colonial and capitalist development, but their very way of life [has been] ridiculed, taken away and replaced by "Western" modes of being. To undermine the role of traditional healers, who are an "outgrowth and expression" of culture, is a part of this process. . . . Traditional healing ... involves the whole person [and is] designed to preserve cultural institutions and to help the patient live at peace with family, clan, village, tribe and inner self.

Source: M. Freeman and M. Motsei, "Planning Health Care in South Africa—Is There a Role for Traditional Healers?" *Social Science & Medicine* 34(11): 1183–1190 (June 1992).

DOCUMENT 110: Life Expectancy Drops in Uganda

Undoubtedly, the greatest problem facing Africa in the last half of the twentieth century has been the runaway population growth—the result of a continuing high birthrate and improved health care leading to a reduced death rate. An annual growth rate of 3 percent, which has been the norm in much of Africa during the last several decades, will lead to a doubling of the population in less than twenty-four years. The population growth rate has been the major factor leading to declining economies, significant stresses on the local environment (depleting large herds of elephants, rhinos, and other large mammals), and internal migration into urban areas of unskilled, surplus laborers. Those who thought that a beneficial by-product of AIDS might be a substantial reduction in population growth have been very disappointed, since it is clear that most HIV-infected adults continue to have many children during their late teens, their twenties, and into their early thirties, before they develop symptoms of AIDS. What has plummeted instead is the life expectancy rate. A healthy nation is one with a stable population growth rate and a stable or increasing life expectancy rate. Uganda (in East Africa) is a country with a too-high population growth rate and a rapidly declining life expectancy rate.

AIDS has caused the life expectancy in Uganda to decrease from 45 years in 1993 to 37 years now, Popcare's Sam Ruteikara reports. The increase in HIV infections, he said, caused the average age at death to be 27 for women and 30 for men. . . . In his report, entitled "AIDS: A Challenge to Church Ministry and National Development," Ruteikara said that the low average dying age, combined with the high number of infants being born with HIV, resulted in the life expectancy being 37. The total number of Ugandans infected with HIV is estimated at 2 million, representing 10 percent of the population.

Source: "Life Expectancy Shortened in Uganda" (Xinhua News Agency, August 18, 1996); CDC National AIDS Clearinghouse (Bethesda, Md.: Information, Inc., 1996).

DOCUMENT 111: Breast-feeding by HIV-Positive Mothers Found More Dangerous Than Thought

Since the mid-1980s, international children's organizations have urged HIV-positive mothers in most of Africa, Asia, and Latin America to continue breast-feeding their infants, even though it is known that there is some potential risk for passing HIV infection to an HIV-negative child through this practice. It has been believed that mixing infant formula with local polluted water is much riskier to the health of the infant than the possibility of HIV infection. In developed nations, such as those in North America and Europe, HIV-positive mothers have been urged not to breast-feed their children, even though the general health benefits of breast-feeding over bottle-feeding have been proven among otherwise healthy mothers. Now, new evidence raises the question of whether it is best for HIV-positive mothers to breast-feed their children even when the water supply is dangerous to the infants.

A new, controversial study by South African researchers suggests that HIV-positive women who breast-feed may be more likely to transmit the virus to their children than was previously thought. Breast-feeding is generally thought to be important to good infant health in poor countries, where children fed formula are more likely to die of respiratory or diarrheal diseases. The United Nations Children's Fund [UNICEF] and the World Health Organization [WHO] have recommended that, in poor countries—where formula is expensive and difficult to prepare properly—even HIV-positive mothers breast-feed their babies. The new findings, by Glenda Gray and colleagues at the Baragwanath Hospital in Johannesburg, may change the current policy, however. According to their report, HIV-positive mothers who breast-feed increase the risk of transmitting HIV to their children by 28 percent. Earlier studies had suggested the risk was 14 percent. In light of the new report, the United

Nations AIDS Program said mothers will be advised of the risks and encouraged to decide [for] themselves whether or not to breast-feed.

Source: "Health: Breast Is Best, but What If the Mother Is [HIV-Positive?]" (IPS Wire, August 16, 1996); CDC National AIDS Clearinghouse (Bethesda, Md.: Information, Inc., 1996).

THE GROWING CRISIS IN ASIA

DOCUMENT 112: Condom Use in Rural Thailand

In the countryside of Thailand in Southeast Asia, perceptions of risk for HIV infection are often inaccurate. Condoms are infrequently used, especially with steady sex partners. This is a risky practice, since people may have more than one partner, and HIV infection rates in Thai cities are already significant. Because of drug use and the large numbers of people working in the sex industry in Thailand, HIV infection in urban high-risk groups can quickly spread to other segments of the population. Already, approximately 3 percent of military recruits are infected. Thailand has become one of the centers of the HIV epidemic in Asia.

The men [questioned] do not view a woman who has had sex before as "promiscuous" even if she currently has another boyfriend, as long as her other relationships did not involve sex for a fee. Once a man determines that his partner is not "promiscuous," the question of whether to use condoms does not arise. . . . Although the definition varies among respondents [the participants in the study], "promiscuous" generally means having many sex partners in short-term, nonselective relationships. No [one] mentioned a need for blood exams to screen potential partners because most believe that they can recognize risky women themselves.

The interviews with women . . . suggest that the desire to have sex without condoms is often mutual. The typical female respondent felt that her sex partners would not spread an STD [sexually transmitted disease] to her. [She feels] she is discriminating in her choice of sex partners. To qualify, her sex partner must be responsible enough not to spread an STD, appear neat and clean, . . . be well educated and have a secure job. . . . No woman reported asking the man to use a condom when it was not his intention to do so, [and] some women felt that the use of condoms suggests that they are not clean and implies that they are commercial sex workers [prostitutes].

Source: Napaporn Havanon, Anthony Bennett, and John Knodel, "Sexual Net-working in Provincial Thailand," *Studies in Family Planning* 24(1): 1–17 (January–February 1993).

DOCUMENT 113: AIDS Spreads Rapidly into Asia

The AIDS epidemic has taken strong hold in parts of Asia. This is be-cause safer sexual practices have not been widespread among individ-uals with multiple sex partners. Commercial sex workers (or prostitutes) in urban centers already have high HIV infection levels, and where injecting drug use is a problem, HIV has spread rapidly. New infor-mation from India, Thailand, and other countries in Asia indicate that HIV is spreading rapidly to the general population. ("Aids" follows the British spelling.)

Asia will be the next big killing field in the Aids epidemic. The pro-verbially dispassionate doctors and scientists gathered for the 10th In-ternational Conference on Aids [during 1994] in Yokohama [Japan] were anything but calm when it came to delivering their prognosis for the region. Prasanta Kumar Choudhuri, president of the Indian Medical As-sociation, foresaw a "holocaust," while the American Medical Associa-tion's James Allen compared Aids in Asia today to the Black Death that devastated Europe in the Middle Ages. . . .

HIV is now affecting Asians from all walks of life . . . at an alarming pace. . . . In South and Southeast Asia, the number of recorded HIV in-fections now [in 1994] stands at 2.5 million, . . . 1 million more than a year ago, [and] . . . an eightfold percentage increase from the previous year.

Source: Jonathan Friedland, "The Coming Holocaust," *Far Eastern Economic Re-view* 157(33): 15–16 (August 18, 1994).

DOCUMENT 114: Tackling the Growing Crisis in China

With over 1.3 billion people, about one-fifth of the world's total pop-ulation, China could eventually have the highest number of persons with HIV infection in any nation. Even if only 2 percent of the total Chinese population were to become HIV-infected, that number would be greater than the total number of HIV-infected persons in the world estimated in 1996. The HIV epidemic in China has been spreading most rapidly among injecting drug users near the "Golden Triangle" north of the Burmese and Thai borders in Yunnan Province (southern China). Not only the drug users, but also their sexual partners and newborn children are becoming infected. HIV has also been spreading, although much more slowly, among China's awakening gay male population in the major cities of Beijing and Shanghai. While the Chinese government may have tripled its AIDS budget to $1.8 million per year, that translates to an average of less than 1 cent for every seven Chinese citizens.

Chinese health officials promised . . . to increase funding for HIV prevention to help slow the rapid spread of the virus. The number of HIV cases in China has tripled each year since 1994. The Ministry of Health will "upgrade laboratory testing techniques and carry out extensive publicity to increase public awareness of the risks," said Dai Zhicheng, director of the ministry's disease control department. Only half of the 30 provinces, autonomous regions, and municipalities have laboratories for confirming HIV, he said. The ministry will hold a national conference in October to increase awareness among local officials, and the government has tripled its AIDS budget to $1.8 million this year.

Source: "China Attacks AIDS Explosion" (United Press International, September 4, 1996); CDC National AIDS Clearinghouse (Bethesda, Md.: Information, Inc., 1996).

DOCUMENT 115: Fighting HIV in Vietnam

In developing countries the message of safer sex is a difficult one to get across, since for most adults the message is not one of celibacy, but of changing the way that they have sex. In Vietnam, for example, it means getting condoms, female condoms, and nonoxynol-9 lubrication into the hands of tens of millions of sexually active men and women, getting information about HIV and AIDS into the minds of the Vietnamese population, and getting those who engage in premarital or extramarital sex to learn to develop the negotiating skills to be able to achieve safer sex practices consistently. Fighting HIV in countries like Vietnam is relatively expensive and a difficult, but necessary, challenge.

Vietnam has launched a number of AIDS awareness campaigns and community projects to deal with its growing AIDS epidemic, the local press reported Tuesday. The country has more than 4,200 reported HIV cases, including 353 people with AIDS and 184 deaths from AIDS. In Ho

Chi Minh City [formerly Saigon], 1,550 people are [known to be] infected with HIV and 200 have AIDS. The government has broadcast information on safe sex and HIV/AIDS prevention through the media, movies, art performances, cultural activities, and family-planning services. In addition, blood test kits have been provided for hospitals, at a cost of $2.7 million. Community projects to care for patients with HIV and AIDS have also been supported by the government.

Source: "Vietnam Launches Anti-AIDS Campaign" (Xinhua News Agency, September 3, 1996); CDC National AIDS Clearinghouse (Bethesda, Md.: Information, Inc., 1996).

DOCUMENT 116: HIV Infection: The Growing Scourge of India

While HIV is relatively new to India, the world's second most populous nation has already become the country with the highest number of HIV-positive persons: about 3 million in 1996. Similar environmental conditions, both cultural and physical, that exist in India and in central Africa continue to promote rapid spread of the virus: extreme poverty, poor sanitation, low status of women, poor rates of literacy, and a tropical, humid environment where potential cofactor disease agents (such as bacteria and other viruses), as well as other genetic subtypes of HIV-1, probably act as triggering mechanisms that make it easier to transmit the virus through sex between men and women.

[In Petrapole, India, across the river from Bangladesh,] thousands of drivers, helpers and hawkers mill about in a vast encampment, in a chaos symptomatic of inefficiencies that have helped to keep India among the world's poorest countries. But there is something here more threatening to India's future than narrow, rutted roadways, entangling paperwork and customs officers exacting bribes from drivers impatient to move on.

The threat comes from AIDS. India's 5 million truck drivers are at the center of an expected explosion of the disease among its 970 million people. At Petrapole, where drivers have little to do, it is common for a man to buy sex every day, sometimes several times a day, from local women and teen-age girls for as little as 10 rupees, about 28 cents. The couples, many of whom meet in truck cabs and roadside bushes, rarely use condoms. . . .

India has shown little inclination to make the AIDS threat a national priority. . . . Many Indian politicians and other opinion makers have argued that the priority in Government health spending should go to diseases like malaria and tuberculosis, which kill tens of thousands of Indians every year. Among these opponents of AIDS spending are nationalists reluctant to acknowledge that India could become the focus of a disease linked to sexual practices and drug use. . . .

The current Indian estimate of three million [persons with HIV] is almost double that of two years ago. . . . India already has more infected people than any other country in the world. . . . Homosexuality . . . accounted for only four-tenths of 1 percent of the infected [about 12,000 gay, bisexual, and transgendered Indian men].

Source: John F. Burns, "Denial and Taboo Blinding India to the Horror of Its AIDS Scourge," *The New York Times*, pp. 1, 10 (September 22, 1996).

AIDS IN LATIN AMERICA AND THE CARIBBEAN

DOCUMENT 117: Good AIDS Knowledge But Poor HIV Prevention Practices

This study of 240 college freshman women in São Paulo, Brazil, is comparable with surveys of young people in the United States. Few thought they were at risk for HIV infection even though the majority did not use condoms. The protective measures they used—for example, selecting a known, steady partner—are not necessarily effective. As in other surveys, their knowledge about HIV/AIDS, modes of transmission, and the epidemic was far greater than their ability to translate this knowledge into effective action or behavior.

The majority of [the sample of female Brazilian university students] interviewed showed knowledge of the forms of transmission of AIDS and the great risk of young people being contaminated with the disease. However, only 6% thought that they themselves were at great risk. Among those who are having sexual intercourse, only 67% stated that they take preventive measures to avoid AIDS contamination. Moreover, it is important to point out that not all the [stated preventive measures—known partners, or a steady, fixed partner] are effective, since only 29% say their partners use condoms. . . .

When these findings were presented . . . [to] medical students, it was sensed that using condoms on a regular basis is still very inhibiting, especially when the partners are known to each other. For some individuals, . . . the use of, or imposition to use, condoms is felt to be an accusation. For others, there seems to be a genuine conviction that having a steady or known partner is a sufficient guarantee against AIDS.

Source: Ruth M. C. Leite, Everardo M. Buoncompagno, Adriana C. C. Leite, Elizabeth A. Mergulhão, and Maria Marta M. Battistoni, "Psychosexual Characteristics of Female University Students in Brazil," *Adolescence* 29(114): 441–460 (Summer 1994).

DOCUMENT 118: Disease Control vs. Freedom in Cuba

The Cuban program for control of HIV infection is unique. Nationwide testing has been combined with quarantine. HIV-positive people live in special residential quarters where their comings and goings are monitored. Although their health care and housing are taken care of, their individual freedoms are restricted. Most residents are either heterosexual soldiers who contracted the virus in Africa or men who had sex with men. While this authoritarian approach has proved effective, it ignores Cubans' civil liberties. Also, since we know that behavioral change programs can change sexual behavior, the presumption that people cannot change their behavior is erroneous. When the quarantine program began in the mid-1980s, the quarantine camps and policies were very much like prisons. Worldwide attention to the quarantine camps liberalized treatment of the incarcerated men and women. The costs of maintaining the camps began to be a burden on the weakened Cuban economy. By 1996, the Cuban government was claiming that all but a few "sexually irresponsible" persons were no longer forcibly confined to the quarantine camps, and internment had become voluntary. With the recent growth of tourism and male and female prostitution in Cuba, it is likely that HIV infection in Cuba will grow rapidly.

The most controversial aspect of Cuba's program for combating AIDS has been the creation of sanitariums for the compulsory isolation of those ... who test positive for HIV antibodies. ... People admitted to a sanitarium have the virus but do not have AIDS. People with AIDS are hospitalized. ...

In the sanitarium, married couples and [gay] couples live together if both have tested positive. Uninfected children ... live with other family members. ... If the children are also infected, they join their parents in the sanitarium. If only one parent tests positive, that parent lives in the sanitarium, and children continue living with the other parent; family members and friends can visit those living in the sanitarium any time they choose.

Residents . . . may also take trips outside. There are occasional organized recreational activities such as an evening at the cinema . . . or an outing to the beach. Residents also return to their communities for visits and meetings. . . . Those who do not live far away can spend weekends with family and friends. If they do live farther away, they can arrange four-day trips home every four to six weeks.

On most of these trips, a senior medical student or intern goes along as [a] chaperone . . . to prevent sexual contacts that could spread the virus. Married couples are allowed passes to leave the sanitarium under more liberal conditions than others and are not required to be chaperoned. . . .

Two assumptions dominate the Cuban quarantine policy. First, people will always be irresponsible in terms of sex, and no policy of safe sex will work that relies on individual control. Second, education cannot change this behavior. Since . . . it is impossible to know which infected people can be trusted to behave responsibly, all must be treated as dangerous. . . .

Source: Marvin Leiner, *Sexual Politics in Cuba: Machismo, Homosexuality, and AIDS* (Boulder, Colo.: Westview Press, 1994).

DOCUMENT 119: Is "Condom" a Dirty Word?

In Buenos Aires, the capital and largest city of Argentina, the government refused to use the word "condom" in its HIV prevention campaign, since it would offend the Roman Catholic Church in this religious South American nation. High school students aggressively protested this decision. Argentina is not alone in allowing religious and political considerations to shape AIDS policy. It was not until about 1993 that the U.S. government's media campaign against AIDS explicitly specified that condoms are effective against HIV, even though they were known to be effective in the mid-1980s.

Last year, scores of high school students in Buenos Aires went on a graffiti-writing rampage to demonstrate their frustration with the Argentine government's refusal to use the word "condom" in its AIDS prevention campaign. "AIDS: For Love, Use a Condom" is scrawled across walls in almost every neighborhood of the city. The government has been criticized by nongovernmental AIDS groups and AIDS activists for what they call "an anti-AIDS campaign from the Middle Ages" because it does not mention condoms. Instead, it notes the modes of transmission. Critics say the federal government has given in to pressure from the Catholic Church not to openly promote condom use. . . . Argentina . . . has the second highest number of [reported] AIDS cases in South America. Government health officials acknowledge the pressure of the Catholic Church and call the control more covert than overt. The Catholic Church, however, says the condom issue is blown out of proportion to make the Church a scapegoat for the government's failure to adequately finance AIDS care and prevention programs.

Source: Calvin Sims, "With Spray Paint, Students Wage 'Safe Sex' War," *The New York Times*, p. A4 (January 19, 1995); CDC National AIDS Clearinghouse (Bethesda, Md.: Information, Inc., 1995).

SUGGESTED READINGS

"AIDS-Free in 1991, Cambodia Tops HIV Rate." *Washington Times*, p. A16 (November 22, 1996).

"AIDS in Developing Nations." *The Futurist* 28, pp. 57–58 (November/December 1994).

"AIDS: Spreading and Fast. . . ." *UN Chronicle* 29, p. 58 (September 1992).

Araújo, M. J. O., and C. S. G. Diniz. "Women, Sexuality and AIDS in Brazil." *World Health*, pp. 14–15 (May/June 1994).

Balter, M. S. "East Europe: A Chance to Stop HIV." *Science* 262, pp. 1964–1965 (December 24, 1993).

Barnathan, J. "The AIDS Disaster Unfolding in Asia." *Business Week*, p. 52 (February 22, 1993).

Biggar, Robert. "The Acquired Immune Deficiency Syndrome in Africa." *Lancet* 1 (8472), pp. 79–83 (1986).

Black, M. "Selling Health from a Roadside Stall." *Choices* 2, p. 31 (September 1993).

Bolton, Ralph, ed. "Special Issue: The AIDS Pandemic: A Global Emergency." *Medical Anthropology* 10 (2–3): 93–209 (1989).

"Church vs. State vs. AIDS." *World Press Review* 40, p. 44 (May 1993).

Conover, T. "Trucking Through the AIDS Belt." *The New Yorker* 69, pp. 56–60 (August 16, 1993).

Cowley, G. "The Ever Expanding Plague." *Newsweek* 124, p. 37 (August 22, 1994).

Farmer, Paul. *AIDS & Accusation: Haiti and the Geography of Blame*. Berkeley: University of California Press, 1992.

Feldman, Douglas A., ed. *Global AIDS Policy*. Westport, Conn.: Bergin & Garvey, 1994.

Feldman, Douglas A., Samuel Friedman, and Don C. Des Jarlais. "Public Awareness of AIDS in Rwanda." *Social Science and Medicine* 24(2), pp. 97–100 (1987).

"Germany's Tainted Blood." *Newsweek* 122, pp. 38–39 (November 15, 1993).

Golden, Tim. "AIDS Rate Low in Cuba, at High Price." *Miami Herald*, p. 7A (October 16, 1995).

Hamilton, David P. "Japan AIDS Scandal Raises Fear That Safety Came Second to Trade." *Wall Street Journal*, p. A1 (October 9, 1996).

"HIV Poised to Ravage Asia." *Journal of the American Medical Association* 276(22), p. 1790 (December 11, 1996).

"HIV-2: A Less Virulent Cousin of HIV-1." *Science News* 146, p. 187 (September 17, 1994).

Jeffrey, P. "Latin America Confronts AIDS." *America* 168, pp. 10–12 (February 13, 1993).

Kalibala, S., and S. Anderson. "AIDS in Africa: A Family Disease." *World Health*, pp. 8–10 (November/December 1993).

Kizito, E., and M. wa Gacheru. "Scared Celibate." *World Press Review* 40, p. 46 (September 1993).

Larsson, T. "NGO's Join Business in the War Against AIDS." *Choices* 2, p. 33 (September 1993).

Lawday, D. "France's Ministers of Bad Blood." *U.S. News & World Report* 114, pp. 69–70 (January 18, 1993).

Mann, Jonathan. "Acquired Immune Deficiency Syndrome (AIDS): A Global Challenge." *World Health*, pp. 12–15 (November 1986).

McNeil, Donald G., Jr. "In Surprising Study, TB Is Found to Be Rampant in South Africa." *The New York Times*, p. A8 (June 26, 1996).

Miller, K. L. "Japan Finds the Silent Treatment Is Poor Therapy." *Business Week*, p. 54 (February 22, 1993).

Miranda-Maniquis, E. "The Silence About Women." *World Press Review* 40, p. 26 (February 1993).

Nau, J. Y. "AIDS: Worse Comes to Worst." *World Press Review* 41, p. 29 (April 1994).

Nesbitt, Jeff. "Dollar's Fall: A Life-or-Death Issue in Africa." *Washington Times*, p. B7 (April 14, 1995).

Purvis, A. "Cursed, Yet Blessed." *Time* 142, p. 67 (December 6, 1993).

Quinn, Thomas C. "Global Burden of the HIV Pandemic." *Lancet* 348(9020), p. 99 (July 13, 1996).

Shenon, Philip. "AIDS Epidemic, Late to Arrive, Now Explodes in Populous Asia." *The New York Times*, p. A1 (January 21, 1996).

"South Africa Fighting Uphill AIDS Battle." *Chicago Tribune*, pp. 1–3 (July 8, 1995).

Stevens, J. "Model Programs Take Aim at HIV Rates in Indonesia." *Science* 264, pp. 24–25 (April 1, 1994).

Tarantola, D., and J. M. Mann. "Coming to Terms with the AIDS Pandemic." *Issues in Science and Technology* 9, pp. 41–48 (Spring 1993).

Ungpakorn, J. "To Defeat AIDS, Stop Preaching." *World Press Review* 41, p. 52 (June 1994).

Vincent, I. "A Port City Battles AIDS." *World Press Review* 40, pp. 36–37 (January 1993).

"World AIDS Day—December 1, 1996." *Morbidity and Mortality Weekly Report* 45(46) (November 22, 1996).

5

The Human Side of AIDS

In *AIDS and Its Metaphors*, Susan Sontag writes that the central metaphor for the AIDS epidemic is "plague." Sickness is believed to be a punishment of individuals and society, rather than a biological process. This way of thinking about the disease is irrational and is based upon fear and prejudice.

Focusing instead on the realities of an illness develops understanding of the disease and creates empathy for people who suffer from it and the people who care for them. By now, nearly everyone in the major metropolitan areas of the United States probably knows of someone with HIV/AIDS—if not a family member or close friend, perhaps an acquaintance. Among the famous people who have died of AIDS or live with HIV, there is someone admired or respected, someone to identify with—Earvin "Magic" Johnson, Arthur Ashe, Rock Hudson, Liberace, Elizabeth Glaser, Ryan White, and many others. The artificial distance between "us" and "them" disappears with the recognition of the similarities of human experience.

Health care workers and volunteers who personally care for patients with HIV disease know in an intimate way what the disease is and how it affects them. But that closeness has a cost. Although the occupational risk of acquiring HIV is very low, it is a real one. Health care workers exposed to blood or body fluids must exercise great diligence and care in maintaining infection control techniques. Despite that risk, they continue their work, and this is evidence of their personal dedication. In addition, there can be a great deal of stress in working with seriously ill or terminally ill patients. Especially vulnerable are psychologists, social workers, counselors, and others providing emotional support to patients. A clinical distance is appropriate, but it does not eliminate empathy for, or concern for, their patients' suffering.

Because of their closeness, friends, families, and partners confront even greater challenges when someone they love has HIV/AIDS. At the same time that they must cope with practical problems related to the illness, they often face other difficult issues, such as learning about a loved one's sexual behavior or drug use for the first time, confronting the unexpected consequences of medical treatment, experiencing the rejection of coworkers, friends, or neighbors, or living with their own HIV infection or illness. The loss of a loved one is painful, and grief can be hard to overcome. In the gay community or in families where more than one person is ill, grief can become perpetual mourning or chronic bereavement. Those who suffer the most may be those who hide their pain out of shame or fear of discovery. While counseling and social support of people experiencing such losses are helpful, the effects of these experiences can be long-lasting. People have found a public outlet for their grief by contributing to the AIDS quilt, which combines personal tribute and remembrance with collective art and political action. The display of thousands of panels together is a powerful statement about the magnitude of these losses.

In this chapter, the first-person accounts of people living with HIV/AIDS are particularly valuable. For those who have not been close to someone who is ill, it is a glimpse into how difficult that experience can be. The epidemic has created an unusual situation in which large numbers of young people and adults in their most productive and creative years suddenly face the possibility of a premature death. This sense of incompleteness is a cause for anger and sadness. Dr. Elisabeth Kübler-Ross writes about the experiences of terminally ill patients in her book *On Death and Dying*. She describes what patients experience—denial and isolation, anger, bargaining, depression, and acceptance. It is comforting to know that at any age there are ways to face death with dignity and courage.

Sources: Elisabeth Kübler-Ross, *On Death and Dying* (New York: Macmillan, 1969); Susan Sontag, *AIDS and Its Metaphors* (New York: Farrar, Straus and Giroux, 1988).

THE MANY FACES OF AIDS: FIRST-PERSON ACCOUNTS

DOCUMENT 120: Kimberly Bergalis

Who are people with AIDS? They are people like Arthur Ashe, African-American tennis star; Pedro Zamora, young Hispanic AIDS educator and star of MTV; Elizabeth Glaser, married mother of two children; Ross Johnson, self-described boy next door; and many, many others. In this section, people with AIDS describe their experiences living with AIDS. In the following selection, Kimberly Bergalis talks about the difficulty of dealing with AIDS while in her early twenties. Ms. Bergalis was one of six persons known to have been infected with HIV directly by her dentist, Dr. David J. Acer. He is the only dentist known to have infected a dental patient. She died in 1991.

I have lived to see my hair fall out, my body lose over 40 pounds . . . I've lived to go through nausea and vomiting, continual night sweats, chronic fevers of 103–104 that don't go away anymore. . . . [D]o you know what it's like to look at yourself in a full-length mirror before you shower—and you only see a skeleton? . . . I slid to the floor and I cried. Now I shower with a blanket over the mirror.

Source: Kimberly Bergalis, quoted in Barbara Kantrowitz, Karen Springen, John McCormick, Spencer Reiss, Mary Hager, Lydia Denworth, Clara Bingham, and Donna Foote, "Doctors and AIDS," *Newsweek* 118(1): 48–57 (July 1, 1991).

DOCUMENT 121: Belinda Mason

In this selection, Belinda Mason eloquently articulates the desires of people with HIV/AIDS: to live free from fear and stigma, and to enjoy the same rights as other American citizens do.

We must learn to practice the justice, freedom, and compassion that we take so much pride in talking about in civics classes and teaching our children about when we tell them what it is to be an American. . . .

I have to say that people living with AIDS and HIV want nothing more or nothing less than what all of you take for granted today—a place to live, the right to have a job, decent medical care, and to live our lives out without unreasonable barriers. We are not asking for extras, only to be included in what America already delivers to her privileged people.

I'm thirty-one this year and my life has been blessed with two healthy children. . . . Relatively speaking, I'm not in bad shape and I used to hope that I would be able to live long enough to see my children, with the help of their father, accept and adapt to the inevitability of my death. More lately I've been hoping that when I'm gone they wouldn't continue to be stigmatized by the shadow thrown by my public life.

But compassion is not going to happen because of a report that we make or an edict that somebody in Washington delivers. It will begin in the small towns, in the quiet country throughout America, when people understand that people living with AIDS and HIV are just like us because they are us.

Source: Belinda Mason, National AIDS spokesperson, quoted in *America Living with AIDS: Transforming Anger, Fear and Indifference into Action*, Report of the National Commission on Acquired Immune Deficiency Syndrome (Washington, D.C.: The Commission, 1991), p. 10.

DOCUMENT 122: Robert Rafsky

Robert Rafsky, an AIDS activist, discusses in this selection why he became politically active and why he strongly supported experimental clinical research on new AIDS drugs.

When I discovered I was infected with HIV, I wasn't worried at first. Maybe I was in denial. My T4 cells, a key measure of immune system health, were high. I wouldn't allow myself to accept the fact that they would drop. . . . It's always possible we'll win. The drug, or drugs, that will turn AIDS into a chronic illness like diabetes will finally be discovered. We'll have years to study the lessons of the fight against the epidemic. As in the old country-western song, the hanging tree will become our tree of life. But it's not likely, at least not in time for me. . . .

There's not much to do except to keep fighting the epidemic, and those whose actions or inactions prolong it, until I get too sick to fight. I'll try to die a good death, if I can figure out what one is. After that, thanks to the epidemic and what it taught me about myself, I expect to rest in peace.

Source: Robert Rafsky, AIDS activist, quoted in "A Better Life for Having Acted Up," *The New York Times*, p. E-11 (April 18, 1992).

DOCUMENT 123: T. H. April

HIV spread rapidly during the early and mid-1980s among people with hemophilia, a blood disorder, when the blood product (called Factor VIII Concentrate) used to control the disorder became contaminated with the virus that causes AIDS. T. H. April, a young man with hemophilia, talks about his experience.

I am twenty-one years old. I have hemophilia and am HIV positive. I found out my HIV status when I was fourteen—when they thought it could mean I was immune. It didn't really matter what they thought then anyway. Death means absolutely nothing to a fourteen-year-old. I thought I was immortal until just about a year ago when my girlfriend at the time and I were going to find out the results of her first AIDS test. Meanwhile, most of my friends still think they are immortal. This is one of the basic tricky aspects of AIDS for the adolescent and the young adult. It is extremely hard to have a mid-life crisis and acknowledge the fact that you are going to die when life has just begun. . . .

Source: T. H. April, quoted in *America Living with AIDS*, Report of the National Commission on Acquired Immune Deficiency Syndrome (Washington, D.C.: The Commission, 1991), p. 28.

DOCUMENT 124: Elizabeth Glaser

Elizabeth Glaser became infected with HIV during a blood transfusion in 1981, a few years before the nation's blood supply was screened for HIV. In her highly publicized speech before the 1992 Democratic National Convention, she attacked political leaders who say they care about AIDS, but do little to help. She died of AIDS in 1994 at the age of 47.

Eleven years ago, while giving birth to my first child, I hemorrhaged, and was transfused with seven pints of blood. Four years later, I found out that I had been infected with the AIDS virus and had unknowingly passed it to my daughter Ariel through my breast milk, and my son Jake, in utero. . . . Exactly four years ago, my daughter died of AIDS. . . . I am here because my son and I may not survive four more years of leaders who say they care, but do nothing. I am in a race with the clock. . . . Once every generation, history brings us to an important crossroads.

Sometimes in life, there is that moment when it's possible to make a change for the better. This is one of those moments. For me, this is not politics. This is a crisis of caring.

Source: Elizabeth Glaser, speaking at the Democratic National Convention, July 1992, quoted in "Messengers on AIDS—Remarks by Elizabeth Glaser: July 14, Madison Square Garden, New York City," *Washington Post* (August 25, 1992); Newsbank 1992 HEA 86:C5–C6.

DOCUMENT 125: Mary Fisher

Not to be outdone by the Democrats, the 1992 Republican National Convention, held one month later, asked a well-known Republican fund-raiser, Mary Fisher, to speak about HIV/AIDS.

I bear a message of challenge. . . . I want your attention, not your applause. I would never have asked to be HIV-positive. But I believe that in all things there is a purpose, and I stand before you, and before that nation, gladly. . . . This is not a distant threat; it is a present danger. . . . My call to the nation is a plea for awareness. . . . Tonight, HIV marches resolutely toward AIDS in more than a million American homes, littering its pathway with the bodies of the young. Young men. Young women. Young parents. And young children. One of the families is mine. . . . [M]y children will inevitably turn to orphans.

Source: Mary Fisher, speaking at the Republican National Convention, 1992, quoted in "Messengers on AIDS—Remarks by Mary Fisher: August 19, Houston Astrodome," *Washington Post* (August 25, 1992); Newsbank 1992 HEA 86:C6–C7.

DOCUMENT 126: Paul Monette

Paul Monette, a well-known writer, tells us what happened when he learned that his male lover (functional same-sex spouse) had AIDS. Monette himself died of AIDS a few years later. More than half of the men who have died of AIDS since the beginning of the epidemic in developed countries have been gay and bisexual men.

"We'll fight it, darling, we'll beat it, I promise. I won't let you die." The sentiments merged as they tumbled out. This is the liturgy of bonding. Mostly we clung together, as if time still had the decency to stop when we were entwined. After all, the whole world was right here in this room. I don't think Roger said anything then. Neither of us cried. It begins in a country beyond tears. Once you have your arms around your [partner] with his terrible news, your eyes are too shut to cry.

Source: Paul Monette, describing the moment he received the news of his male life partner's diagnosis of AIDS, quoted in Paul Monette, *Borrowed Time* (Orlando, Fla.: Harcourt Brace Jovanovich, 1988), p. 77.

DOCUMENT 127: Andrew Ziegler

In this selection, Andrew Ziegler discusses the difficulty that people with AIDS have in accessing and utilizing the health care system.

I feel I am quite fortunate because I know how to access the system. I know all the "right" people. I know how it operates. I know what my rights are. And I know where to go for assistance, because I am part of the system professionally. But I can tell you it is still not very easy. It is particularly difficult when I have to run all over town to see the ophthalmologist, internist, dermatologist, nutritionist, . . . and am not feeling well and trying to hold down a full-time job at the same time. But what about the people who don't have the ability to access the system due to social, economic or educational barriers? How do they access a hostile system, a system designed to discourage their use and participation?

Source: Andrew Ziegler, quoted in *America Living with AIDS: Transforming Anger, Fear and Indifference into Action*, Report of the National Commission on AIDS (Washington, D.C.: The Commission, 1991), p. 46.

DOCUMENT 128: Kim Foltz

Kim Foltz describes how having HIV has affected his life and his thoughts on a daily basis. It is not something he can readily try to forget about.

A few months after I found out I had the virus that causes AIDS, I learned exactly what this disease was going to mean to me. . . . In the following weeks, the virus seemed to tighten its psychological grip on me. . . . [I]t taught me that who I am is irrevocably tied to being HIV positive. . . . I never thought I would be on such intimate terms with death. I am only 43 years old and, like many gay men, have watched a string of friends die. But one of the things I've learned in dealing with HIV is never to give up hope. Each day the first thing I do is get on the scale to make sure I haven't lost weight. Next, I take my AZT [in 1992, it was the primary drug used against HIV]. Then I tell myself I'm ready for the next round.

Source: Kim Foltz, quoted in his "About Men: Testing Positive," *New York Times Magazine* 141, p. 12 (January 5, 1992).

DOCUMENT 129: Arthur Ashe

Arthur Ashe, the famed tennis player, likens his struggle to win on the tennis court to the level of effort he had put into avoiding losing his battle against AIDS. He died shortly after in 1993.

Some people profess to see little purpose to the struggle for life. And yet that is precisely the task to which, in my fight against the ravages of AIDS, I devote myself every day: the struggle for life, aided by science in my fight with this disease. I know that we are all, as human beings, going to our death, and that I may be called, because of AIDS, to go faster than most others. Still, I resolutely do battle with this opponent, as I boldly did battle with my opponents on the tennis court. True, this fight is different. The biggest difference is that I now fight not so much to win as not to lose. This enemy is different, too—dark and mysterious, springing on civilization just when civilization was sure that it had almost rid itself of mysterious beasts forever.

Source: Arthur Ashe, quoted in Arthur Ashe and Arnold Rampersad, *Days of Grace* (New York: Alfred A. Knopf, 1993), p. 221.

DOCUMENT 130: Ross Johnson

Ross Johnson died of AIDS while still in his twenties. This passage contrasts the caring of neighbors when a person gets a nonstigmatized communicable disease or suffers from an unintentional injury with the avoidance that often occurs when someone gets AIDS.

Testing positive was a wake-up call. Since I found out, I've learned how to live. And maybe I've found my life's work—teaching people not to be afraid of who they are or of this epidemic. AIDS is a social disease, and I don't just mean the virus in people's bodies or how it is transmitted, but how society deals with it. It's not like getting the measles or breaking a leg, when all of your neighbors show up at your door with lasagna. People shun you; they are desperately afraid. And of what? It's just Ross Johnson, the boy next door.

Source: Ross Johnson, in Carolyn Jones, George DeSipio, Jr., Ian McKellen, and Michael Liberatore, *Living Proof: Courage in the Face of AIDS* (New York: Abbeville Press, 1994).

DOCUMENT 131: Randolph Winchester King, Jr.

While the period from HIV infection to death from AIDS averages about a decade, the range among those who are not being treated can vary from about two years to two decades or more. Randolph Winchester

King, Jr., points out that with such an unpredictable life expectancy, he will not spend his remaining years preparing to die. Rather, he will spend them living his life to the fullest.

I was tested for HIV virtually as soon as the test was invented. Although I do not recall being alarmed or even very much surprised by the news that I tested positive, it was to change my life profoundly. Projects which were important to me became the all-consuming focus of my energy, as I then believed that I had between one thousand and ten thousand days to live. I applied to several Scottish universities to study Scots law. I recall commenting to my Washington psychiatrist that a university is a good place to die; like a shot he fired back, "A university is a great place to live." On December 5, 1992, the University of Glasgow awarded me my fourth university degree, a Bachelor of Laws in Scots law. Still believing that my physical body is allotted to me for between one thousand and ten thousand more days, I now plan to circumnavigate the world under sail.

Source: Randolph Winchester King, Jr., in Carolyn Jones, George DeSipio, Jr., Ian McKellen, and Michael Liberatore, *Living Proof: Courage in the Face of AIDS* (New York: Abbeville Press, 1994).

DOCUMENT 132: "Meredith"

"Meredith," a woman with AIDS (her name has been changed by the author to protect her anonymity), argues here that, except for her gay friends who have taken the time to learn about AIDS, she is frustrated that her heterosexual friends and relatives have not bothered to educate themselves about her disease.

I'm horrified that I have had to turn to [only] my gay friends for my support system, for my love, for my affection, for an ear, for someone to say, "I'm scared. I'm tired." But I have to constantly educate the people I grew up with who have remained my friends. They haven't taken the time to inform themselves. The responsibility for AIDS education has fallen on me. It's put a strain on my friendships. I say, "Get printed material. Call a hot line. Don't put that strain on my friendship because I don't feel good now. And I need your love. I don't need to be your teacher." I mean, that sounds selfish. It does. But I'm tired. And I'm scared. And I'm sick. I'm losing control of my normal day-to-day functions, both physically and emotionally, and it terrifies me. It's just like being in a void. I can't find the walls.

Source: "Meredith," quoted in Steven Petrow, *Dancing Against the Darkness: A Journey Through America in the Age of AIDS* (Lexington, Mass.: Lexington Books, 1990), p. 68.

DOCUMENT 133: Pedro Zamora

Pedro Zamora learned that he had AIDS while still a teenager. He rapidly became a spokesperson about HIV/AIDS for the Dade County public schools in metropolitan Miami, where he lived. Later, he appeared on an MTV show about the lives of young people, where he portrayed himself as a person with AIDS. His funeral, held in Miami in 1994, was attended by several hundred admirers and friends. It was also picketed by the Rev. Fred Phelps, a minister from Wichita, Kansas, and a few of his followers who carried signs declaring that "God Hates Fags!"

There are two things I hate. I hate it when people tell me that everything is going to be all right. And I hate it when they say they understand what I am going through. Because they really don't understand. They can't.

What I need is somebody to listen to me. Somebody to hug me or hold my hand. Somebody to cry with me, to say it's all right to cry, it's all right to be angry. . . .

Because there is nothing you can do to change how I am going to feel. You don't have a cure, you don't have an answer. All you can do is be there for me. . . .

[D]eath was never a negative thing to me. To me death is just change. What really scares me is the process. It's being sick, being in the hospital, having my family suffer, not being able to take care of myself. That scares me a lot. . . . The way I look at it is today I am pretty healthy, today what I have to do is learn to live with AIDS. If tomorrow death or sickness or a cure comes along, I will deal with that then.

Source: Pedro Zamora, quoted in "Pedro Zamora (1972–1994)," *The Wall Street Journal*, pp. A1, A4 (September 4, 1994).

PSYCHOSOCIAL NEEDS OF PERSONS WITH AIDS

DOCUMENT 134: Gay Men with AIDS Face Discrimination from Their Families

---

Gay people with HIV/AIDS are in a double bind with regard to their families. Families that have difficulty accepting someone's homosexuality may have even greater difficulty once the illness is known. In some cases, gay people "come out" to their families about their sexuality at the same time they reveal their diagnosis. Sadly, some people are abandoned by their families, just when they are most needed.

The experiences of persons with HIV disease who reveal their illness suggest that fears of rejection are warranted. This is especially true for those who are gay. Almost every gay man I interviewed who has told his family reports that at least one family member has ended contact with him, and a few report that all relatives have done so. This rejection largely occurs because diagnosis with HIV disease reinforces families' preexisting repugnance at homosexuality. Families that always had questioned the morality of homosexuality may interpret an individual's illness as divine punishment and proof that they should never have tolerated such behavior. . . .

Because HIV disease makes individuals' homosexuality more concrete to their families, even those whose families previously seemed to accept their lifestyles may experience rejection once the diagnoses become known. . . . [D]iagnosis with HIV disease can force families to recognize that their son or brother is not simply gay in some abstract way, but actually has sex with other men. As a result, families that, despite their moral qualms, once had tolerated their son's or brother's homosexuality may no longer do so.

Source: Rose Weitz, *Life with AIDS* (New Brunswick, N.J.: Rutgers University Press, 1991).

DOCUMENT 135: Loneliness and Social Isolation

The emotional health of people who are ill is important. Unfortunately, people with AIDS must sometimes cope with loneliness as well as a life-threatening illness. They may be without a supportive social network or without a close, emotional relationship. Many AIDS service centers have developed buddy programs where volunteers become "buddies" of persons with AIDS.

[L]oneliness consists of two . . . states, emotional and social isolation. The absence of an attachment figure results in emotional isolation, while the absence of an accessible social network results in social isolation. People with AIDS are at a particularly high risk for either type of loneliness. . . . The person with AIDS either may not have a significant relationship or may have recently lost a partner through death from the disease. . . .

[Gay men and injecting drug users are] particularly vulnerable to breakdowns in social support and [the resulting] loneliness. The gay man may not have previously revealed facts about his lifestyle to his family but a diagnosis of AIDS forces him to face the need to share information about not only his sexual [orientation] but also about the reality that he has a life-threatening disease. His family may react with anger, fear, or revulsion. The [injecting] drug user may also experience rejection. . . . [Some] health care providers [have been reported to be] reluctant to help the person with the dual diagnosis of AIDS and chemical dependency.

Source: Kathleen M. Nokes and Joan Kendrew, "Loneliness in Veterans with AIDS and Its Relationship to the Development of Infections," *Archives of Psychiatric Nursing* 4(4): 271–277 (August 1990).

DOCUMENT 136: Becoming the Primary Caregiver

When patients are ill for months or years, as many AIDS patients are, personal relationships can become strained and more difficult. People with AIDS have great emotional needs but, at the same time, may be asked to comfort and reassure those close to them.

Ill or dying patients are often placed in the role of main comforter to those whom they love and who love them. They may . . . have a deeper, more direct acceptance of their own possible death than those who are placed in the role of most reluctant observers. This can lead to strains and ruptures within close relationships, particularly if the lover is unprepared to accept things the way the patient does. It seems unnatural and unfair to many patients that they have to look after their loved one when the loved one should really be looking after them. Further strains may appear in times of critical illness, when patients appear to turn to their parents, or to those whom they have known since they were small, for more support and sharing than to their lover or spouse. This occurs particularly in younger couples . . . where the bonds of the loving relationship are not as strong or secure as in the older, more established relationships. . . . Perhaps a more universal feature of those who are seriously ill or dying is the feeling of guilt for leaving behind all their responsibilities and burdens, or for the pain they are causing their loved ones.

Source: David Miller, *Living with AIDS and HIV* (London: Macmillan, 1987).

DOCUMENT 137: Uncertainty and AIDS

With a relatively new disease like AIDS, patients face uncertainty with regard to their medical care and treatment as well as their future. New drugs are constantly being developed and tested, and knowledge about the disease itself is expanding. In addition, feelings of guilt or shame about how or when the disease might have been contracted are another source of uncertainty. As a result, anxiety and emotional distress may be greater than with other illnesses.

[U]ncertainty and its ramifications may have an even greater impact on PWAs [persons with AIDS] than on those who suffer from most other illnesses, for several reasons. First, PWAs are more likely than most to know before diagnosis that they are at risk. As a result they suffer difficulties that other ill persons do not experience, because uncertainty and anxiety often sap their emotional energy and physical resources months or even years before they become ill.

Second, PWAs are more likely to feel guilt about the behaviors that led to their becoming ill. Thus, when faced with uncertainty about why they became ill, they are more likely to conclude that it was a deserved punishment. Moreover, PWAs are far more likely to find that their friends, families, and the general public also believe that PWAs cause and deserve their own illness . . . [which] often reinforce[s] the guilt that PWAs feel.

Third, PWAs are more likely to face difficulties in obtaining an accurate diagnosis. . . . AIDS can be difficult to diagnose because it . . . causes multiple symptoms . . . [and because] physicians often . . . avoid questions or actions that would lead to diagnosis.

Fourth, PWAs face greater uncertainty . . . in predicting how their illness will affect their lives; AIDS causes more extensive and less predictable physical and mental damage than most other illnesses.

Fifth, . . . PWAs are more likely to lack answers to their questions about treatment and prognosis. Moreover, because physicians' knowledge about AIDS is developing rapidly and changing constantly, PWAs often are reluctant to trust the answers they do receive.

Source: Rose Weitz, "Uncertainty and the Lives of Persons with AIDS," *Journal of Health & Social Behavior* 30(3): 270–281 (September 1989).

DOCUMENT 138: AIDS and the "Wrath of God"

The influenza and polio epidemics, like other worldwide epidemics, caused the suffering and deaths of many. The HIV/AIDS epidemic differs in that those who suffer from the disease carry the additional burden of the moral judgment of others. Certain religions and moral traditions consider behaviors that put people at risk to be immoral. However, those who argue that AIDS must be the wrath of God do not explain why, if homosexuality is so wrong, lesbians very rarely get AIDS. One could as easily argue that AIDS was placed on Earth by God to test our compassion. If so, have we passed God's test?

Every disease, AIDS included, has symbolic representations, associated words, ideologies, myths, and metaphors. . . . For example, . . . AIDS as evil focuses attention on undesirable groups and away from the blameless, AIDS as sinful allows sermons about the wrath of God. . . . Diseases are understood through the metaphors that describe [them]. For AIDS, "plague" is the principal metaphor . . . whereas cancer phobia taught us to fear polluting environments, AIDS has communicated fears about polluting people. These polluting people are specified in many sources as persons outside the boundaries of acceptable society. . . . [B]lack and Latino media have taken a defensive stance against covering HIV with the excuse that it does not affect them or their readers, who they claim are not [gay men] or drug users.

Source: Beverly A. Hall, "Overcoming Stigmatization: Social and Personal Implications of the Human Immunodeficiency Virus Diagnosis," *Archives of Psychiatric Nursing* 6(3):189–194 (1992).

DOCUMENT 139: The Need for Psychological and Spiritual Counseling

This excerpt discusses the needs of people with HIV disease for counseling, spiritual guidance, and psychological support, which are considerable. The emotional stress of a serious illness, rejection by family or friends, and social isolation are painful and debilitating.

For people living with HIV disease, the stresses of facing a debilitating and possibly terminal illness are compounded by the social stigma that is still attached to the disease. Sometimes shunned by family, friends, and caregivers, persons with HIV disease seek a community of inclusion and need help and understanding to counter the resulting isolation. No one should have to face HIV disease alone.

The psychological needs of those who face HIV disease are enormous. The trauma is particularly acute because HIV disease often strikes in the prime of life. The discrimination that accompanies HIV disease coupled with the stigma of homosexuality or IV drug use may contribute to . . . extreme social isolation. . . . Those unable to work and provide for their families face special emotional, as well as practical, hardships. Women with HIV disease who serve in traditional roles as caregivers for families may have unique needs. They must often struggle, with little outside help, to keep families together. Mothers of children with HIV disease are often sick themselves and can overlook their own needs as they fight to obtain care for their children. Counseling concerning matters of sexuality and intimacy may also be necessary. The specter of HIV disease may prove equally stressful to the sexual partner of an HIV-positive individual. Caregivers must recognize the continued need for sexual expression and intimacy, and the need to limit sexual activities and [to] substitute safer sexual behavior may pose emotional difficulties. Counseling and psychological support services should be available to meet these varied needs. Professional care has the potential to enhance the coping mechanisms necessary for daily living. Such services will . . . [enhance] other facets of care and increase the likelihood that counseling, education and prevention efforts will be successful. . . .

Confronting HIV disease involves coping with illness and pain, loss and death. Many who die of AIDS do so only after months or years marked by physical and emotional suffering. HIV disease can be a catalyst for an examination of the very meaning of life, death, and suffering. . . . A cadre of spiritual counselors, attuned to the needs of persons with HIV disease and able to deal sensitively with sexuality, homosexuality, drug use, chronic illness, terminal illness and cultural differences is needed to meet the needs of people with HIV infection. As with health care professionals, the clergy need special training and may themselves experience stigma in working with people with HIV disease. . . .

Spiritual counseling should be supported not only in the hospital setting, but also in the outpatient and home care environment. Training programs for the clergy, whether based in hospitals or graduate schools, should include curricula designed to prepare trainees to care for people living with HIV disease.

Source: Report of the Working Group on Social/Human Issues to the National Commission on AIDS (Washington, D.C.: National Commission on AIDS, April 1991).

THE ROLE OF FAMILIES, PARTNERS, AND FRIENDS OF PEOPLE WITH AIDS

DOCUMENT 140: Chronic Mourning and Endless Grief

The largest proportion of AIDS cases in the United States has been men who have sex with men. There are probably at least 6 million gay and bisexual men, and probably at least 3 million lesbians and bisexual women, in the United States. In the gay community, many men have been infected with HIV, have developed AIDS, and have died. As a result, the stress on those who survive is tremendous, because so many friends and acquaintances are lost year after year. Grief becomes a state of chronic mourning.

[I]n addition to those actually sick with AIDS, a much larger group is experiencing severe stressors associated with the epidemic, namely, those people who know and have been close to those who have died of AIDS, or who currently have AIDS. . . . It is [someone] who is integrated into a "gay community," that is most likely to have experienced the first ravages of this epidemic, and to be currently experiencing a sense of both personal and collective trauma as the losses and potential illnesses mount. . . . Because of the vulnerability to AIDS shared by almost all gay men, bereavement and illness among gay friends generate powerful reactions. . . . [W]hen friends and associates die, not only in large numbers but in year after succeeding year, without a sufficient interval of time to resolve the grief from one death or set of deaths before the next occurs, the grief reaction may be compounded and contribute to a sense of impending doom and chronic mourning. . . .

[T]he issues are compounded by the high likelihood that chronically bereaved individuals are much more likely to be involved in AIDS activism; assuming leadership positions in gay organizations, taking care of other sick and bereaved men, and putting themselves at higher risk of suffering even more losses.

Source: Laura Dean, William E. Hall, and John L. Martin, "Chronic and Intermittent AIDS-Related Bereavement in a Panel of Homosexual Men in New York City," *Journal of Palliative Care* 4(4): 54–57 (December 1988).

DOCUMENT 141: Gay Marriages Are Still Illegal

Same-sex partnerships are not always appreciated or accepted for being central to the lives of the people involved. When a gay man loses
a partner to AIDS, families and heterosexual friends can be insensitive
and lack understanding. This can add to the survivor's feeling of isolation because a most important relationship is not acknowledged or
honored. Gay marriages are still illegal in the United States, and this
lack of official status helps to make gay permanent relationships appear
illegitimate; thus they are often not taken seriously by the heterosexual
majority.

[The grief of members of the gay male community] is never fully val-
idated by a society that does not understand the grief's intensity. An
example is a father consistently reminding his son that he "only" lost a
friend and that that loss is not as important as losing a family member.
. . . [But] [t]he deceased is often the survivor's only family; the family of
origin may be both emotionally and geographically distant. Also, the
family of origin and nongay friends of the deceased may resent and
refuse to accept the survivor, causing a great sense of abandonment and
isolation. They may not understand the bond between the deceased and
the survivor. . . . Before the actual death, partners [lovers, or functional
same-sex spouses] have . . . been barred from intensive care units and
have been made to feel unwelcome in the hospital. Surviving partners
are often excluded from funeral plans. . . . Abandonment by families of
the deceased [deepens] the survivor's grief and increases the need for
alternative support systems. . . . Survivors feel isolated because the larger
community does not want to know their feelings. No one listens to them
and no one touches them because of a pervasive fear that getting close
to their grief and feelings is equivalent to getting close to the disease.

Source: Ray Biller and Susan Rice, "Experiencing Multiple Loss of Persons with
AIDS: Grief and Bereavement Issues," *Health and Social Work* 15(4): 283–290 (November 1990).

DOCUMENT 142: AIDS Quilt Helps Loved Ones Grieve

The Names Project Foundation sponsors the preservation and display
of the AIDS quilt. For a person who has died of AIDS, friends and family
create a commemorative square, which is then put together with
thousands of others. The quilt, with over 20,000 panels, and the size

of several football fields, has traveled to many cities in the United States. Participation in this unique public monument helps people to express their grief.

[T]he quilt has to be entered in order to be understood; a piece of interactive architecture of both public and private space.... [T]he quilt is a buoyantly colorful, even witty monument.... [It is] a kind of chaotic living room, in which the unkempt [loose fragments] of human beings— their jeans, photographs, glasses, sneakers, letters—are strewn on the ground, as if expecting the people to whom they belonged to return. People walk over this cluttered landscape, looking like tourists, caught between grief and curiosity, saying little, peering intently down at the ground.... The point of it all... is not merely to release grief, but to affirm the dignity of those who have died so young and in the face of unique public disdain.

Source: Andrew Sullivan, "Quilt," *The New Republic* 207(6): 43 (November 2, 1992).

DOCUMENT 143: Women and the AIDS Quilt

The AIDS quilt combines public art and innovative political action, which serves as a reminder that there are people behind the numbers. The quilt makes concrete the deaths of tens of thousands. It should be noted that since there are fewer women with AIDS than men in the United States, there are also fewer panels of the quilt dedicated to women.

The quilt is a great grid, within which there is no hierarchy, no narrative, no start or finish. The sheer number of the panels, with their variety of images and names, is overwhelming.... When there are life dates on the panels, they almost always indicate men who died before their 40th birthday. Relatively few panels commemorate women.... The virtual absence of female names mirrors the situation of women in the AIDS crisis as a whole. Women are less likely to receive adequate treatment and have fewer opportunities to enter trials for experimental drugs. ... But if women's names do not appear very often on the quilt, women's voices were frequently heard as I viewed the quilt—in the repeated laments of mothers calling out the names of their dead children.

Source: Jonathan Weinberg, "The Quilt: Activism and Remembrance," *Art in America* 80(12): 37–38 (December 1992).

DOCUMENT 144: Materials Used in the AIDS Quilt

The materials used to construct panels of the AIDS quilt include personal artifacts, mementos, and pieces of clothing—an endless jumble of bits and pieces. This collage is a unique celebration of people's lives. The following is a list of the items that can be found in the tens of thousands of panels that comprise the AIDS quilt.

[A] 100-year old quilt, afghans, Barbie dolls, bubble-wrap, burlap, buttons, car keys, carpet, champagne glasses, condoms, corduroy, corsets, cowboy boots, cremation ashes, credit cards, curtains, dresses, feather boas, first-place ribbons, fishnet hose, flags, fur, gloves, hats, human hair, jeans, jewelry, jockstraps, lace, lame, leather, love letters, Mardi Gras masks, merit badges, mink, motorcycle jackets, needlepoint, paintings, pearls, photographs, pins, plastic, quartz crystals, racing silks, records, rhinestones, sequins, shirts, silk flowers, studs, stuffed animals, suede, taffeta, tennis shoes, vinyl, [and] wedding rings [can be found in the panels of the AIDS quilt].

Source: *Quilt Facts*, factsheet of the Names Project Foundation.

DOCUMENT 145: AIDS Has Altered the Nature of Grieving

Because so many gay men have died of AIDS, especially in those cities, such as New York, San Francisco, Miami, and Los Angeles, where the disease has hit particularly hard, grieving among gay men in those cities takes on a new dimension. Many survivors can be described as being in a state of perpetual mourning. Chronic bereavement is usually associated with war and other great disasters when many are lost. Indeed, some gay men have grown cynical about death, and have become emotionally numb or neutral when learning about another death among their friends or acquaintances due to AIDS.

When Bill Ceyrolles visits New York he says he feels like a Jew returning to Berlin after the Holocaust. . . . "I walk down the streets and I think that's where so-and-so lived, and there's where another friend lived, and another, . . . so many have died."

Mr. Ceyrolles, who is gay and is himself infected with HIV . . . estimated that he has "known well" 100 people who have died of AIDS in the last five years and that [more than] half of his close friends are sick or dead. . . . "I mourn for so many people. . . . I'm in my early 40's, and it's hard to accept that this is the end of my life and that of my contemporaries. It's overwhelming. It's about 30 years sooner than I'd planned."

. . . For those left behind, conventional bereavement counseling . . . offer[s] little comfort when the losses are so staggering. . . . We have to find ways to handle the experiences of perpetually grieving, of never being out of grief," said Mardi Fritz, a psychotherapist in New York. . . . "[B]y the time you close the circle of grief for one person, [four] others, or 10 others have died."

Source: Elizabeth Rosenthal, "To a Drumbeat of Losses to AIDS, a Rethinking of Traditional Grief," *The New York Times*, pp. A1, A32 (December 6, 1992).

DOCUMENT 146: The Brave New World of AIDS Bereavement

In the United States, hundreds of thousands have died of AIDS. For some people, this has meant the loss of several friends and intimates. Without an elaborate tradition for mourning, participation in political action, volunteer work, and special projects, such as the AIDS quilt and volunteering for a fund-raiser for AIDS research or services, is a way for people to channel their grief into positive action.

AIDS has broken all the rules of modern dying, [and] sabotaged the conventions of mourning. In textbooks, grief is a long journey through stages of denial, darkness, rage. But AIDS permits no such leisure; decimating whole neighborhoods and communities of friends, it allows no time for normal healing. . . . AIDS bereavement bears special burdens. . . . [I]ts grief is often mixed with guilt, anger, or shame. . . . Mourners may themselves be ill and grieving their own impending deaths.

Source: Miriam Horn, "Grief Re-examined: The AIDS Epidemic Is Confounding the Normal Work of Bereavement," *U.S. News & World Report* 114(23): 81–83 (June 14, 1993).

THE ROLE OF HEALTH CARE PROVIDERS AND CAREGIVERS

DOCUMENT 147: Counselors Are Also Affected

Health Crisis Network (HCN) is the primary AIDS services, community-based organization in metropolitan Miami. It was started by a small group of gay male volunteers in 1983. HCN provides a large variety of patient care and support services for people with HIV/AIDS. It offers individual counseling, group counseling, a hotline, addiction services and counseling, a buddy program, food vouchers, an HIV educational program, and legal assistance; it also sponsors an annual Miami AIDS walk (where participants raise money by walking a set distance) and an annual White Party (a fund-raiser where partygoers dress creatively in white clothes or costumes). Counselors at HCN work to support patients suffering from HIV-related illnesses. While it is appropriate to maintain a clinical distance, counselors are themselves inevitably affected by their patients' difficulties and suffering. Today, HCN is a large organization with an annual budget of over $3 million.

"I wonder if he made it through the night." "She couldn't speak but I saw in her eyes that she knew I was there." "I need to go to the hospital to see her today but I have 14 charts waiting for my progress notes for group and the service sheets for the week as well." "One of my team is in shock over the sudden death of a close relative. She needs my support." "I need private time to complete my unit report for the month and to plan. . . ." "My supervisor is coming by to review plans for a Saturday Clinical Services meeting."

. . . These thoughts are not those of a specific counselor. Instead, they represent a composite picture of reactions to events in the work day of any counselor at Health Crisis Network [HCN]. A day in the life of any counselor can begin in this way and often does. It may be a day when he learns that a client died during the night; that she sits with her dying client and there is nothing more to be done except to say good-bye. It is always a day when there is much more to be done, and a day when others are coming to HCN searching for hope and assurance that help is on the way; that something can be done.

A day in the life of an HCN counselor is also filled with moments of joy, spontaneous laughter and shared lunches. Donuts, coffee, nectars and tesayo are passed around the table where Spanish and English intermingle in a sharing of personal experience. [Half the population of metropolitan Miami is Hispanic or Latino/a.]

In this safe and nurturing environment, impatience dissolves with the understanding, honest communication and support of fellow counselors. Tears of sadness mingle with the streams of water supplied to the garden plants and flowers.

His charts are still waiting. Her client is very weak but has made the effort to come in for a counseling session. She wants to be ready for him.

Source: Karin Rhodes, "A Day in the Life. . . . The Counselor," *Update* [*Health Crisis Network Newsletter*]. (Summer 1992).

DOCUMENT 148: On-the-Job Risk to Health Care Workers

For years, the Centers for Disease Control and Prevention (CDC) has studied and investigated the occupational (work-related) risk of HIV infection to health care workers. If proper precautions are taken, the risk is very low. Compared with the number of HIV-infected patients who have been treated, there are relatively few health care workers known to have acquired HIV infection at work. At the end of 1994, forty-two health care workers in the United States were confirmed to be HIV-positive directly from work-related exposure. An additional ninety-one health care workers with no other risks have HIV/AIDS and claim that they were infected on the job, though this has not yet been conclusively confirmed. That is a total of only 133 health care workers nationwide. Nonetheless, HIV infection on the job remains a very real concern to them.

Public health surveillance for and risk-assessment studies of . . . HIV infection provide a basis for formulating measures to minimize the risk for occupational [work-related] transmission of HIV to health-care workers. Data on occupational transmission of HIV have been provided by two CDC-supported national surveillance systems; one initiated in 1981 for . . . AIDS cases and one initiated in 1991 for HIV infections acquired through occupational exposures. . . . [H]ealth care workers are defined as persons, including students and trainees, who worked in a health care, clinical, or HIV-laboratory setting any time since 1978. Persons [who have been] reported . . . have been classified with documented, or possible, occupationally acquired HIV infection. Those classified with documented occupationally acquired HIV infection had evidence of HIV seroconversion, [and] [p]ersons classified with possible occupationally acquired HIV infection did not have behavioral or transfusion risks for HIV infection that could be identified during follow-up investigation. . . . As of September 30, 1992, [the] CDC had received reports of 32 health-care workers in the United States with documented occupationally acquired HIV infection and 69 with possible occupationally acquired infection.

Source: "Surveillance for Occupationally Acquired HIV Infection United States, 1981–1992," *Morbidity and Mortality Weekly Report* 41(43): 823–825 (October 30, 1992).

DOCUMENT 149: The Shanti Project of San Francisco

The Shanti Project has provided support for people with serious illnesses in the San Francisco area since 1974. In 1981, Shanti began
working with AIDS patients, and by 1984 concentrated on serving people with HIV/AIDS. Today, it provides peer and professional counseling, housing for people with AIDS, a home help volunteer program,
educational videos, and a newsletter. The work of the Shanti Project
shows how important volunteers can be. Volunteers help seriously ill
and dying patients manage the practical details of their day-to-day lives
as well as provide emotional support. It is not surprising that counselors
and volunteers taking care of these patients also suffer and can "burn
out" quickly.

Today two of my clients appear in the [obituary] pages—they are both
under thirty. . . . Each is someone's son, someone's brother, someone's
lover, and each will leave a circle of friends and family who will miss
him daily. Recently I lost four clients in one week, and news of the fourth
was almost more than I could bear. Few people stay for more than a few
months in my position, and our lives are different afterwards. Ordinary
words like "love" and "life" take on new meaning. . . .
    There aren't enough of us—staff or volunteers. We burn out; we dream
of death. . . . Friends say, "It must be the work you do. I don't have
dreams like that." . . . I answer, "Maybe not. But maybe you don't have
the memories either."

Source: Carol Cowen, "Real Champions Don't Come Home; One Day at Shanti,"
Whole Earth Review no. 78, pp. 67–69 (Spring 1993).

DOCUMENT 150: Coping On-line

The rapid growth and popularity of the Internet during the mid-1990s
has proven to be a useful source of information and comfort for those
both infected and affected by HIV/AIDS. This reading provides valuable
information for people who readily "surf the net."

Internet news groups provide an important means for the exchange of
HIV and AIDS information, on topics ranging from research and treatment advances to political movements and service organizations. On
"sci.med.aids," users can access daily AIDS news updates, detailed sci-

entific information about drug therapies, and debates about different AIDS drugs. Due to the occasional censorship of posts on "sci.med.aids," James Scutero founded "misc.health.aids," which includes more controversial information. While the dialogue can become extreme, "whatever goes in is going to be tried by fire. It's going to be ground up, analyzed, and reanalyzed. And whatever's true is going to stick," Scutero says. At "alt.hemp-tokers," the legalization of marijuana is advocated, especially for people with AIDS and other illnesses. Another group, "rec.pets. dogs.rescue," posts information about organizations that help AIDS patients care for their pets. AIDS information can also be found on many Web sites, including those developed by AEGIS (AIDS Education Global Information System) at "www.aegis.com," the New York Academy of Medicine at "www.nyam.org," and Medline at "www.healthgate.com."

Source: Howard Gensler, "Coping with AIDS: Together, Online," *Yahoo! Internet Life* 2(7): 24 (December 1996); CDC National AIDS Clearinghouse (Bethesda, Md.: Information, Inc., 1996).

SUGGESTED READINGS

Ball, Steven. "Serostatus and Counseling." *Focus* 11(8), p. 1 (July 1996).

Busby, J. "Your Personal Health: When Someone You Know Has AIDS." *Current Health* 2, 19 (1): 14–15 (September 1, 1992).

Chase, Marilyn. "Tending to Patients with AIDS Teaches Valuable Lessons." *The Wall Street Journal*, p. B1 (July 22, 1996).

Draimin, Barbara H. *Coping When a Parent Has AIDS*. New York: Rosen Publishing Group, 1993.

Feinberg, David B. *Queer & Loathing: Rants & Raves of a Raging AIDS Clone*. New York: Viking Press, 1994.

Glaser, Elizabeth. *In the Absence of Angels*. New York: Berkley, 1991.

Greif, Judith, and Beth A. Golden. *AIDS Care at Home: A Guide for Caregivers, Loved Ones, and People with AIDS*. New York: Wiley, 1994.

Hayes, W. "To Be Young and Gay and Living in the 90's." *Utne Reader*, pp. 94–100 (March/April 1991).

Holzemer, William L., Suzanne Bakken Henry, Cheryl A. Reilly et al. "Problems of Persons with HIV/AIDS Hospitalized for *Pneumocystis carinii* Pneumonia." *Journal of the Association of Nurses in AIDS Care* 6(3), p. 23 (May/June 1995).

Rose, Avi. "HIV and Dying: The Challenges of Caring." *Focus* 11(2): p. 1 (January 1996).

Shirk, Martha. "When Families Live with AIDS." *St. Louis Post-Dispatch*, p. 1C (December 8, 1995).

Stephenson, Joan. "Medical Education Gets Wired: Interactive Media Laboratory Targets Patients and Physicians." *Journal of the American Medical Association* 276(22), p. 1788 (December 11, 1996).

Wiener, Lori, Aprille Best, and Philip A. Pizzo, eds. *Be a Friend: Children Who Live with HIV Speak*. Morton Grove, Ill.: A. Whitman, 1994.

6

The Politics of AIDS

AIDS has had a profound effect upon our society. Before AIDS, sick people were often content to trust the authority of their physician. Very few questioned their doctor about medical care and treatments. People with AIDS (PWAs), however, quickly learned that they need to keep pace with the growing wealth of information about experimental treatments and care strategies in the management of this highly complex disease. PWAs often became more expert about AIDS than their own physicians, since those who survived longest became successful activists for their own medical care. Buyer clubs sprang up in major cities to provide PWAs access, though illegal, to potentially life-supporting treatments that had not yet been approved by the Food and Drug Administration (FDA).

In the early and mid-1980s gay men with AIDS were facing a terminal disease with little or no government support or funding. It became very clear that if HIV-infected gay men were to try to survive for as long as possible, the gay community would have to develop its own health and social service organizations in response to the crisis. Indeed, in the early years of the epidemic it appeared that the entire American gay male community was at risk of annihilation: not just the millions of gay male lives, but the unspoken contributions of the gay community to the larger society would be forever lost.

The earliest U.S. government response to the AIDS crisis at the very highest levels was dead silence. When AIDS was first widely noticed within the medical community in 1981, through public health and epidemiology reports, gay males also learned about it through the gay press and through word of mouth. As the late Randy Shilts's now classic work, *And the Band Played On*, documents in great detail, the politically conservative Reagan administration entered the White House in

1981 with no intention of allowing tax dollars to be used to save the lives of what it saw as "promiscuous homosexuals." When in 1982 it became clear that AIDS affected others as well, the conservative administration was even more reluctant to fund treatment and research for a mysterious disease that attacked mostly stigmatized groups, what was then pejoratively referred to as the "4H Club": "homsexuals, heroin users, hemophiliacs, and Haitian-Americans."

It was not until May 1983, two years after the medical and gay communities learned about the escalating epidemic, that the general public first learned about AIDS. The growth of the gay community during the 1970s had been very much of a secret among the general public in the United States, and not even AIDS was then powerful enough to break the code of silence about homosexuality by the reticent and cautious press. The media did not publicize the disease until after the Gay Men's Health Crisis, the first and largest AIDS service organization, sold out a 20,000-seat arena for a "Night at the Circus" fund-raiser in New York City and a candlelight vigil drew thousands in San Francisco.

The initial reaction of the general public was not a supportive one. Gay men and Haitian-Americans rapidly found themselves the targets of discrimination, as the worried public began to stay away from restaurants with gay waiters, avoided shopping in gay-owned shops, and fired Haitian-American employees. Meanwhile, the lack of government action and significant funding from the president and the Congress continued. Not until 1985, with the death from AIDS of Rock Hudson, no longer just a faceless statistic, did the American public begin to realize the full impact of the epidemic. And it was not until late 1986 and early 1987, as the data began to come in from central Africa of the heterosexual spread of the epidemic, and the growing concern among many U.S. government officials that AIDS might similarly start spreading rapidly through the heterosexual population in the United States, that finally huge expenditures of funds, primarily for HIV testing, surveillance studies, and clinical research, began.

By the late 1980s, as the death toll mounted in the United States, activist organizations such as ACT-UP (AIDS Coalition to Unleash Power) grew rapidly, engaging in street theater, well-attended confrontational demonstrations, and activities such as chaining themselves to the entrances of the FDA and the National Institutes of Health (NIH). Surprisingly, it worked. The FDA shortened its review process for the approval of new drugs and allowed the compassionate distribution of some not yet approved experimental AIDS treatments. The NIH continued to increase its AIDS research budget and developed a sped-up process for its review of AIDS-related research proposals. However, it was not until 1990 that the Congress passed the Ryan White Comprehensive Care Act, which allocated millions of dollars for the care of PWAs. While AIDS political activism was less vocal during the first term of the Clinton administration, by the second term there were signs that a renewed AIDS activism might be emerging.

COMMUNITY RESPONSES TO THE CRISIS

DOCUMENT 151: The Beginning of a Community-Based AIDS Organization: Miami, Florida, 1983

Community-based organizations throughout the United States and elsewhere have been essential in helping people affected by the HIV/AIDS epidemic. They have also served an important political function, reminding people in the larger community of the crisis and showing how local people can take positive action. Emerging out of Network, a local gay professional organization in Miami, Florida, Health Crisis Network was started by a small group of gay men in 1983. Since then, it has expanded and has served thousands of clients with HIV/AIDS. Direct patient services include counseling as well as case management. The HIV hot line provides information and support to thousands in South Florida. Similar primary AIDS service organizations include Gay Men's Health Crisis (GMHC) in New York City, AID Atlanta, AIDS Project Los Angeles, Health Education Resource Organization (HERO) in Baltimore, Howard Brown Memorial Clinic in Chicago, San Francisco AIDS Foundation, Whitman-Walker Clinic in Washington, D.C., and many others (see Resource Directory).

An Open Letter to the Concerned Miami Community:

Due to the rising concern of AIDS in our community it has become evident that there is much to be done in dealing with this situation. As with any chronic or terminal illness, it is important to remember that it is not just the physical condition that needs to be treated. The whole person, as well as their environment, needs to be considered. It is with this in mind that HEALTH CRISIS NETWORK is being brought into existence.

We established some basic goals, and outlined what we feel is necessary to effectively deal with this situation. Our primary concern, of course, will be . . . the person affected with AIDS. For them, we will offer not only access to information concerning this syndrome, but crisis counseling, individual as well as group support systems, financial and legal referral, spiritual counseling and advocacy for the client. For the significant people in the lives of a person with AIDS (i.e., parents, friends, lovers), we will be offering individual and group support, necessary not only for them but for the primary person as well.

We would like to have the opportunity to share more with you. On November 19, 1983 there will be a general meeting to discuss our services further and answer any questions you may have. There will be wine and cheese served at 7:00 p.m. with the meeting following at 7:30 p.m. at the Christ Metropolitan Community Church social hall. . . . We invite and urge you to attend.

Sincerely,
Board of Directors
HEALTH CRISIS NETWORK

Source: Board of Directors, Health Crisis Network, letter to the community (October 1993).

DOCUMENT 152: The Mission Statement of the Health Crisis Network in Miami

Volunteers have carried out much of the work of AIDS community-based organizations. The purpose or mission of AIDS service organizations, such as the Health Crisis Network in metropolitan Miami (Dade County, Florida), is to provide support to people with HIV/AIDS and their families. Services include counseling for people with HIV/AIDS, their partners, friends, and families, as well as practical help, such as transportation, housing, and food delivery. Patient advocacy is another important role; seriously ill patients need help negotiating the health care system. The following is the written mission statement of the Health Crisis Network.

Given the unique diversity of the populations of Dade County, Health Crisis Network . . . is dedicated to meeting the needs of all persons in the community affected by HIV infection as well as its ramifications. Our goals include the following:

1) To provide and facilitate procurement of health, psychosocial, community support services and direct assistance to people with HIV infection and their loved ones so that they may live fully within the limitations of the illness;

2) To provide a comprehensive program of both individual and community education to prevent HIV infection, promote healthy lifestyles and encourage a supportive and accepting attitude towards people with HIV infection;

3) To provide advocacy directly and indirectly for people with HIV infection;

4) To consult, train and assist other groups and organizations addressing HIV infection; [and]

5) To recruit, train, promote, support and empower volunteers to carry out this mission. Health Crisis Network . . . does not discriminate against any member, client, volunteer or employee on the basis of race, age, sex, handicap, religion, national origin or ancestry, sexual orientation, lifestyle, or HIV status.

Source: Mission statement of Health Crisis Network (Miami, Florida, 1986).

DOCUMENT 153: AIDS Can't Wait

Gay Men's Health Crisis (GMHC) is the largest AIDS community-based organization in New York City, well known for its innovative services. In the early 1980s, a small group of gay men started this organization in response to the epidemic. The multifaceted organization provides individual and group counseling, a hot line, case management and social services, legal services, food services, education services and HIV prevention workshops, a newsletter and publication services, recreational activities, special events, a "buddy program," and other services. The buddy program pairs a volunteer with a person living with AIDS; the volunteer helps the client with household chores, medical appointments, and emotional support. This program and others developed by GMHC have been models for community organizations in other cities.

Why our name? It's a question people ask often. If Gay Men's Health Crisis serves men, women and children with AIDS, why continue to call ourselves Gay Men's Health Crisis? AIDS isn't only a gay disease. It never was. We might have an easier time raising money from both public and private sources if we were called say, the "New York City AIDS Foundation," so why not change the name?

The answer lies in the history that we never want to lose. Eleven years ago [in early 1982], before AIDS even had its name, a small group of gay men formed GMHC to help sick friends and lovers cope. What those men pioneered—the world's first buddy program, the first [AIDS-related] medical newsletter, the first AIDS hot line—were one-of-a-kind, ground breaking services that still serve as a model for AIDS care world-wide. The early volunteers chose to name their organization after their community because their community was fighting an epidemic the rest of the world ignored. The rest of the world didn't think it was at risk.

Today GMHC is building on the expertise and experiences of the gay community to reach out to everyone with HIV illness. The name Gay Men's Health Crisis is a reminder of the past and a badge of pride. Our name lets people know that fighting AIDS means fighting the epidemic of discrimination that has helped kill so many so quickly: discrimination not only on the basis of sexual orientation, but also on the basis of race, gender and social status. Our name challenges people to break down stereotypes, put aside narrow definitions of self-interest, stop "us and them" thinking and start saving lives. We're not working to end AIDS because people who get it are gay, or straight, or men, or women, or [persons with hemophilia] or injection drug users. We're working to end AIDS because we are alive and we don't want anyone else to die the way our friends and loved ones have died.

There is another part of our name—Crisis—that people tend to overlook. We work everyday with waiting lists and clogged switchboards and the terrible sense that we need to do more. That urgency never leaves us. We have to do more, and do it quickly. AIDS can't wait.

Source: *We Are All Living with AIDS*, Gay Men's Health Crisis 1991/1992 Annual Report (New York: Gay Men's Health Crisis, 1992).

DOCUMENT 154: Assistance for Communities Often Comes from Within Their Own Ranks

Education is an important tool for preventing the spread of HIV. Unconventional strategies are needed to reach groups such as injecting drug users (addicts who shoot drugs with a needle) and commercial sex workers (prostitutes). AIDS prevention programs have successfully recruited, trained, and employed community outreach workers to bring information to those who may be at greatest risk for infection. Outreach workers are sometimes former members of the population that is being targeted by the community-based organization for education and, therefore, have credibility with people who might otherwise be difficult to reach.

Outreach activities originated in response to some of the social ills of the industrial revolution. It was not until the 1960's, however, that the concept of "outreach worker" emerged as a helping profession that could supplement the efforts of institutionalized systems of assistance. . . . This concept . . . is considered one of the most viable health education techniques that can be applied to the AIDS epidemic. . . . Outreach workers . . . are a new type of professional whose knowledge and abilities are acquired in the school of hard knocks. This new breed of health educator comes to the job already possessing the necessary skills and abilities for successful outreach work. The life experiences and the skills that out-reach workers have developed to deal with their own problems make them uniquely qualified to help community residents help them-selves. . . .

Outreach workers are no longer considered just laypeople; with their expertise, they have proven themselves to be professionals in the field of "involved education." Skilled in the art of grassroots communication, they have demonstrated that they are the key to building and maintain-ing the community support that is vital to program success.

Outreach workers receive intensive training in the problems addressed by their agencies. They learn communication skills, motivational tech-niques, and health education and disease prevention strategies, and they become well versed in the full range of public and private services that are locally available. . . . The natural skills of . . . community health work-ers are essential to successful outreach efforts.

In most areas, outreach workers are recruited directly from the neigh-borhoods where programs are concentrating most of their activities and efforts. The main role of outreach workers has been to serve as the link between the programs and the communities they serve, and their pri-mary task has been to gain community acceptance and encourage in-volvement in these programs. . . . Communication with such groups requires an understanding of various cultural aspects, such as street be-havior and street language. . . .

Often, the target populations [the people you are trying to reach] do not trust outside intervention. . . . In addition, communication between the street population and persons from mainstream American society has been limited and antagonistic.

In response to these reactions, the concept of the indigenous [native to the area] outreach worker has evolved into the most effective way to communicate and transfer intervention methods within the street envi-ronment. Some outreach workers who are ex-addicts are from the same ethnographic, cultural, and street environment as the target population; therefore, they are best equipped to locate and communicate with this population. . . . Armed with . . . a natural commitment and empathy, out-reach workers can implement community programs, which are accepted because they have established credibility.

Concentrated use of community health outreach workers in a specified prevention program is the most effective means of implementing the program for the people who need it. Because outreach workers make contacts on a one-to-one-basis, there is interchange and feedback. This personal contact reaches a variety of people . . . [and] this intervention reaches individuals who do not participate in normal community activities. . . .

Because of the national AIDS crisis . . . community health outreach workers . . . have gained prominence as the most effective means to provide health education, especially among [injecting] drug users . . . Outreach workers are viewed as professionals [involved in] education. . . . [T]asks include educating on AIDS prevention, making activity reports, writing contact descriptions, attending meetings, dispensing condoms or bleach, and providing transportation to outreach sites.

Source: Rebecca S. Ashery, ed., *Program Development for Community AIDS Outreach*, Clinical Report Series (Rockville, Md.: National Institute on Drug Abuse, 1992).

DOCUMENT 155: Attacking AIDS Discrimination

Local governments have responded differently to the AIDS epidemic. In some municipalities, nothing has been done. In New York City, with nearly 200,000 people infected with HIV, the city government has taken an active role in research and prevention, although not as aggressive a role as critics would have liked. This document represents an early attempt at the city level to carve out a humane, antidiscriminatory policy for people with HIV/AIDS.

[New York City] will place heavy emphasis on creating a set of conditions citywide that are likely to *discourage* AIDS-related discrimination. These include:

- A city work force that is largely free of unwarranted fear of HIV infection by co-workers or agency clients, and well-informed about the rights of citizens to be free from AIDS-related discrimination.
- A citizenry sufficiently well-informed about their rights that they are able to demand fair treatment and seek legal assistance when needed.
- City personnel policies that are clear in their rejection of AIDS-related discrimination and that set an example for other jurisdictions and sectors of the economy.
- Well-publicized legal enforcement of human rights laws so that organizations have little doubt that they face risk if they continue to engage in discriminatory practices as employers or service-providers.
- Laws and administrative rules at city and state levels that provide an adequate basis for protecting the human rights of those affected by the AIDS epidemic.

• Laws protecting people from the stigma and discrimination surrounding AIDS by prohibiting disclosure of HIV-related information.

The central focus of the city's actions in this area will be on tackling the *systemic* discrimination that is built into the policies and practices of organizations and industries.... New York City has already begun this effort in its own agencies. Education and training around AIDS will continue in an effort to make city employees and their managers more comfortable serving AIDS clients and patients and to communicate and enforce policies that prohibit all types of AIDS-related discrimination. Information about human rights will be incorporated into the internal training programs of all the AIDS Task Force agencies.

Source: "Action Against AIDS–Related Discrimination," in *New York City Strategic Plan for AIDS* (New York: Interagency Task Force on AIDS, May 1988), section D.8, pp. 1–5.

DOCUMENT 156: Minority Communities and Community-Based Organizations

Many smaller AIDS service organizations focusing on the needs of African-American and Hispanic populations in the United States find it very difficult to raise the funds that are needed. This selection discusses this problem. In early 1997, a multimillion-dollar grant program from the Centers for Disease Control and Prevention (CDC), benefiting mostly minority AIDS community-based organizations, was implemented to assist in helping this problem.

While large AIDS service organizations have become multi-million dollar institutions, smaller community-based groups—created for minority communities—receive a smaller cut of the federal AIDS funding pie. Competition between the two types of AIDS groups has created tension in the AIDS community, despite efforts to give all parties a voice. For example, three African-American board members of the Gay Men's Health Crisis resigned earlier this year, claiming the agency was "not attuned to the needs of minority communities."

Carl Bean, founder of Los Angeles' Minority AIDS Project, says securing funding is the organization's greatest challenge. The group believes that programs should be from the community and by the community, and hires former prostitutes, gang members, and transgendered persons for outreach projects. Meanwhile, Imani P. Woods, who founded Street Outreach Services for people at risk for HIV in Seattle, resigned from the organization last year in frustration over inadequate funding. She says AIDS cases in minority communities are increasing because politicians are not willing to provide the funding needed for community-based AIDS service organizations.

Source: Stuart Timmons, "Blood and Money," *Vibe* 4(6): 98 (August 1996); CDC National AIDS Clearinghouse (Bethesda, Md.: Information, Inc., 1996).

DOCUMENT 157: A Community Responds to the Crisis

The AIDS crisis has forced the gay community to change rapidly during the last two decades of the twentieth century. At first it appeared that AIDS would inhibit the political and social changes that had occurred within the gay community during the 1970s, but by the late 1980s it became clear that the epidemic had accelerated the political and social changes within the community as more gay men and lesbians were compelled to be open about being gay or lesbian. Below are some of the thoughts of several authors and a few others on the enormous impact of the epidemic upon the gay community.

"Ten years ago if some 32-year-old fellow died, his whole friendship circle would be devastated for years. They'd never get over it. Now it's so normal to die at 32."—Sarah Schulman, author

"One of the truths of testing HIV+ is that once you know, you can never not know again."—Michael Slocum, journalist

"Dating (as an HIV+ person) involves a complex set of maneuvers, because the stakes are so much higher. How do you come out for the second time, especially if you really like him? Do you divulge in between the appetizer and the main course, or do you wait until dessert?"—Kiki Mason, author and social critic

"For the friend who still cannot be named—and for all of us who live in a world where secrets must be kept."—an inscription of the AIDS Quilt

"What lengths, what depths they will go in their aversion! The obituaries that refuse to list AIDS as the cause of death—as if there were only one thing worse than being dead and that is being homosexual."—Andrew Holleran, author

"Wouldn't it be great if you could only get AIDS by giving money to television preachers?"—Elayne Boosler, comedian

"As the AIDS crisis has so movingly shown, gay people have built the kind of community that evaporated for many non-gay Americans decades ago. You don't see straight [heterosexual] volunteers queuing up to change cancer patients' bedpans and deliver their groceries."—Jonathan Rauch, author

"They've been going through this for years and they've been really taking care of their own. You have to give the gay and lesbian community a lot of credit for

that. The rest of us have a lot to learn from that."—Magic Johnson, HIV+ basketball player

Source: As quoted in David Blanton, *Queer Notions: A Fabulous Collection of Gay
and Lesbian Wit and Wisdom* (Philadelphia: Running Press, 1996).

POLITICAL APATHY

DOCUMENT 158: The Reagan Years

Presidential leadership sets the tone for issues of national importance.
During Reagan's presidency, it became clear that the AIDS epidemic
was at crisis proportions. At the same time, the administration kept a
low profile and appeared to be acting out of political expediency to
protect its conservative base. Randy Shilts, a San Francisco reporter,
wrote extensively on the epidemic. His book, *And the Band Played
On*, from which this excerpt is taken, recounts the politics and the
public health efforts from 1981 to 1985.

When claiming victory on election night, President Reagan told a
cheering crowd, "America's best days lie ahead." It was during the
month of Reagan's reelection that the nation's AIDS caseload surpassed
7,000. . . .

It was easy to ignore anomalies in 1984. . . . [E]verybody agreed the
future of the United States was bright again. On December 31, the Centers for Disease Control reported that 7,699 Americans were dead or
dying of a disease that had never been heard of when President Reagan
was sworn in during his first term, and nobody paid much attention to
the CDC's warnings that tens of thousands more would be dead by the
time he was done with his second. . . .

In the next twenty minutes, the president laid out his views on AIDS.
There was little talk of education and a lot of talk about testing. There
was no mention . . . of confidentiality guarantees or civil rights protection
for those who tested positive. Reagan's program, of course, would do
very little to actually stop the spread of AIDS. Though testing heterosexuals at marriage license bureaus created the illusion of action, very
few of these people were infected with the virus and very few lives
would be saved. But then saving lives had never been a priority of the
Reagan administration. Reagan's speech was not meant to serve the public health; it was a political solution to a political problem. The words
created a stance that was politically comfortable for the president and

his adherents; it was also a stance that killed people. Already, some said that Ronald Reagan would be remembered in history books for one thing beyond all else: He was the man who had let AIDS rage through America, the leader of the government that when challenged to action had placed politics above the health of the American people.

Source: Randy Shilts, *And the Band Played On: Politics, People and the AIDS Epidemic* (New York: Basic Books, 1987).

DOCUMENT 159: Allowing an Epidemic to Spread Freely and Rapidly

Two years after the appearance of what had then been labeled "AIDS" was a time of government apathy, which allowed the epidemic to spread freely and rapidly, especially through the gay male community of major urban areas in the United States, such as New York City. Since the epidemic is primarily sexually transmitted, it tends to affect clusters of people who know one another. Many clusters of gay men in New York City during these early years were finding their entire friendship networks being wiped out, and the government—it appeared—could not care less.

One look at the numbers—152 reported cases the first year, 1,300 cases the second, 4,156 the third—proved AIDS was gaining speed. The early GMHC [Gay Men's Health Crisis] volunteers had a more personal sense of the epidemic's overwhelming growth. Buddy team leaders found themselves leading teams where fifteen of the . . . sixteen clients died in a week. Intake volunteers started seeing the names of more and more friends on files, and hearing more voices they knew on the phone. An entire generation of gay men and their friends in New York began talking not of how many people they knew who had died, but of how many were still alive. Two years into this crisis, GMHC volunteers and staff looked to their government leaders for help. They found nothing. No money requested by the Reagan Administration for AIDS research. No complete studies on how AIDS was transmitted. The National Cancer Institute had spent less than one-tenth of one percent of its budget funding studies on Kaposi's sarcoma. Total AIDS spending at the Centers for Disease Control was $2 million out of a $202 million budget. By contrast, the CDC spent $9 million on the 1976 outbreak of Legionnaire's Disease and $10 million in the first two weeks of the 1982 Tylenol scare.

In New York City, AIDS leadership was no better. "We couldn't even get near the Mayor," Larry Kramer remembered. "Every time I called, his liaison would either scream at me, hang up on me, or say he was going to call me back and never did." Three years after the first cases of AIDS were reported, New York City had funded absolutely no AIDS education.

Source: "Forcing Government to Act," in *The First Ten Years*, Gay Men's Health Crisis Annual Report, *1990–1991* (New York: Gay Men's Health Crisis, 1991).

DOCUMENT 160: A Belated Realization of the Seriousness of AIDS

When the actor Rock Hudson died of AIDS in 1985, the publicity brought the problem home to many who had previously not been affected. President Reagan was one of those people. Denial of the seriousness of the situation is a natural defense, until a friend or acquaintance becomes ill and dies. What is most alarming about this reading is that the president did not realize the seriousness of the AIDS epidemic until it was explained to him in 1985, at the beginning of his second term in office.

[President Reagan's] former doctor, Brigadier General John Hutton said Reagan had not realized the seriousness of AIDS until July, 1985, when he saw a news report disclosing that the actor Rock Hudson had died of the disease. This was more than [four] years after AIDS had been identified, thousands of Americans had been infected, and AIDS had been the subject of intense national publicity. When Reagan saw the news report about Hudson's death, he asked General Hutton to tell him about the disease. After listening to a long explanation, the General said the President replied: "I have always thought the world might end in a flash, but this sounds like it's worse."

Source: Haynes Johnson, *Sleepwalking Through History* (New York: W. W. Norton, 1991).

DOCUMENT 161: A Belated Tribute for Ryan White

Ryan White, a young man with AIDS and hemophilia (a genetic disease in which the affected person could bleed to death if untreated), was banned from attending school in Kokomo, Indiana, because of his disease. He had become infected with HIV from tainted blood products used to fight his hemophilia during the 1980s. After a well-publicized court battle, he was allowed to attend school. He and his family then moved to Cicero, Indiana. His plight created a great deal of publicity and sympathy for persons with AIDS. Ryan White died in 1990, at age eighteen. Though former President Reagan had expressed his sympathy for Ryan White, the political strategy of his staff in ignoring the AIDS epidemic during the early and mid-1980s, while he was president, was highly detrimental to persons with AIDS.

Ryan White died in an Indianapolis hospital on April 8, 1990, less than a month after his meeting with [then former President] Reagan. He was eighteen years old. Reagan had been moved by White's courage, and he wrote a tribute to him for the *Washington Post* saying, "We owe it to Ryan to make sure that the fear and ignorance that chased him from his home and school will be eliminated." In the op-ed page article Reagan said, "How Nancy and I wish there had been a magic wand we could have waved that would have made it all go away." ... A *Post* reader named David Robinson, who said he was a gay man who had suffered from AIDS for three years, wrote a letter to the *Post* after Reagan's article appeared. "He [Reagan] may not have had a wand, but he had the next best thing: the Presidency of the United States during the first eight years of the AIDS epidemic. ... Reagan could have improved the survival chances of Ryan White and other people with AIDS by speaking out often and forcefully on AIDS. ..."

But Reagan was more distanced in the White House. ... In July 1987, on the same day he visited the National Institutes of Health and held an AIDS-stricken baby in his arms, Reagan appointed an AIDS Commission that included opponents of AIDS education and was devoid of physicians who had treated AIDS patients or scientists who had engaged in AIDS research. The Commission appointments reflected the influence of conservatives who feared not only AIDS, but homosexuals. In naming this body, Reagan sent an unfortunate message to the public that he did not care enough about the AIDS problem to muster the best scientific information available.

Source: Lou Cannon, *President Reagan: The Role of a Lifetime* (New York: Simon and Schuster, 1991).

DOCUMENT 162: A Massive Failure of National Leadership

Founded in New York City in the early 1980s, the Gay Men's Health Crisis (GMHC) is the oldest and largest political advocacy and community-based AIDS organization in the United States. AIDS service organizations have been extremely important in providing services where none were previously available. National leadership and financial support have been late in coming and often are insufficient to meet the enormous and growing demand.

In this election year, it is hard to talk about AIDS without talking about a massive failure of national leadership. We began our fight in 1981, when there was nothing for people with AIDS: No services, no funding, no public information, and no public outcry. Eleven years into this epidemic, we are still a community looking to itself in a crisis. The White House has devoted only one public speech to AIDS in the last four years. Congress slashed funding to the Ryan White Care Act this year, delivering less than a third of the emergency relief promised to the cities hardest hit by AIDS. Government funding of GMHC, once 35% of our budget, has fallen to 15%. That we have done so much with so little should make us proud—and angry.

Source: Jeff Soref and Timothy J. Sweeney, "Letter from the Board President and Executive Director," in *We Are All Living with AIDS*, Gay Men's Health Crisis 1991/1992 Annual Report (New York: Gay Men's Health Crisis, 1992), p. 2.

DOCUMENT 163: Slowly Confronting an Urban Crisis

The AIDS epidemic has had a devastating impact on cities like New York. Not only have the lives of thousands been affected, but the health care system, the courts and government itself have been challenged. New York City, a center of the epidemic in the United States, did not mobilize as quickly as it might have, nor did it anticipate the services or resources needed. The New York City Task Force on AIDS is made up of hospitals, AIDS service organizations, the city government, and the state government. In 1989, the task force revised upward previous estimates of the number of people with HIV disease who would require city services. The cost for providing these services—hospital and ambulatory care, nursing home beds, and special housing—would also be much greater than expected.

One day, historians will describe the Centers for Disease Control's first identification of the AIDS epidemic in the summer of 1981 as both a scientific and social turning point in our nation's history. Few of us then had any idea of the devastating impact these findings would have on a medical care system, a social service network, a set of laws, or, even, on our attitudes and lifestyles. A disease which affected only a handful of New Yorkers then, threatens thousands of New Yorkers today, and absent a cure and a vaccine, for the foreseeable future.

Since then [the late 1980s], historians will also report, the City of New York quantitatively increased and qualitatively improved the range of services it provided to meet both the medical and non-medical needs of those who have AIDS and to prevent its spread to those who do not. And they will report that these efforts were greatly assisted by a host of very dedicated individuals, organizations, and institutions which came forward to assist those of their friends, their relatives and strangers who had the misfortune to suffer from the disease.

In the face of the greatest public health problem of our generation, however, we must leave the writing of history to historians. Though we have done a great deal in the past seven years, this plan clearly demonstrates that we have a great deal left to do.

Source: "Executive Summary," in *New York City Strategic Plan for AIDS* (*New York*: Interagency Task Force on AIDS, May 1988), pp. 1–8.

DOCUMENT 164: The AIDS Commission Speaks Out Against Indifference

People who understand the true magnitude of the AIDS epidemic have a sense of urgency and crisis. This is in contrast to the attitudes of some national leaders. Instead of providing support and comfort, the response has been muted, even indifferent. This is particularly difficult for those who have suffered personally because it feels like an act of abandonment. In the 1991 report *America Living with AIDS*, the National Commission on AIDS criticized national leaders for not putting the epidemic at the top of the country's agenda. The commission believed former President Reagan, then President Bush, and the U.S. Congress were not willing to commit the necessary energy and resources to the crisis. In fact, some members of the Congress, such as Jesse Helms in the Senate and Bob Dornan in the House of Representatives, were actively working against AIDS funding.

Astonishingly, even our most basic efforts to better understand and respond to this new plague have been hampered. Efforts have been made to constrain or forbid behavioral research; in the face of the most deadly sexually transmitted disease ever to confront humanity, some would prohibit even the study of the human behaviors that put our children at risk. Thus we disarm ourselves in the midst of a lethal battle.

Worst of all, the country has responded with indifference. It is as if the HIV crisis were a televised portrayal of someone else's troubles. It has even appeared relatively painless; many of the torments are hidden because so many people do their suffering and grieving in secret, out of fear of stigma, discrimination, or rejection. But the epidemic will not remain painless much longer even for the most indifferent observer; soon everyone will know someone who has died of AIDS. If we are to honor our fundamental social contract with our fellow citizens, with ourselves, and with our children, we must somehow develop a sense of urgency. For there is only a little time left to recognize at a deep and fundamental level that the threat of HIV is all around us and that we must all join in this battle for the sake of future generations. In order to have any chance of winning, we must first energize our nation and transform indifference into informed action. We have used arresting language because Americans readily understand the need to mobilize rapidly for collective action in response to external threats to life. AIDS is a life-threatening disease of global proportions, and it requires the same national resolve and commitment to address it effectively as we exhibit in times of war. . . .

Our nation's leaders have not done well. In the past decade, the [Reagan/Bush] White House has rarely broken its silence on the topic of AIDS. Congress has shown leadership in developing critical legislation, but it has often failed to provide adequate funding for AIDS programs. Articulate leadership guiding Americans toward a proper response to AIDS has been notably absent. We are accustomed to hearing from the "bully pulpit" about national problems and how we should address them, so perhaps the public cannot be blamed for assuming that such a silence means that nothing important is happening. Their false calm is reinforced by politicians who declare that enough has been done about AIDS, since it is "just one disease," and that we should redirect our attention to other diseases that currently kill more people. . . .

There are two destructive attitudes within our borders that hamper these actions. They are a thinly veiled feeling that those who acquire the virus are getting what they deserve and a collective indifference to their fate. As long as these attitudes persist there will be reluctance to engage in the effort required to surmount HIV disease. Overcoming these attitudes will require leadership—leadership from the highest levels of government and the private sector.

Source: "Executive Summary," in *America Living with AIDS*, Report of the National Commission on Acquired Immunodeficiency Syndrome (Washington, D.C.: National Commission on AIDS, 1991), pp. 1–9.

POLITICAL ACTIVISM

DOCUMENT 165: Acting Up for Political Change

Founded in 1987, ACT-UP (the AIDS Coalition to Unleash Power) is a group dedicated to confrontational political action on AIDS issues. ACT-UP's famous logo is a combination of the words "SI-LENCE=DEATH" and an upside-down (inverted) pink triangle, a reminder of the symbol worn by homosexuals in Nazi concentration camps. The group's goals have been to speed up drug development, increase patient access to experimental drugs, and promote effective prevention strategies. The methods for achieving these ends have been nonviolent political action and civil disobedience. Although the group's sophisticated, theatrical protests may have alienated some people, ACT-UP has kept important issues before the public and forced decision-makers to search for solutions. Political pressure has been a decisive factor in bringing about major positive changes in the AIDS policies of drug companies and the government. Although the number of ACT-UP activists had dwindled during the mid-1990s, and the number of active chapters across the nation had declined, in 1997 ACT-UP had a major political action on Wall Street in New York, attacking the high price of the new protease inhibitor drugs and the windfall profits of some pharmaceutical corporations at the expense of people with AIDS.

"Before ACT-UP," says member Mark Harrington, 30, "I didn't have faith in mass political action—in *any* political action. I thought politics was the realm of hypocrisy and shallow platitudes. What impressed me was that I was in a room full of young people who didn't subscribe to the media's view that our generation was apolitical, careerist and materialistic. And anybody could speak, anybody could run for office—it was like ancient Athens."

Although ACT-UP personifies the age-old ideal of town meeting democracy, it is also thoroughly modern, shrewdly blending sixties style activism with the same tactics used by sophisticated political operatives, Spielbergian [referring to filmmaker Stephen Spielberg] spectacle and media manipulation. In an era of short attention spans, ACT-UP has kept its issues in the news with clever, witty and sometimes shocking demonstrations. Whether it's 1,500 people besieging the FDA [Food and Drug Administration] campus in Maryland with smoke bombs or eleven people handcuffing themselves to the New York office of a Japanese pharmaceutical firm, ACT-UP gets results.

ACT-UP has also given activism a fresh look. Its visual-arts collective, Gran Fury, has provided it with an eye-catching graphic campaign centered around the group's maxim, SILENCE=DEATH. In New York City, SILENCE=DEATH stickers—topped by the pink triangle the Nazis used to identify homosexuals, inverted—have become ubiquitous reminders on cash machines, newsstands, tollbooth buckets and pay phones. Gran Fury has also painted outlines of dead bodies in the street; opened *New York Times* vending boxes and wrapped each issue with an all-AIDS mockup called *New York Crimes*; and put politically charged ad parodies in the subways and buses. ACT-UP has developed a behind-the-scenes sophistication that has enabled it to have a major voice in governmental policy . . . [but] [a]long the way . . . [it] has alienated many.

Source: David Handleman, "ACT-UP in Anger," *Rolling Stone*, no. 573, pp. 80–88 (March 8, 1990).

DOCUMENT 166: Faith and AIDS Activism

This is a first-person account of a young theology student's experiences as a member of the AIDS Coalition to Unleash Power (ACT-UP), the AIDS activist group. Religious ideas of social justice and faith are an integral part of her political activism.

This September, instead of returning to Union Theological Seminary, I joined ACT-UP New York. As I learned more about AIDS, it had become a choice between sitting in my room crying and joining an organization that was doing all it could to end the epidemic. . . . And in the outrageously secular, sometimes sacrilegious community of ACT-UP, I'm learning something important about having faith in the face of life and death. . . .

My first action was a political funeral in Washington, D.C. in mid-October, during the display of the massive, ever-expanding Names Project Quilt. . . . It's the fusion of anger and grief enacted ritually in these funerals, enabling us to stick with the action that comes next . . . that I am beginning to understand as faith. Not crying hopelessly in my room, not hoping blindly that a cure and a health care system to make it available will somehow emerge . . . , but acknowledging my anger and grief in community, and acting with others to change history. This faith will keep us going.

Source: Irene Elizabeth Stroud, "Faith and Life (and Death) in ACT-UP," *Christianity and Crisis* 52(19): 420–421 (January 4, 1993).

DOCUMENT 167: As Impolite as the Virus

The writer Larry Kramer has spoken out frequently on AIDS issues and politics. As a leading AIDS activist and cofounder of the Gay Men's Health Crisis and ACT-UP, his opinions are widely followed. Before many others in the gay community, he understood the potential danger of the HIV/AIDS epidemic and worked to mobilize the gay community into action. He has written several books and plays, including *The Normal Heart* and *The Destiny of Me*, which are about experiencing AIDS and gay life. His screenplay for the film *Women in Love* earned an Academy Award nomination in 1969.

I have been fighting this plague for ten years. . . . Gay Men's Health Crisis (GMHC), the world's first service organization for those suffering from this disease, was started in my living room. It soon attracted thousands of volunteers . . . to help us take care of the dying and try to save those still living. We were not successful in either attempt. [Six years later] I founded the AIDS Coalition to Unleash Power (ACT-UP) to perform the necessary screaming and pressuring that GMHC was, and still is, too polite to perform. ACT-UP is impolite, abrasive, rude—like the virus that is killing us. . . .

[N]ow almost all my friends are dead. And my lover. And the odds are, I haven't that much longer myself. . . . I am so tired of screaming to a deaf world. I am so tired of being ignored and being left to die.

Source: Larry Kramer, "Ten Years of Plague: 110,530 Deaths . . . and Counting," *The Advocate*, no. 580, pp. 62–63 (July 2, 1991).

DOCUMENT 168: Proud and Angry

Confronted with the AIDS epidemic and people's anti-gay response, gay men and lesbians are often left feeling angry. ACT-UP and Queer Nation, a gay and lesbian political activist group, are organizations that provide a means to express these feelings in terms of political action. This selection helps the reader understand what it would be like if the same level of bigotry directed against gay men and lesbians were directed against your ethnic group or religion.

If you're straight, it may be hard to understand the need for an . . . in-your-face organization like Queer Nation. It may be hard to imagine the intricate combination of rage and terror that constitutes the gay Zeitgeist [the spirit of the time] of 1992. There's a virus ticking its way through the arteries of people we love. That would be enough to make us crazy, right there. But what's driven some of us around the bend is the fact that, even as our friends keep dying, the hatred of homosexuals flourishes.

Gay-bashing is up all over the country. Homophobia is thriving . . . and it comes as often as not in relatively subtle, nonviolent packages. Take Magic Johnson, for instance. Shortly after announcing he was HIV-positive, he inspired wild applause on the Arsenio Hall show when he said, "I'm nowhere near homosexual." People cheered. If you're a person of color, try to imagine a celebrity telling an appreciative audience, "I thank God I'm white!" If you're Jewish, imagine the same audience clapping and whistling when a celebrity announces, "No way am I a Jew."

If you're gay and you're not angry, you're not paying attention. . . . I believe the AIDS epidemic has taught us that nobody will listen unless we scream. But still, I'm plagued by doubts. At ACT-UP meetings, when members talk about planning a new action that will "show our anger," I find myself asking: What exactly do we expect people to do with our anger once we've shown it to them?

Source: Michael Cunningham, "If You're Queer and You're Not Angry in 1992, You're Not Paying Attention; If You're Straight, It May Be Hard to Figure Out What All the Shouting's About," *Mother Jones* 17(3): 60–68 (May–June 1992).

DOCUMENT 169: Federal Dollars Are Still Inadequate for the Growing Need

With the Clinton presidency, hopes were raised for stronger and more responsive leadership with regard to AIDS issues. Since his first election in 1992, Clinton has indeed proved to be more sympathetic toward AIDS issues. In addition, he created a White House Office of National AIDS Policy and a special panel to speed up the development of new drugs. A campaign to promote the use of latex condoms was started during his presidency. However, critics point out that he has not dramatically changed national priorities or substantially altered the way resources are allocated. All of the national AIDS policy coordinators were persons with little name recognition. AIDS service organizations continue to compete for scarce federal dollars. This passage is taken from a Project Inform publication. Project Inform is a nonprofit information service on drugs and treatment options for people who are HIV-infected and their caregivers.

Sixteen months into the new [Clinton] Administration in Washington, it is clear that the change of political stewardship has not made a major difference for people living with AIDS. High hopes that the sympathetic tone of the new Administration would translate into better policy, faster research, or an improved prevention effort have come crashing back to reality. Whether this is due to any fault of the [Clinton] Administration, or just a consequence of unrealistic expectations, is open for debate. At the very least, there is little evidence that this Administration has made AIDS any more of a national priority than the previous one. . . .

The nightly news, and the President's attention, is dominated by crime, the economy, foreign and military affairs and general health care concerns. While the Administration is struggling to convince the public that a few more million dollars for care and research programs is a big step forward, we learn that $750 million in new money has been allocated to support US companies manufacturing lightweight color computer screens, that billion-dollar military spy satellites are lining up on the launch pad, and that the 1995 budget for nuclear weapons development exceeds $24 billion. There has been no Bill Clinton "Town Meeting on AIDS." The President appeared twice on MTV, but has yet to take questions at an AIDS service organization. Leaders of the automotive industry have been escorted into the Oval Office to collaborate with the government on making more fuel efficient cars, and Hollywood stars have been given phone lines and office space in the White House, but AIDS researchers have had no such access and no such invitation. At best, AIDS has provided an occasional photo-opportunity for a few people to pose with the President.

Source: "AIDS Research & Politics in 1994—Are You Better Off Today . . . ?" *PI Perspective*, no. 14, pp. 1–3 (June 1994).

DOCUMENT 170: The Changing Political Climate

As the political climate grew more conservative after the congressional elections of 1994 and 1996, both the AIDS and the gay/lesbian political communities began to turn to Republican consultants to learn how to interact effectively with politicians who often do not share the same ideas on, and are less supportive of, AIDS and gay/lesbian issues. It has become necessary to shift strategies away from grassroots activism to strategic lobbying.

As AIDS and [gay/lesbian] groups revise their strategies to accommodate the Republican Congress, they are increasingly turning to GOP [Grand Old Party, or Republican] consultants for help. Proponents of the strategy claim that this is how the game is played, and that the use of [public relations] firms and political consultants is a long-overdue step toward making the two movements [AIDS and gay/lesbian] more professional. "People involved in the different movements need to adapt the techniques that work, whether or not they view them as correct," says Andrew Barrer, a former senior advisor in the White House Office on AIDS Policy. But others argue that professional packaging is not a substitute for grassroots activism, and could even divert resources from the unglamorous work involved in AIDS and gay[/lesbian] issues. The new tactics emphasize the general lack of contingency plans that left many groups struggling when the Republicans won last fall. "We had such strong relationships with key congressional offices under the old regime that we might not have done all the work we really needed to do to . . . forge new relationships with a wide range of offices," admits Mike Isbell of the Gay Men's Health Crisis [the nation's largest AIDS service organization].

Source: John Gallagher, "Money Talks," *Advocate*, no. 686, p. 41 (July 25, 1995); CDC National AIDS Clearinghouse (Bethesda, Md.: Information, Inc., 1995).

SUGGESTED READINGS

Altman, Dennis. *AIDS in the Mind of America*. New York: Anchor Press, 1986.

Arno, P. "The Nonprofit Sector's Response to the AIDS Epidemic: Community-Based Services in San Francisco." *American Journal of Public Health* 76, pp. 1325–1330 (November 1986).

"Arthur Ashe AIDS Tennis Challenge Rallies Support of Celebrities." *Jet* 86, p. 48 (September 19, 1994).

Becker, Gary S. "The Painful Political Truth About Medical Research." *Business Week* no. 3486, p. 18 (July 29, 1996).

Berke, R. L. "Time Bomb in the White House." *The New York Times Magazine*, pp. 28–29 (June 6, 1993).

"Black Clergy Gather to Fight AIDS." *The Christian Century* 110, p. 1009 (October 20, 1993).

Carey, J. "What Happened to the War on AIDS?" *Business Week*, p. 34 (July 25, 1994).

"Clinton and AIDS." *The New Republic* 211, p. 7 (December 26, 1994).

Cohen, J. "A 'Manhattan Project' for AIDS?" *Science* 259, pp. 1112–1114 (February 19, 1993).

Coleman, J. A. "ACT-UP vs. the Church." *Commonweal* 118, pp. 533–535 (September 27, 1991).

Cowley, G. "The Angry Politics of Kemron." *Newsweek* 121, pp. 43–44 (January 4, 1993).

Cowley, G., and M. Hager. "The Politics of the Plague." *Newsweek* 122, p. 62 (August 9, 1993).

Decter, M. "Homosexuality and the Schools." *Commentary* 95, p. 1925 (March 1993).

Feldman, Douglas A. "AIDS and Social Change." *Human Organization* 44, pp. 343–348 (Winter 1985).

Fiore, Faye. "White House AIDS Activist Falls into Political Exile." *Los Angeles Times*, p. A1 (September 11, 1995).

Foreman, C. H. "AIDS and the Limits of Czardom." *Brookings Review* 11, pp. 18–21 (Summer 1993).

Gehrke, Donna. "Star Power Pumps Up AIDS Walk." *Miami Herald*, p. 4B (February 24, 1997).

Herczog, M., and S. Hochmann. "Rock Against AIDS, 1993." *Rolling Stone*, pp. 15–16 (April 29, 1993).

"In Search of Unapproved Drugs." *American Health* 12, p. 80 (October 1993).

Kayal, Philip M. *Bearing Witness: Gay Men's Health Crisis & the Politics of AIDS.* Boulder, Colo.: Westview Press, 1993.

Krieger, Nancy, and Glen Margo, eds. *AIDS: The Politics of Survival.* Amityville, N.Y.: Baywood, 1994.

Krim, Mathilde. "Making Experimental Drugs Available for AIDS Treatment." *AIDS and Public Policy Journal* 2 (2), pp. 1ff. (Spring/Summer 1987).

Leo, J. "Tribalism in the Newsroom?" *U.S. News & World Report* 115, p. 18 (December 6, 1993).

Milling, T. J. "A Trek Across U.S. to Help AIDS Children." *Houston Chronicle*, p. 13A (March 3, 1997).

Morgan, L. "AIDS Disinformation." *Seventeen* 51, pp. 73–74 (September 1992).

"The Other Drug War." *The New Republic* 211, p. 9 (October 17, 1994).

Payne, Kenneth, and Stephen Risch. "The Politics of AIDS." *Science for the People* 16 (5), pp. 17–24 (September/October 1984).

Ribadeneira, Diego. "Hands Together Against AIDS." *Boston Globe*, p. B1 (February 24, 1997).

Rosin, H. "Bad Blood: AIDS Activists vs. the HIV Home Test." *The New Republic* 210, pp. 12ff. (June 27, 1994).

Savage, Dan. "The AIDS Crisis Is Over—for Me." *Village Voice*, p. 34 (February 25, 1997).

Schmalz, J. "Whatever Happened to AIDS?" *The New York Times Magazine*, pp. 57–61 (November 28, 1993).

Smith, R. L. "Gays and Bishops: Searching for Common Ground." *America* 171, pp. 12–17 (September 24, 1994).

Viano, E. "Economics: Health and Unequal Opportunity: The Battle for Federal Dollars." *USA Today*, pp. 22–24 (July 1, 1993).

Wadman, Meredith. "NIH Bucks Political Trend to Win Increased Funds from Congress." *Nature* 381 (6584), p. 633 (June 20, 1996).

Winokur, L. A. "Larry Kramer [interview]." *The Progressive* 58, pp. 32–35 (June 1994).

York, B., and J. Johns. "Another AIDS Scam." *The American Spectator* 26, pp. 49–50 (August 1993).

Zuniga, Jo Ann. "Residential AIDS Treatment Program for the Poor to End." *Houston Chronicle*, p. 30A (March 13, 1997).

7

Education and Behavioral Change

In September 1985, dozens of angry parents marched with picket signs in front of a public elementary school in a residential neighborhood of New York City. It had previously been announced that a child with AIDS was attending the school, and the parents wanted the child removed. They were fearful that the child could somehow infect their own children with HIV. Back then, there was much less awareness about how HIV can and cannot be transmitted from one person to another. Clearly, education about HIV and AIDS has dramatically changed how we perceive the risk of the virus, the disease, and people infected with the virus. Today we know, for example, that the child was not a risk to the other children, and there was no reasonable basis for excluding the child from classes.

Since AIDS is a sexually transmitted disease, disproportionately affects gay men, has been until recently a universally lethal disease, and is also transmitted through infected needles during recreational drug use by "drug addicts," it has become a highly stigmatized and greatly feared disease. People often feel "dirty" or "polluted" just touching, or even coming close to, someone with such a highly stigmatized disease. Only intensive and accurate education can dispel the myths that have evolved around AIDS.

Education alone rarely leads to significant and permanent behavioral change. For example, in spite of the dire health warnings on cigarette packages, millions of American teenagers start smoking each year. However, research conducted in the late 1980s and early 1990s definitely shows that risk reduction workshops for persons at high risk for HIV infection will succeed in decreasing the likelihood that the workshop participants will become HIV-positive. The workshops are designed to increase not only the participants' knowledge and awareness about HIV and AIDS, but also their self-esteem, desire to change their risky behavior, capability of changing that behavior, and skills to achieve these goals through role-playing and negotiating techniques for safer sex.

While we know that these HIV prevention workshops will save lives, the cost of providing them to all of the millions of Americans at high risk for HIV infection who would benefit by such an intervention is considered prohibitively expensive. Today, more cost-effective approaches to changing behavior at the community level are being studied by social scientists who are looking at the social networks of people at greater risk for HIV.

PROMOTING AWARENESS AND EDUCATION

DOCUMENT 171: AIDS Awareness Becomes Part of School Programs

Schools now acknowledge that educating children and young people about AIDS and HIV infection is important. Prevention programs for all age groups have been instituted or are being planned throughout most of the country. The majority of states require HIV education in schools. Knowing the facts can help students make decisions to avoid risky behavior and prevent infection. In addition, education programs can help them cope with the reality of classmates, friends, or family members who are HIV-positive.

School systems across the country have sought CDC's assistance in designing, implementing, and evaluating HIV prevention programs that meet the needs of the students and their communities. From 1981 through the end of June 1992, 756 children between the ages of 5 and 12 were diagnosed with AIDS. Most of these cases represent infections the children acquired from their mothers before or during birth. Programs must continue to be implemented in schools to help teachers, parents, and other students understand the disease and deal compassionately with students who are HIV-infected or living with AIDS.

Students who inject drugs and/or are sexually active are just as vulnerable to HIV infection and other sexually transmitted diseases as their adult counterparts.... Since one in five of all reported AIDS cases is diagnosed in young adults 20 to 29 years of age, and the average incubation period between HIV infection and AIDS diagnosis is about 10 years, it's clear that many of those people in their 20's who have AIDS . . . were teenagers when they became infected.

Older teens, males, and racial and ethnic minority teens are disproportionately affected by AIDS. However, the proportion of females among U.S. adolescent cases has more than doubled [from 1987 to 1992]. . . . CDC data indicate that 37 percent of U.S. adolescent females who were reported to have AIDS in 1991 contracted the virus through heterosexual contact, yet most American teens still engage in sexual behaviors that could result in their infection. A . . . national CDC survey showed that 54 percent of U.S. teenagers in grades 9 through 12 had engaged in sexual intercourse.

Even more worrisome, about one in eight 9th graders reported having four or more sex partners, and this proportion increased by grade, reaching one in four among 12th graders. Of these students with multiple sex partners, only 41 percent reported using condoms at last sexual intercourse.

Additionally, 1 in 70 high school students reported illegal drug injection (more boys than girls, and more often among those who also reported multiple sex partners). . . . CDC HIV prevention efforts . . . focus on the 58 million primary, secondary, and college students in the United States . . . [and] encourage programs that begin in elementary school. These programs are designed to help students refrain from initiating unhealthy behaviors in the first place.

For students who engage in unsafe behaviors despite the health risks, CDC helps schools plan and implement HIV prevention programs that meet locally determined standards. These programs are designed to (a) help students stop engaging in sexual activity and/or drug use or (b) teach them effective methods to limit their risks of HIV infection.

Source: "Preventing Risk Behaviors Among Students," *HIV/AIDS Prevention Newsletter* 3(3): 1–2 (1992).

DOCUMENT 172: AIDS Prevention in New York City

Since New York City is one of the key centers of the epidemic in the United States, AIDS education and prevention efforts among young people there are especially critical. The New York City AIDS Task Force, which includes members or staff of hospitals, community groups, medical organizations, and government, developed a comprehensive plan for health education. HIV education becomes part of the broader context of coping with drug use, sex, and human relationships. Prevention programs also need to reinforce students' social skills and

emotional strength. In order to avoid risk, knowledge must be trans-
lated into action.

AIDS education directed to children and young adults must increase
their knowledge of AIDS, their perceptions of risk, their sense of self-
esteem, and the repertoire of social skills that will enable them to protect
themselves against infection. City and State agencies must also expand
drug prevention programs to reduce the chance that a new epidemic of
heroin use might expose an even larger portion of the City's young people to HIV infection.

AIDS education efforts will be directed at children and young adults
as part of a long-range educational plan to discourage their exposure to
health risks. Beyond specific education about AIDS in school science curricula, this effort will take place within and alongside more comprehensive education to shape attitudes about drug use, sex, and human
relationships. With age-appropriate curricula, it will communicate specific risk-reduction information.

Source: "Prevention," in *New York City Strategic Plan for AIDS* (New York: Interagency Task Force on AIDS, May 1988), section D.4, pp. 1–11.

DOCUMENT 173: The Role of Counseling and Testing in HIV Prevention

Counseling and testing programs are major components of federal and
state efforts to educate people whose behavior has put them at risk for
HIV infection. By making anonymous or confidential services accessible, these programs encourage people to step forward, learn the facts
about their risks, be tested for HIV, and be advised and strengthened
as to their future actions. The goals of counseling are to help uninfected
individuals remain HIV-negative and to help people who are HIV-
positive practice safer behaviors. Anonymous HIV test sites have provided services to a growing number of clients. In 1985, 79,000 tests
were done; by 1997, many millions of tests were being conducted.
Home HIV test kits are now sold at drugstores throughout the country.

Human immunodeficiency virus (HIV) counseling and testing services
provided by health departments are a major component of the national
HIV-prevention program. The purpose of HIV [counseling and testing]
is to 1) reinforce perception of risk by those who are unaware or uninformed, 2) help uninfected persons initiate and sustain behavior changes
that reduce their risk for becoming infected, and 3) identify HIV-infected

persons who can be referred for early medical care and counseled to practice safer behaviors. The use of publicly funded HIV [counseling and testing] has steadily increased; in 1991, nearly 2,091,000 HIV-antibody tests were performed, compared with approximately 79,000 [six years earlier].

Source: "Publicly Funded HIV Counseling and Testing—United States, 1991," *Morbidity and Mortality Weekly Report* 41(34): 613–617 (August 28, 1992).

DOCUMENT 174: The Message Must Be Culturally Appropriate

The cultural context of prevention messages is critical for their understanding and acceptance by the target audience. Sensitivity in the selection of the language, images, and suggestions helps avoid misinterpretation. For example, men who have sex with gay men, but think of themselves as heterosexual (not gay), will not respond to messages addressed to the gay community. Advertising executives and market research professionals, who are experienced in fitting messages into the appropriate context, have participated in public health campaigns on AIDS and HIV prevention. In 1994, the Centers for Disease Control and Prevention in Atlanta began a new initiative to prevent sexual transmission of HIV among young adults. This campaign combines techniques of advertising and marketing with those of the social sciences to promote the use of latex condoms or abstinence from sexual intercourse.

No matter how precisely a research or intervention program is targeted towards a specific subgroup, it will not be effective if it fails to communicate in a culturally appropriate manner. For example, a communication that refers to "homosexual" or "gay" behavior may be particularly ineffective in a Latino community in which only the "feminine," passive role in male–male anal intercourse is considered to be homosexual behavior. Similarly, an intervention designed to introduce condom use in married households may not be effective in households in which condom use is not already known. A woman suggesting condom use to her husband would be implying extramarital sexual activity, either by her or her husband. For some women, this would place them in danger of battering or abuse by their husbands. In other households, people may be embarrassed to talk about condoms, and, more [important], they may have misconceptions about how condoms are used that will negatively influence their [receptivity] to the intervention message.

For example . . . many [Latina] women are afraid that condoms will be lost [inside] their bodies.

Interventions that do not take into account the culturally specific dynamics of socio-sexual relations—for example, who has power and how that power is manifested—also will not be effective. . . . The difference in power between men and women in how they negotiate sexual interaction will affect the willingness of each party in a relationship to insist upon the use of condoms. On the other hand, interventions that focus on culturally relevant issues and norms will be particularly effective. . . .

Context [and] cultural [practices are] critical in developing a research or intervention program. Individuals' sexual identity, perception of risk, and willingness to listen to a particular message or to participate in a study will all vary according to context. This, where a study is being conducted or a message is being [spread], will have a profound effect on the amount and validity of the data collected or on the effectiveness of the intervention. . . . Often a message will be most effective if it is [spread] close to the site of sexual activity. Because risk taking may be part of the pleasure associated with some sexual behavior, . . . a message close to the action is more likely to be attended to. In addition, because there are often social norms already operating at the site of the sexual activity, those norms may help to reinforce the message.

Source: Behaviorally Bisexual Men and AIDS: Executive Summary of a Workshop Sponsored by the CDC, October 18–19, 1989 (Washington, D.C.: American Institutes for Research, 1990), pp. 1–22.

DOCUMENT 175: Who Should Determine What the AIDS Curriculum Should Be?

In order to be effective, AIDS education must be factual and straightforward. This is difficult when public health objectives conflict with parents' moral or religious beliefs. Parents and religious groups have often dictated what the sex education and AIDS curricula should be throughout the United States, frequently insisting that these topics be discussed only in high school (if at all), and that only abstinence messages be allowed. Explicit discussions about safer sex practices and role-playing for negotiating skills for safer sex are not permitted in many schools. However, children and teenagers need to think about issues like drug use, sex, and birth control before they find themselves in a situation that might endanger their health. Many teenagers are not only becoming infected with HIV. They are also getting gonorrhea, chlamydia, herpes, syphilis, chancroid, hepatitis, and other sexually transmissible diseases. Perhaps most alarming of all is the increasing rate of teenage pregnancies. Infants are being born to teenage mothers who are financially and emotionally ill-equipped to take care of their new-born child.

AIDS is a public health issue. The school as a representative of the public interest has a responsibility to teach the facts necessary to reduce the spread of AIDS. To properly teach these facts the school must present information that some parents find objectionable on moral and religious grounds.

For example, education about AIDS requires that children be taught the basic facts about sex, birth control, and drug abuse. It is apparent that the most effective approach is to present this information *before* the children become involved in sexual activity and drug abuse. It is not enough for schools to support sexual and drug abstinence. Children need to know the facts so that over time they can make decisions based upon sound knowledge. If this were a perfect society, moral persuasion would be sufficient to reduce the spread of AIDS. The teenage pregnancy rate shows, however, that this is not a perfect society. Public health issues demand a broad, reasoned, educational approach to AIDS. The general adult tendency to want to shield children from unpleasant realities must, in this instance, yield to the imperative of providing children with life-saving information.

Source: Elizabeth P. Lamers, "Public Schools Confront AIDS," in I. B. Corless and M. Pittman-Lindeman, eds., *AIDS: Principles, Practices, & Politics* (Washington, D.C.: Hemisphere, 1988), pp. 175–185.

DOCUMENT 176: Taking HIV Prevention Seriously in the Schools

There are public officials who have taken aggressive action with regard to HIV/AIDS education. For example in Maryland, the Montgomery County Task Force on HIV/AIDS recommended to the Board of Education that comprehensive HIV education begin at an early age and that condom availability programs be part of the overall plan. The school systems of Washington, D.C., and Alexandria, Virginia, already have condom availability programs in place. A realistic approach to intervention treats controversial subjects with sensitivity, but does not avoid effective action. At lower grade levels, basic concepts of good health and hygiene would be taught. Sexual decision-making and risk-taking would be introduced at higher grade levels, or where there is research indicating that many of the students are already sexually active.

Pointing to prevention as the only way around the AIDS crisis . . . [Montgomery County officials] said [they] should focus on a sweeping education program about the disease, including classes [about AIDS] as early as kindergarten. The task force also recommended [a study regarding] the "feasibility of a condom availability program in junior and senior high school."

Source: Arlo Wagner, "Panel Suggests Kindergarten AIDS Classes," *The Washington Times*, p. B1 (July 13, 1993).

DOCUMENT 177: HIV Prevention Materials for Gay Men

Senator Jesse Helms, a strident conservative, and Senator Lowell Weicker, a liberal, represent different views along the political spectrum. In this selection, Senator Helms speaks first, followed by Senator Weicker. Their debate on funding AIDS education focused attention on printed educational materials for gay men. Senator Helms is repulsed by homosexual behavior and particularly upset that federal funds are being used to educate gay men in what he sees as a sexually suggestive way. The concern was that federal funds might have been used to encourage and condone homosexuality. Senator Helms assumes that there is something basically wrong with being gay, but ignores the fact that gay men are citizens and taxpayers, too. Senator Weicker, without challenging Senator Helms's assumption, responds by pointing out that federal dollars fund research and care for other diseases caused by high-risk behaviors, and that AIDS should be no exception. Nevertheless, a version of Helms's amendment passed in Congress, and the Centers for Disease Control and Prevention restricted funding of educational materials that might be considered offensive. In 1992, a federal court ruled that this restriction on educational materials was unconstitutional. Below is the text of the amendment offered by Senator Helms and the transcript of what was said to support or oppose the amendment by the senators.

Amendment No. 956:

Purpose: To prohibit the use of any funds provided under this Act to the Centers for Disease Control [and Prevention] from being used to provide AIDS education, information, or prevention materials and activities that promote, encourage, or condone homosexual activities or the intravenous use of illegal drugs.

MR. HELMS: . . . The amendment I will be calling up shortly will offer some assurance that the hard-earned tax dollars of the American people are not to be used to perpetuate the AIDS problem. Specifically, my amendment states that any funds authorized under this act shall not be used to promote, condone, or encourage sexual activity outside a sexually monogamous marriage, including homosexual activity, or the intravenous use of illegal drugs. . . . This Senator was naive enough at one time to believe that AIDS education meant simply telling people about the deadly AIDS virus. How wrong I was!

About 2 months ago, I received a copy of some AIDS comic books that are being distributed by the Gay Men's Health Crisis, Inc., of New York City, an organization which has received $674,679 in Federal dollars for so-called AIDS education and information. These comic books told the story, in graphic detail, of the sexual encounter of two homosexual men.

The comic books do not . . . change any of the perverted sexual behavior. In fact, the comic book promotes sodomy and the homosexual lifestyle as an acceptable alternative in American society. . . . These comic books, widely distributed, were defended by Mr. Frank Lilly, former vice president and a founding member of the Gay Men's Health Crisis, who currently serves on the President's AIDS commission. Mr. Lilly proclaimed that the comic books are a valid method of educating homosexuals. I do not agree. I think that anybody who would take a look at this material would agree with me. I am restraining myself in describing it. I believe that if the American people saw these books, they would be on the verge of revolt.

I obtained one copy of this book and I had photostats made for about 15 or 20 Senators. I sent each of the Senators a copy . . . in a brown envelope marked "Personal and Confidential, for Senator's Eyes Only." Without exception, the Senators were revolted and they suggested to me that President Reagan ought to know what is being done under the pretense of AIDS education.

So, about 10 days ago, I went down to the White House and I visited with the President.

I said, "Mr. President, I don't want to ruin your day, but I feel obliged to hand you this and let you look at what is being distributed under the pretense of AIDS educational material. Furthermore, Mr. President, this group that produced this book and which is circulating it has received over $600,000 in Federal funds from your Administration."

The President opened the book, looked at a couple of pages, closed it up, and shook his head, and hit his desk with his fist [in anger]. . . .

Some Senators may believe sincerely that the AIDS epidemic has reached such grave proportions that we must disseminate whatever materials anybody wants to produce regardless of the content. . . . But I tell you this, . . . we can talk about condoms and clean needles until we are blue in the face, but until we are ready and willing to discourage and do our dead level best to eliminate the types of activities which have caused the spread of the AIDS epidemic, I do not believe we are ever going to solve it.

Many of the experts . . . tell us that the source of the AIDS epidemic is the AIDS virus. That is like saying that the source of a fire set by an arsonist was the match that the arsonist used, rather than the arsonist who struck the match and set the fire. . . .

MR. WEICKER: Let me present a few remarks, if I might, on what confronts us here. I know of no one who is standing up here and advocating any particular course of personal activity, and I suppose that it would be very easy to get drawn off into an argument as to what is appropriate and what is not appropriate sexual behavior.

Neither I nor the nation has the time to do that. We are confronted with an epidemic, the likes of which this world has never seen, and we do not have time to get into philosophical, academic, or moralistic debates. We better do exactly what we have been told to do by those of science and medicine, which is, No. 1, put our money into research and, No. 2, put our money into education.

This is what we have done traditionally. Whatever the ailment or the hurt was, we did not ask how you got it. If you hurt, if you are down, if you are sick, this nation traditionally has gone to your side without asking any questions.

If we are going to get into the business of moral judgments, then maybe we should ask why we spend money on research insofar as it would help those who have cirrhosis of the liver, which comes from drinking.

Or what about the billions of dollars which have been spent on other sexually transmitted diseases—gonorrhea, syphilis. I can go down a whole list, of federal health research activities, costing in the billions of dollars. When did we ask anyone or when did we try to pass moral judgment on those who acquired one of these particular diseases? Maybe we should ask the question of those who smoke, why should we put our money into cancer research.

I am not equipped to pass moral judgment on my neighbors. I go by a very simple criterion: If somebody is ill, then they deserve the help of their government. . . .

. . . It is also important that the people of this nation understand there is a leadership that leads us toward our best ideals, toward our best instincts, and that we do not wallow in fear and that we do not moralize, we do not point our finger at our neighbor when he or she is hurting. . . .

. . . For the problems that have been caused in this nation by particular types of activity, whether it is drug use or homosexual activity, never before have we rationed our commitment to the cure based on a particular set of values or a particular lecture in morals. I heard the term "God's punishment," but I know what the American response ought to be to a disease.

Source: *Congressional Record—Senate*, pp. S-14202–S-14213 (October 14, 1987).

DOCUMENT 178: Targeting Specific Groups

In the mid- and late 1980s, it was thought that the explosion of AIDS cases in the gay community and among injecting drug users would soon also occur among the total population of the United States. So far, that has not happened. Today, while it is still true that safer sex should be practiced by everyone involved in premarital, nonmarital, or extramarital relationships, it has become clear that HIV prevention campaigns should be targeted to those people who are at greatest risk: men who have sex with men, injecting drug users, crack users, and some minority men and women.

An article appearing in the *Wall Street Journal* on May 1, [1996] entitled "AIDS Fight Is Skewed by Federal Campaign Exaggerating Risks," has stirred concerns among AIDS activists and scientists. The article presented the case that a campaign launched by the Centers for Disease Control and Prevention in 1987 gave the public the alarming misperception that anyone was at risk for HIV. While the article acknowledged that the message was technically correct, it held that the campaign ignored the higher risk of certain groups, including gay men and [injecting] drug users. Most scientists and activists dispute the article's claims that the CDC exaggerated risks or misdirected prevention efforts to secure federal funds. They also say combined prevention and awareness efforts are needed for both those at especially high risk for AIDS and the general population. Ronald O. Valdiserri, deputy director of CDC's National Center for HIV, STD, and TB Prevention in Atlanta, says the article "embodied a simplistic view of HIV prevention." Many scientists say the CDC's campaign was fair in light of the lack of HIV/AIDS information available at the time. But, they add, now that more is known about the virus and the disease, the government's AIDS budget needs to be reallocated to target specific groups.

Source: Steven Benowitz, "AIDS Researchers, Activists Wary of Newspaper Article's Message," *Scientist* 10(12): 1 (June 10, 1996); CDC National AIDS Clearinghouse (Bethesda, Md.: Information, Inc., 1996).

DOCUMENT 179: Educating PWAs About New and Deadly Risks in Managing AIDS Treatments

Today, it appears that AIDS is no longer a universally fatal disease. From preliminary data, it is believed that AIDS can be successfully managed through the use of new medications, including protease inhibitors. One of the protease inhibitors is Ritonavir. However, it is now known that mixing Ritonavir with certain recreational drugs, such as "ecstasy," can result in death. It is important that messages about possible lethal drug interactions reach persons with AIDS (PWAs) who are on the new medications as soon as possible.

Following the death of a British AIDS patient who was taking the protease inhibitor Ritonavir when he died from an overdose of MDMA, or "ecstasy," Ritonavir maker Abbott Laboratories has acknowledged potentially dangerous interactions between the two. The coroner said that Phillip Kay died from an MDMA overdose, with a blood level "nearly ten times that at which we would expect to see serious toxic effects." Kay's partner, Jim Lumb, suspected a drug interaction was the cause because he was sure that Kay would not have taken such an excessive dose. Abbott's Dr. P. Kon wrote to Lumb that "Abbott has not conducted, and does not plan on conducting any drug–drug interaction studies between Ritonavir and any illegal substances, including ecstasy." However, he noted that the lab's researchers had studied the theoretical interactions between the two drugs. They found, according to Kon, that using the two drugs together could result in "a two to three fold increase" in MDMA levels and that in 3 percent to 10 percent of the population, MDMA levels could increase "as high as five to ten fold." Abbott refused to issue a warning, as Lumb had requested, but the company has made a fact sheet available to British doctors who request the information.

Source: Bruce Mirken, "Danger: Possibly Fatal Interactions Between Ritonavir and 'Ecstasy,' Some Other Psychoactive Drugs,"*AIDS Treatment News*, no. 265, p. 5 (February 21, 1997).

PRODUCING BEHAVIORAL CHANGE

DOCUMENT 180: A Psychological Model for Behavioral Change

Education by itself rarely produces behavioral change. What people know about health risks and what they actually do to prevent these risks are often inconsistent. Someone may know that semen can be infected with HIV, and yet not use a condom with a partner whose HIV status is unknown. This gap between knowledge and behavior can be explained by the fact that behavioral change is a complex process, and not usually an instant one. Most often, change occurs gradually, and in stages. The "model" of behavioral change described here is useful as a way of thinking about how best to influence people's sexual and drug use behaviors. Interventions should take into consideration an individual's relationship to these stages. The stages described in this reading include thinking about changing one's behavior, getting ready to change one's behavior, actually making the change, and making sure that the change is permanent. This model, called the "transtheoretical" or "stages of change" model, is psychological, focusing upon the individual. Other models for understanding how changes occur in people are being developed by anthropologists and sociologists who are looking at social networks and changes that occur on a larger scale within communities.

Since the success of HIV prevention programs relies on their ability to change specific behaviors, accurate assessment of behavior change is crucial. . . . Behavioral science research suggests that the process of adopting a new behavior or eliminating a risky one is complex and tends to occur [step by step] as individuals slowly progress through a series of [mental], emotional, and behavioral changes.

Measuring only specific program outcomes, such as rates of condom use, may mask meaningful progress toward making changes in complex behaviors. Some behavioral scientists at [the] CDC have used the stages of change model . . . as a . . . framework for the measurement of behavior change. . . . This . . . model describes health behavior change as a gradual, continuous, and dynamic process. . . . According to the model, people do not move directly from old behaviors to new behaviors, but progress through a sequence of five discrete stages:

Precontemplative: Individuals in this stage have no intention to change their behavior. (They are unaware of the risk, deny the adverse outcome could happen to them, or *are* aware of the risk but have made a decision not to change their behavior.)

Contemplative: People in this stage have formed intentions to change, but have no specific plans to change in the near future.

Ready for action: These people have plans to change their behavior in the immediate future and may have taken some initial actions.

Action: People in this stage have begun changing their behavior, but the behavior change is relatively recent and may be inconsistent.

Maintenance: These people have maintained consistent behavior change for an extended period of time; the newly acquired behavior has become a part of their lives.

The pace of these stages varies greatly. . . . Some individuals may remain in the contemplative stage for months, even years. Also, once a person initiates a behavior change, that person is vulnerable to relapse at any time, and therefore may cycle back through the stages repeatedly. This model has implications for . . . public health interventions . . . [and] suggests that prevention messages should be targeted to the stage of behavior change [that] individuals are in. . . .

Source: "A Conceptual Framework for Evaluating Behavior Change," *HIV/AIDS Prevention* 3(4): pp. 2–3 (1992).

DOCUMENT 181: It Takes "Two to Tango"

At first, simply "getting out the message" about HIV was thought to be enough. This way of thinking proved to be too simplistic. Human behavior, especially with regard to sex and drugs, is highly complex and resistant to change. Even when individuals want to change, their partners and friends may not support this goal and may, in fact, oppose their efforts. Unless you are sexually active within a long-term (meaning several years, not several months), mutually faithful, and monogamous relationship and know for certain that your partner has repeatedly tested HIV-negative, you should always automatically assume that your partner is HIV-positive and act accordingly by practicing safer sex. Nearly half of all Americans who are HIV-positive do not know that they are positive. If you know you are HIV-positive, it is your responsibility to practice safer sex to protect your partner from becoming infected, and to avoid the possibility of getting reinfected with a different strain or of getting a different kind of infection that may interact with HIV to make your health worse. If you know you are HIV-negative, it is your responsibility to protect yourself from becoming infected with HIV or any other kind of sexually transmitted disease. Latex condoms and other forms of safer sex must routinely be used if you are sexually active.

Just as there is no therapeutic "magic bullet," there is no educational panacea. Early optimism, even naiveté, which saw prevention as a simple matter of telling people to stop risky sexual and drug-using behaviors, has given way to a sober recognition of the complexities of changing human behavior. Clearly there is a need for a deeper understanding of intimate, private, and largely unexplored aspects of life. Prevention is a complex problem that calls for changes in deeply rooted attitudes and behavior by individuals, partners in sexual and drug-using relationships, and by society in general. Nothing less than a shift in basic social attitudes is required. . . .

Infected individuals bear the primary responsibility of preventing transmission because only they have the ability to control risky behaviors. But the responsibility does not lie with them alone. By definition risky behaviors involve two people, and the relationship between them. Either partner may initiate behavior change, but it must be mutually acceptable in order to be sustained. Uninfected persons must learn how to protect themselves, since not all those who are infected know that fact or have fully accepted their responsibilities to prevent transmission. . . .

The social climate in which risk-reduction messages are communicated is an important factor in their acceptability. The stigma and discrimination surrounding AIDS must be eliminated not just because of the resultant injustices but because negative attitudes and actions deter prevention efforts. Because of the stigma, those who engage in risky behavior may deny their risk, even to themselves, and may avoid counseling and other educational efforts.

Source: AIDS Prevention and Education: Reframing the Message, Report, Citizen's Commission on AIDS for New York City and Northern New Jersey (New York: *The Commission*, February 1991).

DOCUMENT 182: Increasing Condom Sales to Women

Social marketing, using marketing to produce social and behavioral change, has been used to promote condom use in many nations throughout the world. In the United States, too, the increasing availability of condoms in supermarkets and discount drugstores is doing much to change the attitudes about condoms and increase their use. Today, condoms are rarely hidden on the pharmacist's upper shelf behind the counter, as they often were only a decade ago.

Renewed interest in condoms, which is attributed to increased vendor support, improved products, and studies that promote condom use to prevent pregnancy and sexually transmitted diseases, should thus lead to increased sales of the contraceptives in supermarkets. Hisayuki Naito, of Okamoto U.S.A., says supermarket condom sales stand to increase as more women are buying condoms. Women now buy at least 60 per-cent—and possibly up to 80 percent—of all condoms. Supermarkets command 16 percent of the $270 million condom market. To further their sales, supermarkets are therefore improving their presentation of con-doms, as well as increasing the roles of coupons and advertising in con-dom sales.

Source: "A Resurgence for Condoms?" *Supermarket Business* 52(8): 73 (August 1996); CDC National AIDS Clearinghouse (Bethesda, Md.: Information, Inc., 1996).

DOCUMENT 183: Negotiated Safety: Safer Sex One Can Live With

The concept of "negotiated safety" argues that people at high risk for HIV need to work out with their sexual partner what strategy they will use to practice safer sex. While oral sex without ingesting semen is still risky because of the possibility of unintentionally ingesting pre-ejaculatory fluid, the level of risk for HIV infection is extremely remote. Of course, no one should ever engage in anal intercourse without a condom with a partner who is not proven to be HIV-negative; other much less risky forms of sexual behavior should be discussed prior to sex. What minimal risk, if any, are you willing to take?

Most gay men (and straight men, for that matter) agree that condoms interfere not only with physical sensation but with the spiritual sensation of union. They may also make sex more real than one's romantic illusions can tolerate; just tearing the foil package makes some people feel they are admitting the specter of death into their bedrooms. . . .

Several [young gay men] expressed to me the feeling that they would get AIDS no matter what they did; why even try to be safe? For them . . . contracting the disease seemed almost like a rite of initiation into the gay community. Others were just too ecstatic about coming out of the closet to think about the consequences of their new-found freedoms. These young men . . . felt themselves to be immortal. . . .

Americans have difficulty discussing *any* kind of sex frankly, which may be why our teen pregnancy rate is double the rate of Canada, for instance. But anal sex, which for many gay men is the defining act of gayness, is virtually unmentionable—despite being common among heterosexuals too. [Walt] Odets [a gay HIV prevention advocate] would see this prudishness as another factor in gay men's self-loathing, another way they are "mangled" by a hateful society.

"Most prevention efforts [directed toward gay men] have been based on risk-elimination rather than risk reduction. . . . We don't say to heterosexuals: 'A condom every time' for the rest of their lives," [says Odets]. "We expect them to enter relationships and dispense with condoms when their H.I.V.-negative status is confirmed. It's a very old story, telling gay men how to have sex; publicly they're complying, privately they're doing something else. We're the only country in the Western world that is continuing to even *discuss* the issue of oral sex in gay men. Oral sex *can* transmit HIV, but the risk is comparable to everyday, ordinary risk in modern life, like driving a well-maintained car at moderate speeds on the superhighway with a lap belt and shoulder belt on. Not to acknowledge the low risk is to deny the value of sex between men."

Source: Jesse Green, "Flirting with Suicide," *The New York Times Magazine*, pp. 39–45, 54–55, 84–85 (September 15, 1996).

DOCUMENT 184: Using Negotiated Safety

The concept of "negotiated safety" discussed in the previous reading may be an effective way of coping with AIDS. Many of the earlier ardent restrictions of safer sex practices developed in the 1980s were designed as temporary measures for a disease that was thought to be more infectious than it in fact is, and for a disease that we had thought would have a vaccine and/or cure by now.

Research shows that negotiated safety among HIV-negative homosexual men in relationships may help them remain uninfected. Susan Kippax of Macquarie University in Sydney, Australia, and colleagues report in the February issue of *AIDS* that "a significant number of men used negotiated safety as an HIV prevention strategy." Among a study group of 1,000 men, Kippax found that 62 percent of subjects who claimed to be in a regular seroconcordant HIV-negative relationship [where both partners are HIV-negative] reported having unprotected anal sex within a relationship with an HIV-negative partner. Some 91 percent of these men said that [they] did not have unprotected anal sex outside of that relationship.

Source: " 'Negotiated Safety': Common HIV Prevention Strategy Among Homosexual Men" (Reuters, March 4, 1997).

SUGGESTED READINGS

"ABC's of AIDS Education Slow in Reaching Workplaces." *American Medical News* 40(7), p. 17 (February 17, 1997).

Aggleton, Peter, et al. "Risking Everything?: Risk Behavior, Behavior Change, and AIDS." *Science* 265, pp. 341–345 (July 15, 1994).

Alter, J. "The Power to Change What's 'Cool.'" *Newsweek* 123, p. 23 (January 17, 1994).

DiClemente, R. J., and J. L. Peterson, eds. *Preventing AIDS: Theories and Methods of Behavioral Interventions*. New York: Plenum, 1994.

"Drinking Increases HIV Susceptibility." *USA Today*, p. 7 (February 1994).

Ford, Michael. *One Hundred Questions and Answers About AIDS: What You Need to Know Now*. New York: Beach Tree Books, 1993.

Friedman, D. R. "How Clean Needles Are Saving Lives." *U.S. News & World Report* 114, p. 24 (March 29, 1993).

Hammett, T. M., and R. Widom. "HIV/AIDS Education and Prevention Programs for Adults in Prisons and Jails and Juveniles in Confinement Facilities—United States, 1994." *Morbidity and Mortality Weekly Report* 45(13), p. 268 (April 5, 1996).

Jaret, P. "Should You Be Tested for the AIDS Virus?" *Glamour* 91, p. 41 (June 1993).

Johnson, F. "Safe Sex." *Mother Jones* 17, pp. 47–49 (September/October, 1992).

Kirp, D. L. "Needle Exchange Comes of Age." *The Nation* 256, pp. 559–560 (April 26, 1993).

Locke, L. "Bars, Condoms, and AIDS: Three Cities, Three Answers." *Governing* 6, pp. 14–15 (February 1993).

Madaras, Linda. *Linda Madaras Talks to Teens About AIDS: An Essential Guide for Parents, Teachers and Young People*. Rev. ed. New York: Newmarket, 1993.

Massaquoi, H. J. "Ten New Dating Rules in the Post-Magic Johnson Era." *Ebony* 47, p. 126 (February 1992).

Nelson, S. "Talking Smart, Acting Stupid About AIDS." *Glamour* 90, pp. 174–175 (February 1992).

"A New Safe Sex Method for Women Needs Your Attention." *Glamour* 92, p. 132 (May 1994).

Norris, Michele L. "Taking Control." *Emerge* 8(5), p. 57 (March 1997).

Nourse, Alan E. *Teen Guide to AIDS Prevention*. New York: Watts, 1990.

Painter, Kim. "Program's Focus on Sexual Abstinence Questioned." *USA Today*, p. 1D (February 25, 1997).

Philipson, T. J., et al. "Why AIDS Prevention Programs Don't Work." *Issues in Science and Technology* 10, pp. 33–35 (Spring 1994).

Radetsky, P. "Is Married Sex Safe Sex?" *Redbook* 178, pp. 92–94ff. (March 1992).

Roberts, Sally. "Addressing AIDS at Work." *Business Insurance* 30(18), p. 14 (April 29, 1996).

"Take the Money and Shun." *POZ* no. 13, p. 27 (April 1996).

Yarber, William. *STD and HIV: A Guide for Today's Young Adults*. Reston, Va.: American Alliance for Health, Physical Education, Recreation, and Dance, 1992.

8

Legal and Ethical Issues

AIDS is a highly stigmatized disease that can bring out either the best or the worst in people. In the United States, the courts have ruled that the Americans with Disabilities Act legally protects people with AIDS or HIV, persons suspected to have AIDS or HIV, and even persons associated with persons with AIDS or HIV. However, we do legally discriminate against potential immigrants with AIDS or HIV, insurance companies can turn down persons with preexisting medical conditions such as AIDS or HIV, and some people still shun and avoid persons with AIDS or HIV. In the workplace, many large corporations have excellent programs to assist their employees with HIV/AIDS and to educate their HIV-negative employees about successfully working with their coworkers who are HIV-infected. The Centers for Disease Control and Prevention (CDC) has produced a comprehensive manager's kit on AIDS in the workplace, as part of its America Responds to AIDS campaign. However, most employers still do not have an AIDS program in place.

AIDS, by the sheer nature of the disease, has raised numerous ethical questions and concerns. All states confidentially report diagnosed AIDS cases to the federal government, but should they also report all persons who test positive for HIV? Should commercial sex workers (or prostitutes), pregnant women, and perhaps everyone else in the country, for that matter, be required to be tested for HIV? Should people with HIV/AIDS, as had occurred in Cuba, be forcibly quarantined until a cure can be found? What about their human rights? Should condoms be distributed free in high schools to sexually active students? If yes, are you sending the wrong message to high school students who are not having sex that sex at such a young age is OK? If no, are you willing to risk the lives of sexually active students just to make a point? And where would you draw the line: What about free condoms in middle schools also? Should condoms be distributed in prisons or jails? Should condom makers be allowed to advertise on television?

Should needle exchange programs be developed for injecting drug users? Who should notify sexual partners of persons with HIV/AIDS if their partners do not do it? Should the medical use of marijuana be legalized to prevent the "wasting syndrome" in persons with AIDS? Should the federal government pay for the expensive new drugs of persons with HIV who have no or inadequate insurance and could not otherwise afford to take them? How much money should the developed nations of the world donate to the poorer nations of the world, where 90 percent of the world's AIDS cases live? These and many other ethical and legal concerns have been raised by politicians, health administrators, government officials, and the concerned public. Most of these issues are discussed in the readings of this chapter. How would *you* answer these questions?

AIDS, THE WORKPLACE, AND THE LAW

DOCUMENT 185: The Americans with Disabilities Act

When the Americans with Disabilities Act (ADA) became effective on July 26, 1990, people with HIV/AIDS were included as disabled; therefore, their rights and opportunities became protected by federal law. Broad in scope, the law covers employment, public services, public accommodations, transportation, and telecommunications. With regard to employment, every aspect is protected: from the hiring process, salary, benefits, and promotion to termination. The law also protects people with HIV/AIDS from being excluded from public accommodations, such as schools, hospitals, doctors' offices, and restaurants, on the basis of their medical condition. The ADA protects not only people with HIV or AIDS but also people who are believed to be HIV-infected, as well as people who associate with HIV-infected people. Local and state laws may differ from the ADA, and the ADA does not supersede local laws when they provide greater protection. Prior to passage of the ADA, protection for people with HIV depended upon a patchwork of local and state regulations and other federal laws, such as the Rehabilitation Act of 1973. The city of Los Angeles, for instance, developed strong anti-discrimination regulations for people with AIDS or HIV-related symptoms. However, many other cities did not provide such protection. With the ADA, the federal government now provides the same protection for everyone throughout the country.

The Americans with Disabilities Act (ADA) protects the handicapped against discrimination in the delivery of goods and services and in the employment sector. Protection is extended to public and private organizations, whether they receive federal funds or not. The ADA definition of a "handicap" or "disability" is:

(1) a physical or mental impairment that substantially limits one or more of an individual's major life activities;

(2) a record of such impairment; or

(3) being regarded as having such an impairment.

The ADA does not specifically mention protection against discrimination of people infected with HIV. However, in September 1988, the U.S. Attorney General expanded the accepted definition of a handicapped person to include: "a person with AIDS, AIDS-related conditions, or someone perceived as having AIDS."

The Act further defines discrimination as not making reasonable accommodations to the known physical or mental limitations of a qualified individual with a disability who is an applicant or employee, unless the [business or organization] can demonstrate that the [change] would impose an "undue" hardship on the operation of this [business or organization]. Some examples of reasonable accommodations include:

1) making existing facilities handicap accessible;

2) job restructuring;

3) change from full-time to part-time work;

4) modification of work equipment;

5) change in physical location of work;

6) provision of qualified readers or interpreters; [and]

7) other similar accommodations for individuals with disabilities.

The term "undue hardship" is defined as a significant difficulty or expense taking into consideration the cost of the accommodation, the size and resources of the [business or organization, and] the fiscal impact of the expense. . . . There are five titles to the Act, but the three with the greatest impact on people with HIV disease are Titles I, II and III.

I. *Title I—Employment*

Title I protects employees [and] job [applicants] against discrimination because of their handicap or the perception of a handicap [or] disability. Protected areas include discrimination in "job application procedures, the hiring or discharge of employee, employee compensation, advancement, job training, and other terms, conditions and privileges of employment." Organizations with 15 or more employees are covered under the Title.

A. Illegal Drugs

The ADA excludes *current* users of illegal drugs from handicap [or] disability protection. However, a person who has successfully completed a drug rehabilitation program, and is no longer using drugs, or who is currently enrolled in a recovery program, and no longer using drugs, has disability protection under this Act. An employer is permitted to conduct drug screening tests on applicants [and] employees, and to make employment decisions based on [the] test results.

B. HIV Testing/Screening

The ADA does not specifically mention HIV screening tests, but it does address medical examinations, employment tests and selection criteria. The ADA defines as discrimination "using employment tests or other selection criteria that screen out or tend to screen out an individual with a disability or class of individuals unless the test or other selection criteria [are] shown to be job-related for the position in question and is consistent with business necessity." Further, it is prohibited to "conduct a medical examination or make inquiries of a job applicant or employee as to whether [the] applicant [or] employee is an individual with a disability, or as to the nature or severity of the disability, unless such [an] examination or inquiry is shown to be job-related and consistent with business necessity." Based on the [above] criteria, HIV testing/screening for employment purposes would appear to be discriminatory. . . .

C. Food Handlers

Again, the ADA does not specifically discuss HIV-infected food handlers. However, the Congress did consider allowing the transfer of HIV-infected food handlers to non-food handling jobs. This provision was deleted in the final bill upon the advice of the Centers for Disease Control and other health authorities who have determined that HIV is *not* spread through casual contact, or handling [or] eating food.

II. *Title II—Public Services*

According to this Title, no qualified individual with a disability shall, by reason of [this] disability, be excluded from participation in or be denied the benefits of the services, programs or activities of a "public entity," or be subjected to discrimination by any such "entity."

A "public entity" is defined in the law as:

1. any state or local government; [or]

2. any department agency, special purpose district, or other [organization acting on behalf] of a state or local government.

III. Title III—Public Accommodations and Services Operated by Private Entities

Title III prohibits discrimination in entities that affect commerce, known as "public accommodations." The Act states that "no individual shall be discriminated against on the basis of disability in the full and equal enjoyment of the goods, services, facilities, privileges or advantages of any place of public accommodation by any person who owns, leases or operates a place of public accommodation."

Examples of "public accommodations" are as follows:

1) an establishment for serving food or drink;
2) a place of exhibition or public entertainment, such as a movie theater or stadium;
3) a place of public gathering, such as an auditorium or convention center;
4) a general store for commerce, such as a grocery store, clothing store, shopping center or other establishment for the sale of goods;
5) a place of public display or collection, such as an art gallery or library;
6) a zoo or amusement park;
7) a private school or place of education;
8) a place of lodging, such as a motel or inn where there are at least five rooms to let;
9) a public establishment for exercise or recreation, such as a spa or golf course;
10) a social service center, such as a day care center, senior citizen center, homeless shelter or adoption agency; and
11) a public accommodation also includes service establishments, such as the office of a lawyer, insurance office, pharmacy, hospital or professional office of a health care provider. This last category includes a private physician's office. . . .

Public accommodations must be handicap-accessible with physical barriers removed. If removal is not possible or too costly, then alternate methods of providing the service must be offered.

Source: Joe Geoffrey, *Summary of the Americans with Disabilities Act as It Applies to HIV/AIDS* (Atlanta: Georgia Department of Human Resources, Division of Public Health, Epidemiology and Prevention Branch, April 19, 1995).

DOCUMENT 186: People with Asymptomatic HIV Also Protected Under the Americans with Disabilities Act

The Americans with Disabilities Act is continually challenged, only to be upheld in federal appeals courts. In the following case, a dentist refused to provide care to a patient because she was HIV-positive. The

judges ruled that it did not matter whether she had AIDS or was merely
HIV-positive without any symptoms; discrimination is still discrimination, and that is illegal.

People who are HIV-positive but have no AIDS symptoms are protected from discrimination under the Americans with Disabilities Act,
ruled a federal appeals court. The ruling came in the case of Sidney
Abbott, who was refused dental care because she is infected with HIV.
The dentist, Randon Bragdon of Bangor, Maine, said he feared the "direct threat" of transmission, which he claimed was supported by recommendations from the Centers for Disease Control and Prevention to
use increased precautions such as eye shields and double gloves. A three-
judge panel of the 1st U.S. Circuit Court of Appeals decided Thursday
that "HIV-positive status . . . whether symptomatic or asymptomatic,
comprises a physical impairment under the ADA."

Source: Frank J. Murray, "Disability Act Protects HIV-Positive People, Court
Rules," The Washington Times, p. A3 (March 7, 1997); CDC National AIDS Clearinghouse (Bethesda, Md.: Information, Inc., 1997).

DOCUMENT 187: The American Medical Association's Policy on Treating AIDS Patients

The American Medical Association (AMA) reminds physicians that during epidemics and health crises, they are needed more than ever, despite risks to themselves. According to traditional ethics of the
profession, a physician cannot refuse to treat patients infected with
HIV. This responsibility remains even though health care workers have
accidentally been infected with HIV in the course of caring for patients.
These cases are, however, relatively few in number.

The Council on Ethical and Judicial Affairs of the American Medical
Association recognizes the growing AIDS crisis as a crucial health problem involving the physician's ethical responsibility to his patients and to
society. . . . AIDS patients are entitled to competent medical services with
compassion and respect for human dignity and to the safeguard of their
confidences within the constraints of the law. Those persons who are
afflicted with the disease, or who are seropositive, have the right to be
free from discrimination.

A physician may not ethically refuse to treat a patient whose condition
is within the physician's current realm of competence solely because the
patient is seropositive. The tradition of the American Medical Associa-

tion, since its organization in 1847, is that: "When an epidemic prevails, a physician must continue his labors without regard to the risk to his own health." That tradition must be maintained. A person who is afflicted with AIDS needs competent, compassionate treatment. Neither those who have the disease nor those who have been infected with the virus should be subjected to discrimination based on fear or prejudice, least of all by members of the health care community. Physicians should respond to the best of their abilities in cases of emergency where first aid treatment is essential, and physicians should not abandon patients whose care they have undertaken.

Source: Current Opinions of the Council on Ethical and Judicial Affairs (American Medical Association, 1986), sec. 8.10.

DOCUMENT 188: Protecting Health Care Professionals Through Infection Control Procedures

> Since physicians are indeed bound by their duty to treat all patients who visit them, they need to be extremely knowledgeable about methods to protect themselves from infections. The AIDS epidemic has raised the awareness of health care workers, including doctors, of infection control techniques. These methods include the use of barriers, such as gloves, goggles, and masks, and careful handling, cleaning, and disposal of syringes and other sharp instruments.

Many have argued that the practice of medicine is inherently virtuous and that medical ethics involves a duty to treat patients with HIV infection. Others . . . find fewer special obligations [inherent in] the occupation and emphasize the liberty of physicians. For them, the relationship between a doctor and a patient is contractual, and the doctor's rights . . . are [equal] to those of the patient. . . .

[However], medical ethics entails obligations that extend beyond those usually expected of citizens in our political system. Physicians recognize that as doctors they have duties that are greater . . . than those of others. This sense of obligation must translate to a willingness to treat all sick patients.

Hospitals should therefore focus not on transmission but on policies for reducing transmission. . . . In 1987, the Occupational Safety and Health Administration and the CDC issued joint recommendations that emphasized the use of gloves and other barrier methods to prevent viral transmission. Today, health care workers need more information about methods for preventing infection.

Source: Troyen A. Brennan, "Transmission of the Human Immunodeficiency Virus in the Health Care Setting—A Time for Action," *The New England Journal of Medicine* 324(21): 1504–1507 (May 23, 1991).

DOCUMENT 189: The Risk of Occupational HIV Infection

While nearly one in twenty persons with AIDS in the United States are, or have been, employed in health care, only a relative few became HIV-infected from their work environment. By 1995, only forty-four health care workers had unquestionably become infected through their workplace, usually by an accidental puncture or cut with an HIV-infected needle or sharp implement. An additional ninety-seven persons may have been infected on the job, but the evidence is not clear.

Of the persons reported with AIDS in the United States through June 30, 1995, 15,719 had been employed in health care. These cases represented 4.8 percent of the 324,158 AIDS cases reported to CDC for whom occupational information was known (information on employment in the health care setting was missing for 146,130 reported AIDS cases).

The type of job is known for 14,870 (95 percent) of the 15,719 reported health care workers with AIDS. The specific occupations are as follows: 1,359 physicians, 94 surgeons, 3,515 nurses, 375 dental workers, 301 paramedics, 2,139 technicians, 770 therapists, and 3,129 health aides. The remainder are maintenance workers, administrative staff, etc. Overall, 75 percent of the health care workers with AIDS, including 1,077 physicians, 75 surgeons, 2,589 nurses, 291 dental workers, and 213 paramedics, are reported to have died.

CDC is aware of 46 health care workers in the United States who have been documented as having seroconverted to HIV following occupational exposures. Twenty have developed AIDS. These individuals who seroconverted include 18 laboratory workers (15 of whom were clinical laboratory workers), 16 nurses, 6 physicians, 2 surgical technicians, 1 dialysis technician, 1 respiratory therapist, 1 health aide, and 1 housekeeper/maintenance worker. The exposures were as follows: 40 had [a] ... puncture/cut injury ..., 4 had ... mucous membrane and/or skin exposure, 1 had both ... exposure[s], and 1 had an unknown route of exposure. Forty-one exposures were to HIV-infected blood, 3 to concentrated virus in a laboratory, 1 to visibly bloody fluid, and 1 to an unspecified fluid.

CDC is also aware of 97 other cases of HIV infection or AIDS among health care workers who have not reported other risk factors for HIV infection and who report a history of occupational exposure to blood, body fluids, or HIV-infected laboratory material, but for whom seroconversion after exposure was not documented. The number of these workers who acquired their infection through occupational exposures is unknown.

Source: "Facts About HIV/AIDS and Health Care Workers," in Centers for Disease Control and Prevention, *HIV/AIDS Prevention* (Atlanta: CDC, August 1995).

DOCUMENT 190: Murder in the Dentist's Chair

Only one dentist with AIDS has ever been proven to have infected a patient. Actually, Dr. Acer of South Florida infected at least six of his patients. The following article argues, given what we know about HIV epidemiology and transmission, as well as the evidence available, that these infections could not have been accidental. With the nearly universal use of gloves, masks, and sterilized or disinfected equipment in the dental office, there is no reason to fear going to one's dentist today. Dr. Acer was apparently the only health professional who ever purposely attempted to infect his patients.

It has been over five years since the death of Dr. David J. Acer, a Stuart, Florida dentist. And yet the HIV-related deaths of at least six of his former patients still remain a mystery. . . . The Centers for Disease Control and Prevention had previously compared Dr. Acer's HIV-infected blood with the blood of the six patients, including Kimberly Bergalis, who became HIV positive, and found that in all cases they were genetically linked directly to the dentist. Clearly, they were infected by the dentist. But research among many other HIV-positive dentists throughout the United States shows not a single instance where a dentist infected his or her patients. The only dentist proven to infect a patient with HIV is Dr. Acer, and he infected not just one but at least six patients over an 18 month period in 1988–89. Actually, he probably infected 11 or 12 patients, but we don't know about the others yet.

The State of Florida HRS investigative team did not perform a very comprehensive investigation with the pool of dentist patients. Two letters were sent out to all 2,500 patients, but only 1,100 came in for an HIV test. No door-to-door contact tracing was conducted. Of the 1,100, seven tested positive, and five of them were genetically linked to the dentist. A sixth patient recently was discovered when she tested HIV positive while enlisting in the Navy. Among the 1,400 untested former patients, it is probable that either five or six additional patients were infected with HIV by Dr. Acer. Eventually, it is likely that the identity of most of these additional patients will become known as they develop AIDS-related symptoms.

So how could so many of his patients become so easily infected? It has been pointed out that Dr. Acer was inconsistent at best in sterilizing his dental equipment and in using gloves. But this would only contribute to transferring HIV from one patient to another. This is not what happened here. The patients were being infected with the dentist's HIV, not with each other's. Some people have speculated that he may have been using the dental equipment on himself and then used it on the patients. But if this would have happened, we should expect that the infections would occur rapidly in succession. The evidence, however, shows that the known infected patients were chronologically scattered throughout the 18 month time frame. It would also demonstrate blatant disregard for the health of his patients, since he knew he had AIDS at the time and he was fully aware of how HIV can spread.

Others argue that the six infected patients may have been infected from sexual behavior or injecting drug use. Kimberly Bergalis, some say, may not have been the virgin that she told her parents and the public she was. But the truth is that it really does not matter at all how sexually active the six patients were, since the evidence is certain that their HIV is genetically linked directly to the dentist. Unless they were having sex with the gay dentist, and there is absolutely no evidence of this, they had to have been intentionally infected directly by Dr. Acer in his dental chair.

Since it had to have been intentional, how could this have occurred? The dental assistant who worked most closely with Dr. Acer during this time period is refusing to answer any questions. [Dr. Acer's former male] lover is also refusing to speak with anyone. So we can only speculate. It is possible that he prepared the Novocain syringes mixed with his own HIV-infected blood and then directly injected the mixture into the mouths of his intended victims. This procedure may have weakened the effect of the anesthetic, and some of the infected patients have indeed reported that the dentist frequently gave ineffective injections which required him to repeat the injection.

But what motive could he have to perform such an horrific act on his own patients? A former friend of the dentist has claimed that he was trying to show the world that even straight, white women can get AIDS—that it is not "just a gay disease." But I don't think this is the reason. If he was trying to make a political statement about the universal transmissibility of HIV, why didn't he simply come out and say so on his deathbed? If he was trying to make a point, he had an excellent opportunity to tell the investigators shortly before his death. I suspect instead that it was nothing more than a series of personal attacks against particular patients that, for whatever reasons, he just didn't like.

Barbara Webb, one of the six known victims, told me a few months before her recent death that she had a very bizarre incident with Dr. Acer one day. He was having some difficulty extracting her tooth, and she innocently said to him, "This must be very difficult for you." Apparently misinterpreting her statement to mean that she was questioning his professional competence, he glared at her, gritted his teeth, and replied, "No, it's just a matter of leverage." Dr. Acer rarely let his emotions show. A few days later, when he learned that his assistant had sent Ms. Webb a small vase with a single flower in it to compensate for the trouble she had during her tooth extraction, the dentist insisted that her insurance be billed for the vase, even though he knew that her insurance would not fully cover the cost. Ms. Webb ended up paying for part of the cost of her unexpected gift from the dentist office. She also told me that she began to notice that his Novocain injections seemed weaker after the incident.

Where then do we go from here? The district attorney in Stuart has told me that they do not have the authority or resources to conduct an investigation into the Dr. Acer case at this point. Only a grand jury investigation would have the authority to subpoena those persons who may know what really went on, and obtain the private files of the dentist. To initiate such an investigation against someone who died over five years ago would be quite exceptional. The one thing that I believe must be done now is to re-contact those 1,400 former patients who previously refused to be HIV tested. If ever there was a valid justification for HIV-related contact tracing, this is it. We need to find those five or six other patients who were deliberately infected by Dr. Acer, and to find out what they have in common with the six known victims. Only by locating and interviewing these hidden other victims, will we have any hope of finding out the complete truth to what really happened inside Dr. Acer's dental chair.

Source: Douglas A. Feldman, "Murder in the Dentist's Chair," *She Times*, p. 12 (November 1995).

DOCUMENT 191: Secondhand Discrimination

The Americans with Disabilities Act prevents employers and others from discriminating against people who are associated with a person who has AIDS or HIV. In this case, an owner of a restaurant fired an employee because his male life partner had AIDS. The owner claimed that he was afraid that business might be hurt if he did not fire him.

The owner was forced by the court to pay the fired employee not only his back pay but compensatory damages.

The owner of an Oklahoma restaurant has been ordered to pay damages to an employee he fired because the employee's domestic partner had AIDS. In the first ruling of its kind, Terry Turner was ordered, under the Americans with Disabilities Act, to pay Paul Saladin $6,548 in back pay and compensatory damages. Evidence in the trial showed that Turner knew Saladin was gay and that his life partner, Ed Gaudin, had developed AIDS. Turner suspended Saladin for 30 days and then later, would not allow him to return to work. Testimony indicated that Turner feared that Saladin's association with someone who had AIDS would hurt his business. This was the first time an employer was found liable under the ADA provision that prohibits discrimination against a qualified individual due to that person's association with a person with a disability.

Source: Frank Baran, "HR News: Employer Liable for Firing Worker Whose Partner Had AIDS," *Human Resource Executive* 10(9): 16 (August 1996); CDC National AIDS Clearinghouse (Bethesda, Md.: Information, Inc., 1996).

DOCUMENT 192: The Workplace Responds to AIDS

Because of the large numbers of Americans infected with HIV, corporations have to face the reality of employees who are infected or ill. A corporate AIDS program is a practical necessity, especially for large corporations or organizations. Unlike other diseases, HIV can cause disruption, fear, panic, and prejudice among employees. Comprehensive programs have a number of components, including education and training, information and referrals, and counseling. Among the larger companies, many have AIDS policies in place. For example, Levi Strauss and Company, Fuddruckers Restaurants, and Digital Equipment Corporation are known for their programs that are considered successful models for other corporations.

AIDS is different from other diseases and needs to be treated as such. Because it is both deadly and transmittable (though not through casual contact), fear about catching HIV can run rampant. The virus' association with [gay men] and drug users can inspire scorn and prejudice [that] other diseases don't. . . . Rule [number 1] in the best corporate AIDS programs is that you have to expect trouble and be proactive in educating workers about the issues AIDS raises. That requires a comprehensive program that is clearly endorsed from the executive suite down. . . . Ignorance and secrecy are by far the most disruptive factors when it comes to AIDS in the workplace. As soon as someone shows signs of illness or starts to miss work, rumormongering among co-workers can fan irrational responses. Managers, meantime, have no context within which to evaluate a sick employee's sagging performance. . . . And the person with AIDS—afraid of losing health benefits, being harassed, or even being fired—may put off disclosing the illness as long as possible.

Education usually takes the form of videos, seminars, and literature. The idea is to dispel myths, present the company's policy, and discuss ways to prevent the spread of the disease. Some companies . . . make the sessions mandatory for all employees. Others . . . don't force the issue, but are well-regarded for the wealth of information they provide. . . . While most policies prohibit moving a co-worker away from an employee with AIDS, many programs will provide counsel to those who are upset over the idea of working next to someone with a deadly disease.

Source: Ron Stodgill II, "Why AIDS Policy Must Be a Special Policy," *Business Week* no. 3303, pp. 53–54 (February 1, 1993).

DOCUMENT 193: The Ten Principles for the Workplace

Since HIV/AIDS is a reality in the workforce, employers are motivated to act. In addition to legal and financial incentives, well-run companies recognize the importance of facing the situation in a reasonable and humane way. The "Ten Principles for the Workplace" in this selection were written by the highly regarded Citizens Commission on AIDS for New York City and Northern New Jersey. Over 400 companies and organizations have endorsed these ten principles, which have served as models for businesses in the United States and abroad. The National Leadership Coalition on AIDS, a group of private corporations, labor organizations, and others, supports progressive and proactive policies on AIDS in the workplace. In 1991, seventy CEOs of U.S. companies, including Robert Haas of Levi Strauss and John Aker of IBM, joined the coalition in endorsing the ten principles and pledged to make AIDS in the workplace a priority concern.

Undoubtedly, the presence of people with AIDS or HIV disease in the workforce has been a major motivation, perhaps the greatest one, for employers to address this issue. . . . The prolonged life span and improved quality of life that is now available to many employees with AIDS or HIV infection, coupled with . . . legal protections, will lead to more productive and longer working lives but will also create more need for flexibility in scheduling and other workplace accommodations. The cost of health care benefits and reimbursements for drugs and outpatient services will be major issues for employers, employees, and unions, particularly among smaller businesses that lack health care benefits or have inadequate coverage. . . .

The *Ten Principles for the Workplace* are:

1. People with AIDS or HIV . . . infection are entitled to the same rights and opportunities as people with other serious or life-threatening illnesses.

2. Employment policies must, at a minimum, comply with federal, state, and local laws and regulations.

3. Employment policies should be based on the scientific and epidemiologic evidence that people with AIDS or HIV infection do not pose a risk of transmission of the virus to coworkers through ordinary workplace [contact].

4. The highest levels of management and union leadership should unequivocally endorse nondiscriminatory employment policies and educational programs about AIDS.

5. Employers and unions should communicate their support of these policies to workers in simple, clear, and unambiguous terms.

6. Employers should provide employees with sensitive, accurate, and up-to-date education about risk reduction in their personal lives.

7. Employers have a duty to protect the confidentiality of employees' medical information.

8. To prevent work disruption and rejection by coworkers of an employee with AIDS or HIV infection, employers and unions should undertake education for all employees before such an incident occurs, and as needed thereafter.

9. Employers should not require HIV screening as part of general pre-employment or workplace physical examinations.

10. In those special occupational settings where there may be a potential risk of exposure to HIV (for example in health care, where workers may be exposed to blood or blood products), employers should provide specific, ongoing education and training, as well as the necessary equipment, to reinforce appropriate infection control procedures and ensure that they are implemented.

Source: "The Ten Principles for the Workplace," in *AIDS: Is There a Will to Meet the Challenge?* (New York: Citizens Commission on AIDS for New York City and Northern New Jersey, February 1991), p. 19.

DOCUMENT 194: Creating a Compassionate Workplace Through Education

The cost to business of ignoring the rights of employees who have HIV disease can be considerable—in terms of both legal costs and disruption in the work environment. The remedy is education and training programs, particularly for supervisors, who set the tone for their work group. For example, DAKA International, which runs cafeterias and Fuddruckers restaurants, has an AIDS program that includes education, confidential counseling, and an anonymous hot line. When employees are no longer able to work, they can take paid leaves of absence.

HIV has a direct effect on business in that it places a drain on the pool of healthy adults of working age. . . . In addition, businesses are accountable for indirect costs of HIV, including possible decreases in productivity of HIV-infected employees. Companies may also incur hefty legal fees and litigation costs if they ignore laws that protect HIV-infected employees. . . .

In every workplace, it is only a matter of time before an employee . . . steps forward to say, "I am infected with HIV." . . . Education is the recommended response to the social and financial issues presented by AIDS and HIV . . . [and] is particularly important for supervisors, who may have to manage employees who have AIDS or test positively for AIDS. . . .

The best HIV training and communication programs for creating a compassionate workplace give employees two information sources: a company official and an external field expert. The "insider/outsider" arrangement is a practical one. The insider knows the educational needs of the company and its employees; the outsider provides factual medical information about AIDS.

Source: Laura B. Pincus and Shefali M. Trivedi, "A Time for Action: Responding to AIDS," *Training & Development* 48(1): 45–51 (January 1994).

DOCUMENT 195: Earning Employee Loyalty

The pragmatic reasons for developing good workplace policies on AIDS include avoiding legal battles, managing health care costs, and keeping workers healthy and productive. Perhaps a more important reason is that it helps to create a good work environment. An employer who treats employees with respect and compassion earns their loyalty. Pacific Bell exemplifies a company that treats its employees well in terms of its AIDS policy. A special AIDS education task force within the company helps educate workers. Employees who become ill with HIV disease work as long as they are able; their medical coverage is continued for the length of their illness.

[T]he real reason companies should concern themselves with AIDS has less to do with . . . income and more to do with caring. . . . AIDS attacks the immune system of personal relationships and organizations like businesses, making them even more vulnerable to weaknesses already there. . . . A company that already treats its employees well will respond compassionately when one of its own has AIDS. . . . All employees . . . look to see how the company treats an employee with the virus—because they . . . wonder . . . if it will act with integrity about, say, cancer, . . . or drug addiction, . . . or homosexuality.

Source: Tom Ehrenfeld, "The Business Lessons of AIDS," *Inc.* 16(4): 29–30 (April 1994).

DOCUMENT 196: Understanding AIDS Discrimination

Fear and ignorance lead to discrimination against people who are infected with HIV, are assumed to be infected, or associate with people who are. People have been fired from their jobs, excluded from school, evicted from their homes, and threatened. Legislation on the local, state, and federal levels has defined what discrimination is, and the courts have clarified this further by ruling on specific cases. As a counter to discrimination, legislation has helped to set firm limits for behavior. However, the law is reactive and not the best remedy for discrimination. Education programs, advocacy groups, and positive actions of individuals are other ways to influence people and effect change.

HIV-related discrimination is most often directed against three groups of people: those who "have AIDS," those who are assumed to "have AIDS," and those who live with or associate with people who have or are assumed to "have AIDS" (including health care professionals). The first two groups include persons who are (or are perceived to be) [gay] men, [injecting] drug users, persons with hemophilia, some ethnic minorities, and prostitutes. The assumption that is often made is not simply that these persons are at an increased risk of HIV infection, but that "they all have it," are infectious, and—therefore—pose an immediate risk to others. . . . HIV-related discrimination has its origins in misinformation and fear. It is based more on incorrect knowledge about HIV and its means of transmission, than on total ignorance. The resulting fear is a logical outcome of a belief that life may be at stake.

Source: Brett Tindall and Gregory Tillett, "HIV-Related Discrimination," *AIDS* 4 (supp. 1): S251–S256 (1990).

DOCUMENT 197: Company in Japan Faces Criminal Charges over Tainted Blood

Randy Shilts's book and film, *And the Band Played On*, document how blood banks in the early 1980s refused to screen their blood for hepatitis B, prior to the discovery of HIV, even though it was known that this was a good predictor of tainted blood drawn from persons with AIDS. During the mid-1980s, blood banks in Canada, Japan, France, and elsewhere were slow to screen blood and blood products given to persons with hemophilia, and in need of a blood transfusion, for HIV, in order to cut costs. Multimillion-dollar court settlements have since been paid by blood banks, and blood bank directors face criminal penalties, including time in prison. In the following reading, cost-effectiveness has led one manufacturer of blood products in Japan to possibly be charged with professional negligence resulting in deaths.

Recent raids at Green Cross, Japan's leading manufacturer of blood products, marked the start of an investigation that could lead to criminal charges of professional negligence. Former Green Cross executives are suspected of allowing the distribution of non-heated blood products, knowing of the risk of HIV involved. The office raids were made to investigate a homicide complaint against former Green Cross President Renzo Matsushita that was filed by the family of a [person with hemophilia] who died of AIDS complications after receiving blood products made by Green Cross. Prosecutors said Matsushita could be charged with professional negligence resulting in death. Takeshi Abe, the former director of a government AIDS study team, has also been questioned by prosecutors in connection with criminal complaints related to the deaths of [people with hemophilia] who had been given HIV-tainted blood products. The scandal has already hurt the company's sales; hospitals managed by local governments had boycotted the company before the raids, and sales were expected to fall even more. Green Cross shares dropped 10 percent in the two trading days that the raids took place.

Source: "Drug Companies Probed on Knowledge of Risk in Blood-Related AIDS Deaths," *Nikkei Weekly* 34(1737): 2 (August 26, 1996); CDC National AIDS Clearinghouse (Bethesda, Md.: Information, Inc., 1996).

ETHICS AND AIDS POLICY

DOCUMENT 198: HIV and Immigration Policy

From a public health perspective, highly restrictive immigration policies are not necessary. Particularly in the case of temporary visitors
who can obtain waivers if needed, the increased risk to the public is
negligible. The National Commission on AIDS recommended a review
of immigration policy on people with HIV/AIDS. President Clinton tried
to change the ban on HIV-positive immigrants, but was not successful
with Congress. The current policy excludes persons who test positive
for HIV from entering the United States, or from staying in the country,
even if they are otherwise fully eligible to obtain a green card to become an immigrant. Those who are HIV-positive may, through their
attorney, try to get a waiver if they have an immediate family member
in the United States and if they are seen by immigration authorities as
"unlikely to spread HIV." Those who fail to get a waiver, and fail to
win an appeal, are excluded from entering or are deported if already
in the United States. Ironically, some of those deported may have been
infected with HIV after they arrived in the United States. Since HIV is
preventable through safer sex practices and other methods, the logic
for discriminating against HIV-positive immigrants to the United States
is not supportable.

BE IT RESOLVED, that the National Commission on Acquired Immune Deficiency Syndrome recommends and calls upon the Administration to immediately implement the following:

1. The Department of State, the Department of Justice and the Department of
   Health and Human Services should conduct a comprehensive review of immigration policies as they regard communicable disease, particularly HIV infection, focusing on public health needs.
2. Nonimmigrants, such as conference participants, should not be questioned
   regarding their HIV status as a condition for entry into the United States or
   for issuance of a visa. Similarly, persons carrying medications or products
   associated with HIV infection or hemophilia should not be subject to detention
   or questioning.
3. The following practices should also be implemented pending the comprehensive overall review of immigration policies recommended above:

A. For applicants who otherwise qualify for legalization, asylum, or refugee status and who may be infected with HIV, standards for waivers should be liberally applied and they should be routinely granted particularly where family unity, humanitarian and or public interest grounds may exist.

B. For applicants who otherwise qualify for permanent residency and who may be infected with HIV, similar waiver procedures should be adopted to the extent permitted by law.

C. The Department of State, the Department of Health and Human Services and the Immigration and Naturalization Service should engage in cooperative efforts to institute policies and disseminate information targeted at notifying relevant [immigrant] groups of the availability of waivers and the circumstances under which they are granted.

D. To the extent that HIV testing is part of any medical examination of applicants for permanent residency, refugee status or legalization, the Immigration and Naturalization Service and the Centers for Disease Control should carefully monitor training and compliance with their Instructions to Designated Physicians. Particular attention should be paid to pre- and post-test counseling, confidentiality and appropriate referrals of persons for medical care and follow-up counseling.

E. Confidentiality should be protected where HIV testing is part of the medical examination of applicants for visas, permanent residency, asylum, refugee status or legalization. Permanent markings in passports (including the use of codes which may become known) which in any way suggest that a person is infected with HIV or any other designated communicable disease should be prohibited. Where medical examinations take place, steps should be taken to safeguard all medical information (including HIV status), particularly from staff recruited locally in foreign countries.

Source: "Resolution on U.S. Visa and Immigration Policy" (Washington, D.C.: National Commission on AIDS, December 1989), pp. 1–2.

DOCUMENT 199: Mandatory HIV Testing of Commercial Sex Workers

This selection is written by a female commercial sex worker (CSW, a less pejorative term than "prostitute") and head of COYOTE (Call Off Your Old Tired Ethics), a CSW organization. Since prostitution is currently illegal in the United States, except in Nevada, mandatory HIV testing would include only those CSWs identified by the legal system and would not effectively reach this population. Peer education has been useful in helping to educate and to support safer sex practices among these women. Interestingly, the lowest HIV rates among CSWs occur in Nevada.

If prostitutes were effectively transmitting the virus, by now . . . we would have seen more than 30,000 straight, white, middle-class, middle-aged men in the New York metropolitan area diagnosed with the disease, most of them married. Yet we have not seen these kinds of figures. . . .

Mandatory testing may identify a few prostitutes who have been infected with HIV, but it will not prevent AIDS. Condoms and other safe sex practices are how STDs, including AIDS, are prevented. It is highly important . . . that prostitutes across the United States be encouraged to use condoms consistently. The California Prostitutes Education Project (CAL-PEP) in San Francisco has been a model AIDS prevention program, based on the assumption that prostitutes, who know best what the job is like, are the best people to provide education and motivation to other prostitutes. CAL-PEP's staff is almost entirely made up of current and former prostitutes, a model that is being followed in many other communities. CAL-PEP distributes condoms, spermicides, bleach, and information to street prostitutes in the San Francisco area.

Source: Priscilla Alexander, "U.S. Prostitutes Are Less Likely to Spread AIDS Than IV Drug Users," in C. C. Abt and K. M. Hardy, eds., *AIDS and the Courts* (Cambridge, Mass.: Abt Books, 1990), pp. 132–140.

DOCUMENT 200: Mandatory HIV Testing of Pregnant Women

Now that it has been proven that AZT treatment of HIV-positive pregnant women can significantly reduce the likelihood that their infants will become HIV-positive, should HIV testing of pregnant women become mandatory? Whose rights are more important? The pregnant woman who does not wish to be cajoled into taking AZT, which frequently has serious side effects? Or the newborn child, who would be at greatly increased risk of becoming HIV-positive and probably dying if the mother does not get tested for HIV and take AZT?

The issue of mandatory HIV testing for pregnant women and their infants has become increasingly controversial as the rate of AIDS among females has risen. Women [in 1996] account for 19 percent of all AIDS cases, up from [7] percent in 1985. Moreover, an estimated 6,000 to 7,000 HIV-positive women gave birth in 1993, according to the Centers for Disease Control and Prevention. A clinical trial by government researchers showed in 1994 that, with early detection, AZT could reduce perinatal [around the time of birth] transmission by two-thirds, heightening the

importance of HIV testing. By a close vote, the American Medical Association agreed to endorse mandatory testing in June.

However, other medical groups oppose mandatory testing on the
grounds that it could keep the women most at risk from seeking any
prenatal [before birth] care. For its part, Congress has passed legislation
to urge the states to reduce the rate of perinatal HIV transmission—by
mandatory testing or other means—or risk losing federal funds for AIDS.
New York has passed a law to require that all newborns are tested and
that results be "unblinded" [so that the mothers would be informed if
their child tests positive for HIV]. Advocates of voluntary testing, including the CDC, cite high rates of testing when pregnant women were
counseled about HIV as part of prenatal care.

Source: Deborah L. Shelton, "Is It the Time . . . ?," *American Medical News* 39(33):
13 (September 2, 1996); CDC National AIDS Clearinghouse (Bethesda, Md.: Information, Inc., 1996).

DOCUMENT 201: Promises Broken in Chicago

Does a large municipal government need to know if its teachers are
HIV-positive before hiring them? Certainly, it could contain its health
insurance costs by screening out those who would likely need expensive medical treatments. It would also ease the unfounded fears of parents who may wrongly believe that the HIV-infected teacher might
somehow infect their children in the classroom. Further, having a
teacher around with an illness frequently contracted through unprotected gay sex is likely to make some homophobic educational administrators feel uncomfortable. But the Americans with Disabilities Act
mandates that no one may discriminate against persons with HIV or
AIDS. Teachers with HIV—and everyone else with HIV, for that matter—have the fundamental right of freedom from discrimination based
on their medical condition. Unless the medical condition is one that
can be casually transmitted by touch or through the air, such as the
ebola virus, there is no justification for discrimination.

The Chicago Public School system continues to require individuals
applying for teaching positions to reveal whether they have HIV, despite
promising to delete the question from medical forms six months ago.
The school system is also asking other potentially illegal, highly personal
questions as part of its medical examination form for job applicants. The
school system has called the questioning "an oversight" and "improper."
However, a spokeswoman for Lambda Legal Defense, a New York-based

gay rights law firm, suggests that the schools have a credibility problem, having agreed to remove the question from forms in March but not appearing "to have exerted a lot of energy to follow through on what they promised." Two years ago, Chicago Mayor Richard M. Daley ordered the city agencies not to question job applicants about their HIV-status after the city had to pay $90,000 in legal costs for testing police applicants for HIV.

Source: Greg Hinz, "City Schools Still Screen Illegally for AIDS," Crain's Chicago Business 19(37): 3 (September 9, 1996); CDC National AIDS Clearinghouse (Bethesda, Md.: Information, Inc., 1996).

DOCUMENT 202: Television Squeamish About Running Condom Ads

Latex condoms used properly are highly effective in preventing transmission of HIV. In 1987, U.S. Surgeon General C. Everett Koop was outspoken on the issue. He criticized the television networks for refusing to air condom advertisements. Since then, public service announcements on the subject have been broadcast.

Criticism has been heaped on the three major TV networks for their refusal to [reverse] . . . prohibitions on condom ads. . . . Among [them] . . . was U.S. Surgeon General C. Everett Koop . . . [who said that condoms are] "the best method of reducing or preventing [AIDS] infection known at this time for those who . . . will not practice abstinence or monogamy. If television networks peddle all the attractive parts of sex, then they should be willing to also peddle something that might prevent the transmission of a sexually acquired disease."

Source: Julie Rovner, "TV Networks Resist Push for Condom Ads," Congressional Quarterly 45, p. 267 (February 14, 1987).

DOCUMENT 203: Should Condoms Be Given Out in the Schools? In Prisons and Jails?

Condom availability programs in schools and prisons are very controversial. Opponents argue that these programs may actually encourage sexual activity rather than discourage it. Is this a proper role for these institutions, and are they equipped to handle this responsibility? People who are in favor of these programs point out that, in any case, unprotected sexual activity occurs in both groups. Why not take the opportunity to provide information and skills to protect those who are at risk? Schools and prisons have taken on health education efforts before, and in a crisis situation can respond again.

In general, both opponents and supporters of condom availability programs agree that abstinence is the best and only surefire means of preventing HIV infection. They part company, however, over how to prevent transmission when the abstinence message goes unheeded.

Opponents argue that distributing or increasing access to condoms condones and may encourage sexual activity among teens as well as among prisoners, who by law are prohibited from having sex during incarceration. Proponents counter that condoms are a vital means of protecting the lives of teenagers and inmates who, despite the abstinence message or legal prohibitions, will still engage in sexual activity. They caution, however, that condom availability programs must be part of a larger HIV/AIDS education and prevention effort. . . .

Opponents of condom availability programs question the necessity of making condoms available in schools, given the fact that sexually active teenagers can already buy them. Despite the availability of condoms for sale, however, only 47% of females and 55% of males report using condoms when they first have sex. Perhaps for that reason, the HIV infection rate among teens continues to soar.

While most of the public and media attention has focused on schools, some public health officials and advocates are also calling for condoms to be made available to prisoners, another population hard hit by the HIV/AIDS epidemic. Generally, the rate of HIV infection among prisoners is much higher than that of the non-incarcerated population [due to greater incidence of injecting drug use and sexually transmitted diseases]. . . .

[F]ive jurisdictions—New York City, San Francisco, Philadelphia, Vermont, and Mississippi—make condoms accessible to prisoners, although not [generally] on request because of the prohibition on sexual activity in prisons. Rather, inmates *can request* condoms [only] when they visit sick hall, prison physicians, or in conjunction with HIV/AIDS education efforts. . . .

Despite their potential to reduce HIV transmission within prisons, . . . it is unlikely that . . . [condom availability programs] will catch on . . . [due to] prohibitions on sexual activity in prisons, fears of condoning homosexual behavior, and concerns about security (for example, condoms may be used to store drugs or [to attempt to] strangle other inmates). . . . Denial—first, that prisoners are having sex and, second, that HIV is being transmitted within prisons—best explains why many health

officials and policy makers view condom accessibility programs as a misguided or immoral policy approach.

Source: "Condom Programs in Schools and Prisons: Lessons in Policy and Controversy," *Intergovernmental AIDS Reports* (September 1992).

DOCUMENT 204: The Call for Needle Exchange Programs

Needle exchange programs are often criticized because some people
believe that they encourage drug use. Their effectiveness in controlling
the spread of HIV is considered secondary. Philadelphia faced this argument when the city decided to initiate a needle exchange program
that would also help place drug users in treatment programs.

Mayor Rendell, citing an "alarming" spread of the AIDS virus in Philadelphia, yesterday authorized a citywide clean-needle-exchange
program for [injecting] drug users.... Rendell contends that needle-
exchange programs reduce the spread of [HIV] while also helping drug
addicts enroll in treatment programs. But state officials say they are concerned about other possible consequences—namely, that the city's program would promote illegal drug use. [The city's health commissioner]
dismissed such arguments, contending that anyone who believes the
availability of clean needles promotes drug use "doesn't understand the
disease of addiction."

Source: "Rendell Frees the Way for Drug Needle Swap," *Philadelphia Inquirer*, July
28, 1992.

DOCUMENT 205: Developing a Workable Needle Exchange Program Is Not That Easy

New York City's pilot needle exchange program was relatively struc-
tured. Participants were frequently monitored and tested. They were
also encouraged to enter drug rehabilitation programs. Fewer people
than expected, however, entered the pilot program. Efforts to attract
drug users to program sites are less effective than bringing services to
them.

The "clinical trial" began on November 7, 1988 ... after [two] years of
planning and redesign.... [F]or a large-scale trial to be feasible, the pilot

study would have to attract enough volunteers, who would have to exchange their used needles regularly for clean ones and be prepared to enter drug treatment programs when vacancies occurred. Another important [factor] for success was community support. . . . The number of [injecting] drug users that could be enrolled was . . . limited to 400. To participate, addicts (18 years and older) had to register at the Health Department's headquarters in lower Manhattan, where they would be interviewed and examined by doctors, sign consent forms, and be tested for tuberculosis, sexually transmitted diseases, and HIV infection. These tests were to be repeated regularly throughout the trial. Only drug users who had applied to a drug rehabilitation program and been turned away because it was full were eligible for the study. . . .

Participants could exchange injection equipment between 10 AM and 3 PM Monday through Friday at the lone distribution site in downtown Manhattan, where they also received counseling and education. Each participant had an identification card with a photograph attached, to prevent others from getting access to the clean needles. Furthermore, the researchers planned to check the returned needles and syringes to make sure the blood in them was the same type as the participant's. If it wasn't, the participant would be warned, [and perhaps] dropped from the study. . . .

After [two] months, only 56 addicts had enrolled, and only 76 needles had been dispensed. Health officials decided to alter the experiment so they could concentrate more on getting drug users into rehabilitation programs. [It was] conceded that the number of addicts so far enrolled would be too few to draw any valid scientific conclusions.

Source: Warwick Anderson, "The New York Needle Trial: The Politics of Public Health in the Age of AIDS," *American Journal of Public Health* 81(11): 1506–1517 (November 1991).

DOCUMENT 206: The Importance of Outreach Workers in HIV Prevention

San Francisco's approach to AIDS prevention for drug users was based upon outreach workers bringing services directly to this population. Bottles of bleach, condoms, and educational materials were distributed where drug users congregated, rather than waiting for them to come to a specific site. Evaluation of this program showed that efforts to educate this difficult-to-reach group were helping to reduce high-risk behaviors.

San Francisco's model for managing the HIV/AIDS epidemic has become world famous. . . . Under the leadership of the YES Project, a San
Francisco agency that specialized in applied ethnographic research, the
Mid-City Consortium to Combat AIDS pioneered an effective street-
based strategy. It consisted of . . . sending outreach workers into the natural hangouts of drug users, where they provided AIDS education and
distributed condoms and one-ounce bottles of bleach to disinfect needles.
During the time data for this study were being collected, the YES Project
deployed some thirty outreach workers and field supervisors and passed
out bottles of bleach with such regularity and consistency that on the
street bleach may have been better known for its capabilities of disin-
fecting potentially contaminated needles than it was for doing laundry.
Other agencies added to the prevention effort and provided posters,
pamphlets, comic books, billboards, and videotapes addressing the connection between sharing contaminated hypodermic needles and HIV infection. . . . [T]he term CHOW—the acronym for "community health
outreach worker"—had worked its way into the street idiom and become
as well entrenched as the slang for crack. . . . [T]here was hardly a hidden
population of injection drug users in the city of San Francisco that had
not been targeted for street-based intervention. . . .

As a result of intensive health outreach strategies, respondents had
acquired a working knowledge of the HIV epidemic and generally put
into practice those measures that would protect them against infection.
One of the significant findings of [the] research . . . is that where AIDS
educators penetrate drug-using networks and establish positive, helping
relationships, members of the target groups [the people the program is
trying to reach] will practice risk-reduction methods.

Source: Harvey W. Feldman, Frank Espada, Sharon Penn, and Sharon Byrd,
"Street Status and the Sex-for-Crack Scene in San Francisco," in M. S. Ratner,
ed., *Crack Pipe as Pimp: An Ethnographic Investigation of Sex-for-Crack Exchanges*
(New York: Lexington Books, 1993), pp. 133–158.

DOCUMENT 207: Needle Exchange Programs *Do* Work

New Haven's needle exchange program has proved to be so successful
that it has become a model for other programs. Needles distributed to
drug users are coded so they can be tracked upon their return. It is
estimated that the program has reduced new HIV infections by 33 percent. This decrease means substantial savings to the health care system.
Most important, the program did not lead to increased injecting drug
use. In fact, just the opposite happened. Drug use declined. In the past,

it was illegal in Connecticut to buy syringes or carry them without a prescription. The law has now been changed.

On the basis of the contamination rates, the circulation time of the needles, and other data, the mathematical model estimated that the program reduced HIV transmission rates by 33 percent among those who participated. . . . The model indicated a drop in new HIV infections from six per year to four per year for every 100 drug injectors in the program. On that basis, [it was estimated] that 20 infections had been prevented over the first two years of the program, . . . while saving at least [two million dollars] for the health-care system [in avoided treatment costs].

Other results of the program, however, may ultimately prove as important as the savings in lives and money. . . . [T]here was no evidence of any increase in injecting drug use in New Haven as a result of the program, [and] one of every six addicts who joined the program subsequently entered drug treatment.

Advocates of needle exchange often contend that it reaches people who are ordinarily wary of official government programs, including drug treatment. The New Haven experience appears to bear that out. The implication is that a well-run needle-exchange program can serve an outreach function, attracting addicts who distrust the establishment system and usually shun it.

Source: "Can Clean Needles Slow the AIDS Epidemic?" *Consumer Reports* 59(7): 466–469 (July 1994).

DOCUMENT 208: Ten Years Too Late?

We have known from research studies conducted in Europe in the mid- and late 1980s that needle exchange programs work. In the United States, however, needle exchange programs faced considerable political opposition from those who felt that the government was just giving up on the war against drugs in the inner city. Some conservatives did not like the government spending any money on a program that appeared to encourage or tolerate injecting drug use. Some African-American political and religious leaders were also opposed to the idea that the government was abandoning the inner cities, and using needle exchange programs as an excuse for cutting down on funding law enforcement and drug treatment centers. Ten years after a needle exchange program in Washington, D.C., was first proposed but not implemented, health officials there recognize that hundreds of lives have probably been lost in that one city alone due to this delay. In

1997, a needle exchange program was finally begun in Washington, D.C.

On the heels of a report that Washington, D.C. health officials could have prevented as many as 650 HIV infections among injection drug users had they started a needle-exchange program 10 years ago, [the District of Columbia's] Whitman-Walker Clinic [the primary AIDS health and service organization] will announce today [March 5, 1997] that it has received a contract for [the] City's first large needle-exchange program. Research published this week in the *Lancet* [a well-respected British medical journal] suggests that because drug use plays an especially significant role in the Washington AIDS epidemic, a needle-exchange program would have been particularly beneficial. Under the new program, 100,000 sterile syringes will be distributed during the next year from Whitman-Walker's site in Anacostia [a section of Washington, D.C.] and from four mobile units near areas of high drug activity. Clinic Director Jim Graham predicts that the program, along with . . . a new oral HIV test that can be used in city neighborhoods, will begin to control the epidemic among injection drug users.

Source: Amy Goldstein, "Study Finds Needle Swap Is Imperative," *The Washington Post*, p. B10 (March 5, 1997); CDC National AIDS Clearinghouse (Bethesda, Md.: Information, Inc., 1997).

DOCUMENT 209: What Is the Physician's Responsibility to Prevent His or Her Patient from Infecting Others?

While all states report their AIDS cases to the Centers for Disease Control and Prevention (CDC), a U.S. government agency in Atlanta, confidential reporting of HIV-positive cases to the CDC is required in thirty of the fifty states. Three of the thirty states require reporting of HIV-positive children only. Some of the states with the largest numbers of HIV-positive persons, such as New York and California, do not require reporting of these persons, unless they are diagnosed with AIDS, at all. Reportable "AIDS" is defined by the CDC as an HIV-positive person with a T-4 cell count of less than 200 (an indicator of weakened immunity) or a diagnosis of one or more of the many opportunistic infections and a few kinds of cancer that frequently occur among AIDS patients. The question raised in this reading is whether a doctor has the responsibility to prevent his or her patient from infecting others. How far should he or she go? What do *you* think?

In states where [HIV] reporting is not required, doctors may still do so when a patient's behavior is putting someone else in danger. Once a case is reported, the health department can then decide to initiate contact tracing. Contact tracing is a public health strategy for controlling the spread of sexually transmitted diseases. Sexual contacts of the case are interviewed, counseled and offered treatment or referrals, in an attempt to prevent others from being infected.

Physicians have a responsibility to prevent the spread of contagious diseases, as well as an ethical obligation to recognize the rights to privacy and to confidentiality of the AIDS [sufferer]. These rights are absolute until they infringe in a material way on the safety of another person or persons. Those who are not infected with the virus are entitled to protection from transmission of the disease. Thus, the societal need for accurate information and public health surveillance must also be respected. As the Board of Trustees stated in its [1987 report], "A sound epidemiologic understanding of the potential impact of AIDS on society requires the reporting [on an anonymous or confidential basis to public health authorities] of those who are confirmed as testing positive for the antibody to the AIDS virus."

In those jurisdictions in which the reporting of individuals infected with the AIDS virus to public health authorities is not mandated, a physician who knows that a seropositive patient is endangering a third party faces a dilemma. The physician should attempt to persuade the infected individual to refrain from activities that might result in further transmission of the disease. When rational persuasion fails, authorities should be notified so that they can take appropriate measures to protect third parties. Ordinarily, this action will fulfill the physician's duty to warn third parties; in unusual circumstances when all else fails, a physician may have a common law duty to warn endangered third parties. However, notification of any third party, including public health authorities, without the consent of the patient may be precluded by statutes in certain states. . . .

Source: Reports of the Council on Ethical and Judicial Affairs (American Medical Association, 1987).

DOCUMENT 210: Sex and Injecting-Drug-Using Partners of HIV-Infected Persons Need to Be Told

The Centers for Disease Control and Prevention (CDC) has recommended that partner notification be incorporated into HIV prevention programs. Partner notification most often refers to telling sexual partners that their sexual partner (lover, husband, wife, or one-night stand) is HIV-positive or has AIDS and that they may have become infected. Partner notification may also include needle-sharing partners. HIV-positive people should be encouraged and trained to discuss the situation with their partners. Otherwise, physicians and public health personnel may take on this responsibility.

The Centers for Disease Control and Prevention [CDC] currently recommends the following: "Persons who are HIV-antibody positive should be instructed in how to notify their partners and to refer them for counseling and testing. If they are unwilling to notify their partners or if it cannot be assured that their partners will seek counseling, physicians or health department personnel should use confidential procedures to assure that the partners are notified...."

Notification of unsuspecting partners is especially important because it enables persons who may not have been reached through other AIDS education programs to receive risk-reduction education. For example, the partner notification process can identify female and male partners of [injecting] drug users or female partners of bisexual males who may have been exposed to HIV infection but who may be unaware of their risk. Partner notification activities targeted toward women of childbearing age contribute additionally by potentially preventing the perinatal [around the time of birth] transmission of HIV.

Source: "Partner Notification for Preventing Human Immunodeficiency Virus (HIV) Infection—Colorado, Idaho, South Carolina, Virginia," *Morbidity and Mortality Weekly Report* 37(25): 393–402 (July 1, 1988).

DOCUMENT 211: The Process of Counseling, Testing, and Partner Notification

As part of an overall HIV prevention plan, partner notification is a component of counseling and testing programs. Properly conducted, it is a way to reach people at greatest risk while protecting the confidentiality of all parties. In counseling sessions, informing and protecting sex and needle-sharing partners is a principal objective.

Since 1985, [the Centers for Disease Control and Prevention (CDC)] has collaborated with federal agencies, state and local health departments, and national and community organizations to implement a comprehensive HIV prevention program. An important component of this prevention program is counseling, testing, referral (for additional medical and other services), and partner notification ... activities. These activities are interrelated and benefit infected individuals as well as uninfected persons at high risk for HIV infection.

HIV-antibody testing is coupled with two sessions of individual counseling, one before testing and one after receipt of test results. Counselors review with the client appropriate health and support services, how HIV transmission occurs, and methods for preventing future transmission. For persons who are HIV-positive, the counselor also reviews the importance of notifying sex and/or needle-sharing partners of the potential risk of infection. Partner notification for HIV infection is a form of outreach, targeting prevention activities to those at highest risk—sex and needle-sharing partners of HIV-infected individuals . . . [and] provides an opportunity to offer prevention, medical, and support services . . . to these individuals.

There are two models for partner notification . . . : Patient referral and provider referral. In the patient referral model, HIV-infected individuals . . . are encouraged to inform sex or needle-sharing partners of their exposure to infection without the direct involvement of health department staff. With provider referral, the health department—with the full knowledge and agreement of [the HIV-positive person]—notifies some or all sex or needle-sharing partners voluntarily identified by [that person]. [HIV-positive individuals], whose names are never revealed to partners, voluntarily provide names, descriptions, and addresses so provider referral can be carried out by trained health department staff.

[Partner notification] is a service offered to individuals with HIV infection at the time of post-test counseling or at a later counseling session. The process is always voluntary, and the confidentiality of the information is always maintained. Counseling partners who are already infected can prevent potential transmission to others. In addition, high-risk but as yet uninfected partners are identified, potentially preventing new infections if behavior change can be initiated and sustained. . . .

An assessment of long-term behavior change after the notification process is . . . a second component of these projects, . . . [which will] determine whether behavior change is adopted and maintained up to a year after notification among [the HIV-positive persons] and [their] counseled partners.

Source: "Partner Notification: Possibility for Behavior Change and Early Care," HIV AIDS Prevention, pp. 9–10 (February 1991).

DOCUMENT 212: Should Persons with AIDS Be Allowed to Smoke Marijuana?

In 1996, voters in California voted to legalize marijuana for medical use only by AIDS, cancer, glaucoma, and other selected seriously ill patients. Some people with AIDS who had been losing weight rapidly noticed that their appetite returned when they smoked marijuana. Some have argued that smoked marijuana is better in combating the "wasting syndrome" than Marinol, a drug that has the same active ingredient as marijuana but not the euphoric effect. Should persons with AIDS be allowed to legally use marijuana? In healthy persons, while marijuana does produce a euphoric effect, increases appetite, enhances visual acuity, and may have a role in temporarily augmenting some cognitive abilities, it also impairs concentration and memory, verbal and reading abilities, and judgment while carrying out specific activities (such as driving), and may cause respiratory problems, paranoid thoughts, and possibly other serious medical problems when used on a daily basis.

As the national debate over the medical use of marijuana continues, eight people across the country are receiving 300 joints a month as part of a federal program. Cancer patient Irvin Rosenfeld of Boca Raton, Florida, is one of the eight and says he feels that "without the marijuana, I would be dead. And I'm still a good and productive member of society." The federal government has opposed state initiatives to legalize marijuana for medical use—a policy that has been criticized by the *New England Journal of Medicine*, which called federal prohibitions "misguided, heavy-handed, and inhumane." A synthetic form of THC, the major active ingredient in marijuana, has been found to be beneficial for patients with AIDS and cancer. Although THC is available as the medicine Marinol, advocates of medical marijuana say that smoked marijuana is more effective.

Source: Stephen Smith, "Facing the Questions of Medical Marijuana," *Miami Herald*, p. 1A (March 3, 1997); CDC National AIDS Clearinghouse (Bethesda, Md.: Information, Inc., 1997).

SUGGESTED READINGS

"AIDS and Ethics." *The Futurist* 26, p. 57 (July/August 1992).
Arnesen, I. "HIV Prisoners (II)." *The Nation* 256, pp. 4–5 (January 4–11, 1993).
Bacon, John. "Nationline: AIDS Confidentiality." *USA Today*, p. 3A (October 10, 1996).
Bayer, Ronald, et al. "HIV Antibody Screening: An Ethical Framework for Evaluating Proposed Programs." *Journal of the American Medical Association* 256 (13), pp. 1768–1774 (October 3, 1986).
"Exchange the Program." *Richmond Times-Dispatch*, p. A10 (March 12, 1997).
Gelman, D. "The Young and the Reckless." *Newsweek* 121, pp. 60–61 (January 11, 1993).
Gorman, C. "Opening the Border to AIDS." *Time* 141, p. 45 (February 22, 1993).

"Gynecologist with HIV Barred in Britain." *The Washington Times*, p. A16 (March 12, 1997).

"Home Drug Test Kits." *The Washington Post*, p. A20 (October 10, 1996).

"Insurer Is Ordered to Pay, Despite Fraud." *The New York Times*, p. A22 (February 26, 1997).

Kliger, Craig. "When It's Ethical to Withhold AIDS Drugs." *The New York Times*, p. A30 (March 7, 1997).

Kronemyer, B. "AIDS and the Workplace." *Career World* 22, pp. 26–30 (November 1993).

"Lawmakers Prepare HIV Prevention Act." *The Washington Times*, p. A9 (March 14, 1997).

London, William M. "Medical Marijuana, Distinctively Speaking." *The Washington Post*, p. A18 (March 3, 1997).

McCombie, S. "The Cultural Impact of the 'AIDS' Test: The American Experience." *Social Science and Medicine* 23:(5), pp. 455–459 (1986).

"Men Plead Not Guilty in AIDS Data Leak." *The Washington Times*, p. A6 (March 7, 1997).

Mintz, John. "Reversal on Military HIV Issue Is Rare Hill Victory for Gay Rights Activists." *The Washington Post*, p. A9 (April 26, 1996).

Osborn, June. "Widespread Testing for AIDS: What Is the Question." *AIDS and Public Policy Journal* 2(4), pp. 3ff. (Fall/Winter 1987).

Plummer, W. "Dr. Acer's Sixth Victim." *People Weekly* 39, p. 107 (May 24, 1993).

"Politically Inconvenient." *The Nation* 256, p. 289 (March 8, 1993).

"Possession of a Dangerous Weapon." *Time* 140, p. 23 (December 14, 1992).

Roush, C. "Profits and Good PR?" *Business Week*, p. 87 (May 17, 1993).

Shenitz, B. "Patients Left Out in the Cold." *Newsweek* 120, p. 48 (November 23, 1992).

Sontag, Deborah, and Lynda Richardson. "Doctors Withhold HIV Pill Regimen from Some." *The New York Times*, p. 1 (March 2, 1997).

Sullivan, R. E. "The AIDS Monster." *Mademoiselle* 98, pp. 82–84 (April 1992).

Terl, Allan H. *AIDS & the Law: A Basic Guide for the Nonlawyer*. Washington, D.C.: Hemisphere, 1992.

Thompson, D. "Getting the Point in New Haven." *Time* 139, pp. 55–56 (May 25, 1992).

"To the Point." *Philadelphia Inquirer*, p. A10 (March 11, 1997).

Wolfe, Sidney M. "Lift the Federal Ban on Needle Exchange." *The Washington Post*, p. A20 (February 27, 1997).

9

The Future of AIDS

In this volume, we have seen how people in the United States and around the world have responded to the AIDS crisis. We have seen humankind both at its best and at its worst. We have seen those who would volunteer their time, donate their money, and speak out about an effective policy for HIV prevention and for the needs of persons with HIV and AIDS. We have also seen those who would manipulate AIDS, sometimes under the guise of religion, as a political tool to reinforce their own prejudices and bigotry. Perhaps our greatest enemy is not quite so obvious: it is apathy. The AIDS crisis will continue to deepen if we accept AIDS as a normal condition of life, if we become indifferent to the needs of persons with AIDS and HIV, if we fail to reinforce what we have learned so far about HIV prevention, if we no longer care about what AIDS does to people.

As we enter the twenty-first century, the rate of technological and social change on a global level continues to accelerate, as it has done throughout the twentieth century. Each new generation brings with it not only a new technological reality but also a new social reality that meets the needs of the technological innovations. However, many prefer a world that is unchanged and traditional, often forgetting the weaknesses of that prior time and relishing only its advantages. They prefer a world where diseases were not discussed, where sex education did not exist, where homosexuality "dared not speak its name," where condoms were not needed, where the poor and the minorities stayed in their place. But if we were to apply the elements of such a world to the existing one, AIDS and HIV would have easily flourished, and the progress against AIDS that has occurred would never have happened. We need to be watchful of the social consequences of AIDS on our lives and the lives of everyone in each of the 191 nations on this earth.

In addition to discussing some of these issues, this chapter looks at some of the recent trends in the areas of vaccine research, home HIV testing, the future of AIDS hospices, the increasing spread of AIDS among the elderly, the new optimism that has grown from the development of the new protease inhibitor drugs which have already extended thousands of lives, a possible "morning-after" drug treatment, the failure to meet the needs of the poor and the homeless with AIDS, and new research on a gene that protects one from becoming HIV-positive. The chapter ends intentionally on a cautionary note. Though the number of new HIV cases each year appears to have stabilized in the United States, we must not allow ourselves to become too complacent. New HIV-1 subtypes, from international transmission and from local mutations developed through resistance to the new drugs, may grow and change the trajectory of HIV transmission into populations currently at lower risk for HIV. The global spread of HIV throughout the developing world is continuing at an alarming rate, and not nearly enough is being done or funded to sufficiently slow the pace.

AIDS requires everyone's concern and assistance. It requires our commitment to volunteer in AIDS service organizations: serving as a buddy in a "buddy program," working on an AIDS hot line, helping to deliver meals to homebound persons with AIDS. It requires our desire to learn about how to abstain from sex, to learn about how to practice safer sex when we are truly ready, to tell others about the basics of AIDS and HIV, to support World AIDS Day every year. Unfortunately, AIDS is not going away in the near future. Everyone needs to live in a world where AIDS is honestly confronted and earnestly challenged, and to do what they can to ensure that it does not thrive.

DOCUMENT 213: Political Apathy and the Challenge for America

The bipartisan National Commission on AIDS was created by Congress to develop an overall strategy to combat the epidemic. Appointments to the commission were made both by Congress and by President Bush. The commission heard testimony throughout the country, gathered information, and issued a series of transcripts and reports, beginning in 1989 and ending in 1993. Although spending on AIDS increased significantly during President Bush's administration, the commission felt President Bush, like President Reagan before him, largely ignored the situation and was not willing to take the lead. The commission wanted to convey to the national leadership and to the country a sense of

urgency; without dramatic action, the number of people infected
would only increase.

With the election of President Clinton, there was a change of tone
in Washington and hope for stronger leadership. Clinton established
the Office of National AIDS Policy within the White House and promised to carry out the commission's recommendations. However, while
spending for AIDS research and care continued to climb under President Clinton, and he held the first White House Conference on AIDS
in December 1995, he failed to give his several appointed national
AIDS coordinators much real power and he only very occasionally
talked about AIDS. While the new drugs that became available in 1996
have so far proved to be very beneficial, they are neither a vaccine nor
a cure.

The people of the United States have arrived at a crossroads in the
history of the HIV epidemic. In the months to come they must either
engage seriously the issues and needs posed by this deadly disease or
face relentless, expanded tragedy in the decades ahead. In just ten years
. . . HIV, the causative agent of AIDS, has claimed more American lives
than did the Korean and Vietnam wars combined. If, from this day forward, there were never another instance of new infection, the upcoming
decade would still certainly be much worse. The amount of human suffering and number of deaths will be much greater.

The face of AIDS will change as well; thus far it has focused its dev-
astation [in North America and Europe] predominantly on young [and
middle-aged] men. In addition, it is also a disease that affects an entire
family—now, all too often, mothers, fathers, and children die swiftly,
one following the other, leaving a few orphans as a grim reminder of
what was once a family.

Workers on the front lines are struggling heroically to cope with illness
and death, but their tools have been too few, their resources too constrained, and their logistics too crippled by the sabotage of disbelief,
prejudice, ignorance, and fear.

Nor has the virus followed rules of fair play. Gay and bisexual men
still bear much of the burden of HIV disease. Disproportionately and
increasingly the epidemic has attacked segments of society already at a
disadvantage—communities of color, women and men grappling with
poverty and drug use, and adolescents who have not been effectively
warned of this new risk to their futures. And with these shifts have come
new anger, mistrust, and attempts to assign blame, which have drowned
out the warnings that should signal the magnitude of the mounting crisis. Sadly, this has permitted too many Americans to detach [themselves]
from the fray, to feel the problem is that of others different from themselves, and to retreat into resentful indifference. Diversity, which should

be our greatest strength as a nation has for the moment become a weakness, and has sanctioned a begrudging and sometimes callous response. Even the language of prevention, which should be tailored to the myriad subcultures and ethnicities of people at risk, is constrained in the name of morality, withholding potentially lifesaving information and devices in order to avoid offending a public presumed to be in agreement with such constraints. . . .

In war, we tend to look for a human enemy to attack, and . . . thus far this tendency has been all too evident in our response to HIV. But in confronting AIDS, our response must be just the opposite. Compassion and concern for human suffering must direct our efforts. It is against the virus, not those infected, that this war must be waged. Tragically, to date, too many of us have failed to understand this fundamental distinction or acknowledge what a massive national effort is needed to contain the epidemic.

The sapping of our collective strength comes from many directions. There has been a dominant undercurrent of hostility toward many people with HIV disease, as if they are somehow to blame. But no one gets this virus on purpose. We do not withhold compassion from people who suffer from other diseases related to behavior. As [former] President Bush stated in his single speech about AIDS, "Other diseases strike and we don't blame those who are suffering. We don't spurn the accident victim who didn't wear a seat belt; we don't reject the cancer patient who didn't quit smoking. We try to love them and care for them and comfort them." We must replace the innocent/guilty mindset with sympathy and care for people with HIV disease. . . .

[W]e cannot turn away from what is coming, lest we be blind-sided. There are at least one million Americans silently infected with HIV. Most of them will get sick during the next decade. And in the absence of a national effort, the virus continues to spread. . . . AIDS is already the leading cause of death for young men and women in many parts of the country and is climbing relentlessly up the list of causes of "years of potential life lost."

What makes these numbers particularly tragic is that there is so much that we *can* do to turn the tide of HIV through prevention of further spread, and so much that we *must* do to provide more humane and compassionate care to those who have already been caught in the path of the virus. . . . To accomplish the tasks that loom ahead, we must, as a society, find a way to convert anger, fear, and indifference into informed action. We must deal effectively with discrimination and prejudice, overcome present governmental inertia, rededicate ourselves to maintaining a necessary intensity of research endeavor, educate the public to replace panic with informed awareness of what is needed to prevent infection, and coordinate our resources to meet the urgent health care needs of the

sick in cost-efficient ways that take full advantage of our powerful science. We must recognize our obligations to future generations in these
tasks, for further indifference or misdirected efforts spells doom for millions. . . .

Source: "Executive Summary," *America Living with AIDS*, Report of the National
Commission on Acquired Immune Deficiency Syndrome, 1991 (Washington,
D.C.: U.S. Government Printing Office, 1991), pp. 1–9.

DOCUMENT 214: How Has AIDS Affected Our Culture?

The author of this selection argues that, in many respects, we have not
responded well at all to the AIDS crisis. And the author has an important point. Too many have used AIDS to reinforce their justification for
a strict, traditional moral code that may be anachronistic at the turn of
the twenty-first century, or to promote a rigidly conservative political
agenda, or to foster an anti-sex stance. Yet, it is possible that these
reactions to AIDS may have elicited within our culture a new perspective on some of the assumptions that we have traditionally taken for
granted. Ironically, the advent of AIDS may not cause a return to cultural orthodoxy but, rather, a hastening of culture change.

The AIDS epidemic has brought out the best in many, and there are
a lot of unsung heroes and heroines out there. But in our establishment
world—the world that largely determines public attitudes, the development of national priorities, and the allocation of major resources, human and financial—we have not done well at all. The reasons are many
and complex. This disease, transmitted by behaviors so intimate, evokes
passionate feelings . . . [that] connect closely to attitudes often unexplored . . . and to beliefs about what is "right" and "wrong." So AIDS
has often evoked emotions and responses not so laudable. And these
responses have fostered denial that we have a problem and seem to have
legitimized a reluctant response to this human catastrophe all over the
world. . . .

[W]e have failed to develop an overarching, well-articulated national
plan for dealing with the epidemic, . . . [and] have allowed arguments
about taste or morality or propriety to block the delivery of potentially
lifesaving information and devices to our teenagers, to drug users, and
to the American community at large. . . . [W]e have not developed the
medical care or social support systems necessary to care . . . for those ill
with HIV. . . .

Source: David E. Rogers, "Report Card on Our National Response to the AIDS Epidemic—Some A's, Too Many D's,"*American Journal of Public Health* 82(4): 522–524 (April 1992).

DOCUMENT 215: Moving Along the Fault Lines of Our Society

How our society "handles" AIDS reveals much about our society. How the diverse societies of the world differently "handle" AIDS reveals the fundamental differences among the world's societies. Look at how a people treats its members with HIV or AIDS, and you can learn much about the humanity, or the selfishness, or the caring, or the apathy of that people. The authors of the following selection, a prominent anthropologist and a biologist, examine how AIDS, like an earthquake, moves along the fault lines of our society.

AIDS highlights processes of social change: . . . changed sexual mores for heterosexuals as well as homosexuals; the economic dislocations and prejudice that are increasingly turning some minority communities in America into an underclass. The history of failure to heed the early warnings of the epidemic is a statement of our priorities as a society. Now that we know how to prevent the disease from spreading, its continued spread must advertise the ways in which, in this interconnected and interdependent world, we fail to communicate to individuals the very knowledge they need to survive. AIDS moves along the fault lines of our society and becomes a metaphor for understanding that society.

Source: Mary Catherine Bateson and Richard Goldsby, *Thinking AIDS: The Social Response to the Biological Threat* (Reading, Mass.: Addison-Wesley, 1988).

DOCUMENT 216: It's Not Too Late to Start Controlling HIV Infection

When we consider that AIDS is a preventable disease, we need to ask ourselves if we have done enough on a global level to prevent it. As we enter the turn of the twenty-first century, it is clear that AIDS, especially in much of Africa and Asia, is out of control and we have not done enough to prevent it. Tens of millions of people have already become infected with HIV. Millions have already died of AIDS. The author of the following segment of an editorial in a medical journal states what he feels we need to do.

We have obviously failed to prevent the global spread of AIDS.... Our response to the HIV epidemic is now at a time of crisis.... It is now reasonable to consider dropping the term "AIDS" in favour of "advanced HIV disease".... [O]ur highest priority must be prevention of sexual transmissions of this virus, as well as of other STDs that facilitate spread of HIV.... HIV must be prevented among drug users ... [with] innovative strategies to avoid exposure to blood contaminated needles and syringes.... [P]revention programmes must be planned, evaluated and revised.... Prevention strategies must be culturally relevant, understandable, and targeted towards the needs of ... specific populations.... [T]here is a need for comprehensive and forceful global leadership during the second decade of this epidemic.... The world will continue to live with HIV into the next century. However, our inability to eradicate HIV does not preclude our making substantial progress in controlling the infection.

Source: Alan R. Lifson, "Preventing HIV: Have We Lost Our Way?," *The Lancet* 343(8909): 1306–1307 (May 25, 1994).

DOCUMENT 217: Promoting an End to Global AIDS Discrimination

Even in a city like Lusaka, the capital of Zambia in south central Africa, where about 180,000 of its 1 million men, women, and children are HIV-positive, AIDS is still a stigmatizing disease and AIDS discrimination is still commonplace. In India, squeamishness about the disease among government officials has led to a deadly delay in tackling the rapid growth of HIV infection in that nation of nearly 1 billion people. Back in the 1980s, it took many years before the governments of Burundi and the Congo allowed researchers in to freely study the disease. Reports in the late 1980s of executions by the Burmese (Myanmar) government of HIV-positive female commercial sex workers returning from Thailand and of anti-gay suppression to "combat AIDS" in Singapore show us how far AIDS discrimination can go in nondemocratic and repressive societies.

The HIV pandemic flourishes where an individual's capacity to learn and to respond is constrained. Belonging to a discriminated against, marginalized, or stigmatized group reduces personal capacity to learn and respond.... [T]o the extent that societies can reduce discrimination and promote respect for rights and dignity, they will be successful in preventing HIV transmission, caring for those who are infected and ill, and advancing the health of all people. By viewing AIDS in this manner . . . we can better understand and respond to the pandemic. The common ground is health, in its full, modern definition of physical, mental, and social well-being. . . .

The central insight from a decade of hard work against AIDS is that societal discrimination is at the root of individual and community vulnerability to AIDS—and to other major health problems of the modern world. This links HIV/AIDS work to the larger global movement for health.

Source: Jonathan Mann, Daniel Tarantola, Jeff O'Malley, and the Global AIDS Policy Coalition, "Toward a New Health Strategy to Control the HIV/AIDS Pandemic," *Journal of Law, Medicine & Ethics* 22(1): 41–52 (Spring 1994).

DOCUMENT 218: Anonymous HIV Testing in the Privacy of Your Own Home

For years it was hotly debated whether or not funds should be spent on more HIV testing centers, whether or not pretest counseling was as essential as posttest counseling, and whether or not HIV-positive test results should be reported by the states to the CDC. In many respects, this has now become a moot issue with the introduction of anonymous home HIV test kits that can be purchased for about $40 at discount drugstores and elsewhere. The home test kits are opening up HIV testing to millions of Americans who otherwise would have stayed away from HIV testing centers, feared losing their ability to get health insurance if their HIV-positive results were reported to the government, or were simply uncomfortable asking their doctors for the test. The tests are highly accurate, clear HIV information is given, and counseling and referrals are anonymously provided over the phone.

Johnson & Johnson, facing competition from Home Access Health in the home HIV test kit market, has decided to begin national direct mail sales of its test, called Confide, immediately and to increase national retail availability. . . . The company [began] national advertising of Confide's 800-number in [1996]. J&J is also facing a legal battle with Elliott Millenson, a former executive who developed the test and was hired by J&J to head its Direct Access Diagnostics Division. An arbitrator has ruled that the company should return the product rights to Millenson. Home Access Health, meanwhile, has launched a $5 million to $7 million advertising campaign for its test kit. A similar test by ChemTrak is awaiting approval from the Food and Drug Administration, and SmithKline

Beecham will seek approval to market to consumers its saliva-based HIV test, now approved for use by doctors.

Source: Michael Wilke, "J&J's Confide Faces Legal Battle, New Rival," *Advertising Age* 67(32): 3 (August 5, 1996); CDC National AIDS Clearinghouse (Bethesda, Md.: Information, Inc., 1996).

DOCUMENT 219: The Growth of AIDS Hospices

The trend toward outpatient care for AIDS is a positive one. For patients, having good options gives them a sense of control. Some people choose to die at home, in familiar surroundings. In the past, nursing homes or other long-term facilities were hesitant to admit AIDS patients, who need specialized care and, as a result, are less profitable. As a consequence, most AIDS patients have received care in hospitals or at home. As communities become more understanding of the nature of the disease and the needs of patients, special outpatient facilities or hospices are created. In Seattle, for instance, a $7 million hospice, specially designed for AIDS patients, was built using private and city funds. The design incorporated suggestions and ideas of people with AIDS. The hospice has room for thirty-five residents and places for thirty-five day patients. Not only does the Bailey-Boushay House have beautiful views and greenhouses throughout, but the cost is modest, an estimated $200 per day, approximately one-third the cost of comparable care in a hospital or regular nursing facility. In Chicago, a combination of city and private funds has established a hospice program for families in which at least one member has AIDS. Services include a furnished apartment, twenty-four-hour staff, food for five days, and volunteer support. Hospice care for AIDS patients can be a humane and cost-effective alternative to the hospital. However, as more people with AIDS respond well to the new protease inhibitor drugs that are now available, it is not clear if this will lead to a decreased use of AIDS hospices.

Outpatient care for AIDS patients is . . . increasingly being provided by hospices, nursing homes, and residence care services. Hospice and nursing home care, traditionally established for terminally ill cancer patients and chronically ill aged persons, have become more available for persons with AIDS nationwide. San Francisco, one of the first cities to make hospice programs available to persons with AIDS, has been viewed by other cities and nations as a model for community care for HIV-infected persons.

Source: Janet J. Kelly, Susan Y. Chu, James W. Buehler, and the AIDS Mortality Project Group, "AIDS Deaths Shift from Hospital to Home," *American Journal of Public Health* 83 (10): 433–437 (October 1993).

DOCUMENT 220: HIV Among the Elderly

While most people with AIDS are diagnosed when they are in their early thirties, 10.5 percent of all reported AIDS cases through December 1996 were among people fifty years old or over. Many middle-aged and elderly men and women are still quite sexually active, and the myth that somehow they are protected from becoming HIV-positive is wrong and dangerous. Men over fifty are more likely than younger men to use the services of female or male commercial sex workers (CSWs). In some cities where "crack" is commonly sold for sex, such as Miami, about 25 percent of all female streetwalking CSWs and 62 percent of all male streetwalking CSWs are HIV-positive.

In Florida's Broward County, the number of AIDS patients over 50 has more than doubled in the last two years. Health workers suspect that many older people with AIDS are not diagnosed because doctors mistake the symptoms for signs of aging or [Alzheimer's disease]. Older people do not think they can be at risk for HIV, and therefore often forgo testing and safer sex practices. They are also less likely to use condoms because they are unconcerned with birth control. The thinning of tissues with age, however, makes older people more vulnerable to infection.

Source: Karen Rafinski, "AIDS on Rise in Americans over 50, Officials Warn," *Miami Herald*, p. 3B (September 6, 1996); CDC National AIDS Clearinghouse (Bethesda, Md.: Information, Inc., 1996).

DOCUMENT 221: No Vaccine Yet Available

The HIV/AIDS epidemic is global in scope; therefore, successful vaccine development requires nations to cooperate in this effort. Vaccine trials with human subjects have already begun in the United States, Thailand, Brazil, Uganda, and other countries. While developed nations control the scientific technology and resources, developing countries are concerned about cost and availability. The principal political issue is one of fairness. Will poor nations be able to afford the vaccine? If they cannot, who will help them? During the first half of the 1990s, vaccine development in the United States slowed down following some initial failures, while the World Health Organization continued its vaccine work in a few developing countries.

Although many AIDS experts agree that a vaccine is the best solution to the AIDS pandemic, [not enough] research is focusing on this goal. [Numerous] HIV vaccines have undergone preliminary human trials, but few have moved forward. Furthermore, a vaccine being developed against the strain of HIV prevalent in the United States and Europe may not be effective against the forms common in the developing world. By the year 2000, an estimated 40 million people will be infected with HIV, and 90 percent of them will live in developing countries. The International AIDS Vaccine Initiative has received a $7 million grant from the Rockefeller Foundation to pursue an AIDS vaccine, and medical director Margaret Johnston says that individual countries should decide what efficacy of a vaccine is acceptable for their people. These countries also need to educate their people about HIV prevention, she added.

Source: Ruth SoRelle, "15 Years into Pandemic, and Still No AIDS Vaccine in Sight," Houston Chronicle, p. 6D (September 9, 1996); CDC National AIDS Clearinghouse (Bethesda, Md.: Information, Inc., 1996).

DOCUMENT 222: The New Optimism About Vaccines

A vaccine that will protect people from HIV infection is the hope for the future. By the mid-1990s there was growing optimism for an effective vaccine, but nothing is certain. It may be years before a successful vaccine is developed and becomes available for the general population.

Currently three dozen preventive HIV vaccines are being tested in small-scale clinical trials around the world. The National Institute of Allergy and Infectious Diseases (NIAID) is poised to move into large-scale efficacy trials as soon as a suitable product is identified, according to Jack Killen, M.D., director of NIAID's Division of AIDS. . . . Since 1988, more than 1,900 healthy, non-HIV-infected adults have voluntarily enrolled in 25 Phase I and II experimental AIDS vaccine trials conducted in the United States by the NIAID-sponsored AIDS Vaccine Evaluation Group (AVEG). AVEG consists of six university-based clinical testing sites, two central immunology laboratories, and a data coordinating and analysis center. . . . The AVEG trials have involved 16 experimental AIDS vaccines, 10 adjuvants [a substance that enhances the immune responses stimulated by a vaccine], and a variety of delivery vehicles and routes, dosages and schedules of immunization.

Source: Laurie K. Doepel, *AIDS Vaccine Research Highlights*, National Institutes of Health press release (July 8, 1996).

DOCUMENT 223: Do You Have the Gene That Protects You from HIV?

Since 1983, when it was first known that HIV (then called LAV, and later HTLV-III) causes AIDS, through a discovery of Dr. Luc Montagnier of the Louis Pasteur Institute in Paris, people have been wondering why some people who are repeatedly exposed to HIV do not become infected. Some gay men who had engaged in unprotected sex with other men in the early days of the epidemic, before the value of using condoms was known, found themselves the lone survivors of a sexual network that had developed HIV, then AIDS, and died. Is it just good luck? Why were they spared? Research now shows that a mutant gene, called CKR-5, fully protects (when two copies are present) about 1 percent of the population from becoming infected with HIV even after repeated unprotected exposures to the virus. However, for the rest of us, the gene is ineffective. Since the genetic test is not commercially available, and since so few are likely to have two copies of the gene, it should always be assumed by everyone that they are susceptible to infection upon unprotected HIV exposure.

A genetic mutation protects some people from infection with the AIDS virus even when they are repeatedly exposed to it through sex. . . . The findings by researchers working independently at the Aaron Diamond AIDS Research Center in New York City and the Free University of Brussels provide a genetic explanation for a phenomenon that has long perplexed epidemiologists: Some people do not get infected despite having [repeated] sex with partners who die from AIDS. . . . The findings might lead to the development of pills or injections to prevent HIV infection or to additional AIDS treatments. The mutant gene controls production of a protein that is needed to allow the entry into cells of HIV-1. . . . The gene is called CKR-5 . . . [and] HIV-1 remains harmless in . . . people [who inherit two copies of the mutant gene].

Source: Lawrence K. Altman, "Genetic Mutation Protects Some People from HIV Infection, Researchers Say," *The New York Times*, (August 9, 1996).

DOCUMENT 224: Can HIV Transmission Be Blocked?

Some of the new approaches to HIV vaccine research are using innovative ways to block the transmission of the virus. It appears that some
people may have immune cells that do not permit HIV to replicate,
even after the person is infected with the virus. This, and other promising avenues of research, may soon yield an answer and an effective
vaccine.

At the recent meeting of the American Association for the Advancement of Science, researchers presented new clues to the mystery of why
some people remain uninfected with HIV despite repeated exposures to
the virus. Miles Cloyd of the University of Texas presented findings that
suggest that some HIV-resistant individuals may have immune cells that
do not allow HIV to replicate, even after being infected. Last year, scientists reported that HIV could not infect the immune cells of some individuals because they carried a gene for a defective co-receptor required
by the virus. Cloyd and his colleagues found that when they added HIV
to samples of CD4 cells from 50 healthy individuals, the virus could not
replicate in up to 15 percent of the cells. The virus would cease repro-
duction after entering the cells and copying its RNA into DNA. It is
unknown whether the mechanism would protect people from HIV infection, but preliminary data from two men who seemed to clear the
virus suggest that it may. CD4 cells taken from these men seemed to
show the same reaction as the cells in the study. Further research will
test the CD4 cells from 50 HIV-negative men who are at risk of contracting the virus from their infected partners.

Source: Jocelyn Kaiser, "A New Way to Resist AIDS?" *Science* 275 (5304): 1258
(February 28, 1997); CDC National AIDS Clearinghouse (Bethesda, Md.: Information, Inc., 1997).

DOCUMENT 225: Could HIV Be Prevented *After* the Exposure?

If you engage in risky sexual behavior, such as failing to use a condom
during vaginal or anal sex, and the next day you realize that you have
done a "really dumb thing," imagine if there were some pills you could
take that would significantly lessen the chance that you would "sero-
convert" (become HIV positive). Well, that is exactly the purpose of a

study begun in 1997, which attempts to see whether two well-known AIDS drugs (AZT and 3TC) can help prevent HIV infection after exposure to HIV during sex. We know that this strategy is usually, though not always, effective after HIV exposure to infected blood in medical settings. Could it work after a mistake made in the bedroom, as well?

A study to test the efficacy of "morning-after" drug therapy for people who are accidentally exposed to HIV is slated to begin soon in San Francisco. As part of the trial, researchers at the San Francisco General Hospital will recruit individuals exposed to HIV as the result of one incident of risky behavior. The study participants will receive a 30-day supply of AZT and 3TC [two common drugs that attack the virus], with the hope that the treatment could prevent the virus from taking hold. AIDS prevention advocates warn that the therapy could reverse the trend toward safe behaviors, but the researchers say the strategy is worthwhile. Studies of similar preventive therapy for health care workers who are accidentally exposed to HIV on the job have shown that the drugs dramatically reduce the risk of infection.

Source: Lidia Wasowicz, " 'Morning After' Pill for AIDS," United Press International (March 3, 1997); CDC National AIDS Clearinghouse (Bethesda, Md.: Information, Inc., 1997).

DOCUMENT 226: Can the New Drugs Eradicate HIV?

The new protease inhibitor drugs have raised the level of optimism about the future of AIDS. Some feel that these pharmaceuticals, and even better drugs still in the experimental stages, may herald not just a new shift in AIDS from a mostly terminal to a mostly chronic medical condition, but even to a possible cure. Others are not so optimistic. They fear that the rapidly mutating virus may simply develop a resistance to each and every improvement that modern medicine can offer.

AIDS experts reported last week that it may be possible, using combinations of HIV drugs, to "eradicate" HIV from an infected person's body. The promising news was reported last week from a meeting convened by the medical journal *Antiviral Therapy* and the University of Amsterdam. AIDS experts reviewed unpublished data from trials taking place in the United States, Europe, Canada, and Australia which tested various drug combinations, and showed that, in some patients, the amount of HIV can be reduced to undetectable levels for up to two years. Thus far, no patients have taken the drug combinations for more than two years, so researchers say more time is needed to determine how effective the therapies are. Researchers also noted that getting treatment soon after infection was important to reducing the viral level.

Source: "'Eradication' of HIV Seen as Possible," *The Washington Post*, p. A12 (June 16, 1996); CDC National AIDS Clearinghouse (Bethesda, Md.: Information, Inc., 1996).

DOCUMENT 227: Will the New Protease Inhibitor Drugs Help Everyone?

The new protease inhibitors have already begun to prolong the lives of many people with HIV and AIDS. Thousands of Americans with AIDS would have certainly died if it were not for these new drugs. Some have virtually recovered from their deathbeds. But some people cannot tolerate the side effects of the drugs, and can no longer take them. Others, who take the drugs on an irregular basis, find that they have developed a resistance to them, and they are no longer effective. The new drugs require a strong commitment and an accurate watch to ensure that the sequence of twenty-two or more pills a day is taken at precisely the correct hour and exactly an hour after or before having a meal. The treatment regime is very complicated, requiring patients to have or develop good self-discipline and planning skills.

Not everyone has equal access to these new and expensive drugs. Some physicians who care for the homeless, "crack" users, and injecting drug users with AIDS are refusing to put these patients on protease inhibitors, because they feel that they do not have the personal capacity to self-administer their drug intake as scheduled and to time their meals with their pills. The physicians argue that it is better that the drugs should be withheld from them. If they take them sporadically, they will develop a permanent resistance to the drugs and be worse off than before. The author of this selection believes that the new protease inhibitor drugs are less likely to be used to help the poor, the homeless, and minority women.

Despite the recent report that AIDS-related deaths in the United States decreased last year, health groups warn that the AIDS risk remains a threat for many people, especially the poor. Michael Isbell, director of the Gay Men's Health Crisis, notes that although AIDS deaths did decline overall, "mortality related to HIV continues to grow in certain populations, particularly women and racial and ethnic minorities." The Centers for Disease Control and Prevention [CDC] reported last week that while AIDS deaths among men decreased 15 percent, the figure rose by 3 percent among women between early 1995 and early 1996. The agency also said that the rate of AIDS progression from HIV infection among African Americans is seven times higher than it is for whites and three times higher for Latinos. "Homeless people, poor people of color—these people are going to die" if they contract HIV, said Keith Cylar of Housing Works, a New York agency for poor or homeless AIDS patients.

Source: "U.S. Health: AIDS Deaths Decline, But Groups Warn," IPS Wire (March 3, 1997); CDC National AIDS Clearinghouse (Bethesda, Md.: Information, Inc., 1997).

DOCUMENT 228: Is AIDS Nearly Over? Or Is This Just the Beginning?

With the successes of the new protease inhibitor drugs, with some hopeful signs about the possibility of a vaccine on the distant horizon, and even with some evidence that teenagers are increasingly remaining abstinent or are having safer sex with condoms, some people in the United States and other developed nations are beginning to become smug about AIDS. But this may be the wrong time to be too smug! For one thing, the ten major subtypes of HIV-1 may spread to the United States and proliferate throughout the population. Since it is believed that each of the major HIV subtypes has its own unique pattern of transmissibility, at least one of the subtypes may spread much more easily within the nondrug-using heterosexual population. For another thing, since the virus mutates more rapidly when it develops resistance against new drugs, the round of new drugs may promote a speeding up of the pattern of mutation, resulting in new subtypes of the virus. These new subtypes not only would be impervious to the effects of the new drugs, but also may be more easily transmitted to the total population. Clearly, we must maintain our strong vigilance.

Researchers studying the mutability of HIV warn that the development of drug-resistant strains or more infectious strains of HIV could have a serious impact on the epidemic. Ten major subtypes of HIV have been identified so far, but researchers "know very little" about the implications of the virus's diversity, notes HIV expert Francine McCutchan. The variation is advantageous for the virus, she says, because it allows the mixing of different subtypes to create new and potentially stronger strains. While many subtypes have been found in countries like Uganda and [in several countries in] Asia, where the epidemic is running rampant, new evidence from New York HIV patients reveals the emergence of strains never before found in the United States. In a study of 43 HIV-positive Bronx residents, the U.S. Centers for Disease Control and Prevention's Kathleen Irwin found that at least two, and up to eight, patients were infected with HIV subtypes previously found almost exclusively in Asia, Africa, and South America. HIV easily invaded the South Bronx, where poverty, drugs, and homelessness give the virus several routes of transmission. Research suggests that injection drug users are especially susceptible to re-infection and recombination. The failure among HIV patients to stick to an anti-HIV drug regimen or to practice safer sex or safer drug use can also contribute to drug resistance and increased variation.

Source: Mark Schoofs, "The HIV Melting Pot," *Village Voice* 42 (7): 43 (February 18, 1997); CDC National AIDS Clearinghouse (Bethesda, Md.: Information, Inc., 1997).

SUGGESTED READINGS

"AIDS Mortality Alters Population Projections." *1996 World Population Data Sheet.* Washington, D.C.: Population Reference Bureau, June 1996.

Carey, J. "AIDS: Maybe There Isn't a Magic Bullet." *Business Week*, pp. 108–109 (October 24, 1994).

Cohen, J. "Are Researchers Racing Toward Success, or Crawling?" *Science* 265, pp. 1373–1375 (September 2, 1994).

Collins, Huntly. "AIDS-Related Deaths in Philadelphia Drop 23.5 Percent." *Philadelphia Inquirer*, p. B1 (March 7, 1997).

Cowley, G. "What If a Cure Is Far Off?" *Newsweek* 121, p. 70 (June 21, 1993).

"High-Powered Support for AIDS Vaccine." *Science* 275, p. 1055 (February 21, 1997).

Marlink, M., et al. "Reduced Rate of Disease Development After HIV-2 Infection as Compared to HIV-1." *Science* 265, pp. 1587–1590 (September 9, 1994).

Merson, M. H. "Slowing the Spread of HIV: Agenda for the 1990's." *Science* 260, pp. 1266–1268 (May 28, 1993).

Montagnier, Luc, and Marie-Lise Gougeon. *New Concepts in AIDS Pathogenesis.* New York: Dekker, 1993.

"The NAMES Project AIDS Memorial Quilt." In *Always Remember: The NAMES Project AIDS Memorial Quilt.* New York: Simon & Schuster, 1996.

National Academy of Sciences. *Confronting AIDS: Directions for Public Health, Health Care, and Research.* Washington, D.C.: National Academy Press, 1986.

" 'Provide' Services." *POZ*, p. 28 (March 1997).

Radetsky, P. "Are There Any More Out There?" *Discover* 14, pp. 64–65 (January 1993).

"Researchers Say Drug Helps AIDS Patients Live Longer." *Baltimore Sun*, p. 2A (March 4, 1997).

Sakson, Steve. "AIDS Drugs Cloud Future for Buyers of Life Policies." *Houston Chronicle*, p. 1C (July 20, 1996).

Salk, J., et al. "A Strategy for Prophylactic Vaccination Against HIV." *Science* 260, pp. 1270–1272 (May 28, 1993).

Sturgis, Ellen. "We Won a Battle, but AIDS War Must Go On." *Boston Globe*, p. A14 (March 4, 1997).

"A Two-Minute Test for the AIDS Virus." *Maclean's* 110(7), p. 70 (February 17, 1997).

Glossary

AIDS: acquired immunodeficiency syndrome. A condition, first described in 1981, that results in a gradual weakening of the body's immune system, leaving it vulnerable to many opportunistic infections and certain types of cancers; the final stages of HIV disease; defined by HIV seropositivity and a T4 count below 200 and/or specific opportunistic infections or cancers.

AIDS activist: a person or group that attempts to increase people's awareness of AIDS, to educate about preventive methods, to further the efforts of researchers in finding a cure and of pharmaceutical companies in devising new drug therapies; works to increase funding for AIDS services, and to grant rights to and achieve social justice for people with AIDS.

AIDS community-based organizations: local organizations that address the psychological, emotional, and practical needs of people with HIV and AIDS, and their families. They provide such services as bereavement counseling, AIDS awareness education, and substance abuse programs. Also known as AIDS service organizations.

Antibody: a protein produced by the body in reaction to an antigen (such as a virus or bacteria). The antibody neutralizes the antigen and produces an immunity to it. The human immunodeficiency virus (HIV), which causes AIDS, destroys antibodies.

Antigen: a microorganism that produces a response from the immune system when it is introduced into the body. Viruses, bacteria, and various proteins are antigens that elicit the production of T lymphocytes, the immune system's response to a foreign organism.

ARC (AIDS-related complex): a term used in the early years of the AIDS epidemic to describe the variety of symptoms that occurred in individuals before they were diagnosed as having AIDS. This term became archaic in 1993, when the Centers for Disease Control and Prevention (CDC) revised the definition of AIDS to include more of the conditions that were previously included under ARC.

Asymptomatic: not having any symptoms of disease; appearing and feeling healthy while infected.

AZT (also known as zidovudine): a drug that has been shown to be very therapeutic for many or most patients when used in combination with another anti-retroviral drug, such as ddI, 3TC, D4T, or ddC, and a protease inhibitor drug. It was the first drug widely used against HIV, but has been shown to be ineffective in most cases when used without other drugs over a prolonged period.

Behavioral change: the modification of sexual or drug-taking behavior to lessen the risk of becoming infected with HIV.

Biological false negative: a negative result of a laboratory test for a condition that is in fact present.

Biological false positive: a positive result of a laboratory test for a condition that in fact is not present.

Bisexual: a male or female who engages in sexual relations with, or is attracted to, persons of the same sex as well as persons of the opposite sex.

Blood transfusion: direct injection of whole blood or plasma into the bloodstream. Until 1985, donated blood was not tested for HIV in the United States.

Candidiasis: a yeastlike fungus infection that is a common opportunistic infection of those with HIV.

Caregiver: one who tends to the medical or emotional needs of people with HIV or AIDS. Caregivers can be either professionals, such as home attendants, or volunteers, such as friends or relatives.

Casual contact: day-to-day contact between people at home, school, work, or in the community that does not involve sexual contact or the sharing of drug needles.

CDC: the Centers for Disease Control and Prevention, a government research and administrative agency located in Atlanta, Georgia. A major role of the CDC is to promote HIV prevention in the United States.

CD4: an infection-fighting white blood cell that is gradually destroyed by HIV.

Chlamydia: a sexually transmitted disease that results in a painful whitish discharge from the penis in men and presents no symptoms in women until the late stages. Chlamydia may result in sterility (a person would be unable to have a child) if it is not treated.

Clinical trial: an impartial investigation of a new drug conducted by a research institution, using human subjects.

Cofactors: biological or social conditions affecting a person with HIV or AIDS that will delay or accelerate either the likelihood of infection upon exposure or the onset of the symptoms of the disease.

Condom: a sheath, usually made of latex, used to cover the penis during sexual intercourse to prevent pregnancy or sexually transmitted diseases, including AIDS. It is highly effective in preventing HIV transmission.

Cytomegalovirus (CMV): a virus, similar to herpes, commonly found in the general population. While causing no harm in most healthy individuals, CMV can produce serious illness, including blindness, in persons with AIDS, some infants, weakened persons, and people whose immune systems are suppressed by drugs or cancer.

ddC (dideoxycitidine): a drug that works to delay the onset of AIDS in people with HIV infection, when used in conjunction with AZT and a protease inhibitor drug.

ddI (dideoxyinosine): a drug that works to delay the onset of AIDS in people with HIV infection, when used in conjunction with AZT and a protease inhibitor drug.

Elisa test (enzyme linked immunosorbent assay): a laboratory procedure that detects the presence of HIV antibodies in blood. Two Elisa tests and a confirmatory Western blot test are usually conducted before an HIV seropositive test result is given.

Endemic: a condition of disease commonly found among a population.

Epidemic: an outbreak of a disease among a population that is not normally found in a large segment of that population.

Epidemiology: the systematic study of the occurrence and spread of diseases.

Ethnography: a qualitative research method developed by anthropologists to learn about the sociocultural aspects of human behavior through observing, participating in, and discussing lived experiences in a social setting.

FDA (Food and Drug Administration): the federal organization that is responsible for the testing of drugs before they are approved for public use in the United States.

Gay (homosexual): a male or female who engages in sexual relations with, or is attracted to, persons of the same sex. A female homosexual is also referred to as a lesbian.

Gay bathhouse: a commercial business visited by gay men, where sex between men often occurs in rented rooms or the steamroom. Some gay bathhouses are quite elaborate, with gym facilities, a sauna, a recreation room, a barbecue area, a swimming pool, and a sundeck. Today, free condoms are available at most gay bathhouses.

Genital herpes: a sexually transmitted disease caused by the herpes simplex virus type 2, which results in painful sores on the genitals or anus. There is no cure, but there are effective treatments.

Gonorrhea: a sexually transmitted disease that causes a painful yellowish discharge from the penis in men and often has no symptoms in women until the late stages of the disease. If untreated, gonorrhea can lead to sterility and many other serious complications.

Hemophilia: a rare, inherited disorder, usually in males, that keeps blood from clotting normally. There are about 20,000 persons with hemophilia in the United States. Many persons with hemophilia became infected with HIV when the blood products used to treat hemophilia became contaminated during the early and mid-1980s.

Heterosexual: a male or female who engages in sexual relations with, or is attracted to, persons of the opposite sex. In the United States, about 95 percent of the adult sexually active population is heterosexual.

High-risk behavior: behavior that permits bodily fluids carrying HIV to pass from one person to another, such as sharing needles or unprotected sexual activity (penetrative sex without using a condom).

HIV (human immunodeficiency virus): the retrovirus that causes AIDS. It was previously known as LAV or HTLV-III. There are two types: HIV-1, which is the more common and dangerous type and includes several subtypes (or clades), and HIV-2, which is found mostly in West Africa and is less lethal.

HIV-related dementia: loss of memory, or intellectual impairment, due to the destruction of neurons by HIV.

Hospice: a facility for the care of the physical and emotional needs of terminally ill patients.

HTLV-III: an early name for HIV; no longer in use.

IDU: an injecting recreational drug user.

Immune system: the body's defense system against disease and infection.

Immunosuppression: the weakening of the immune system.

Infected person: a person who is infected with HIV and may or may not have developed symptoms of AIDS, but who can spread the virus through bodily fluids even if he or she does not appear sick.

Intercourse: intimate sexual contact between the penis and vagina or anus.

IVDU (intravenous drug user): a person who uses drugs intravenously, by injecting them into a vein. Today, the broader term IDU (injecting drug user) is more often used.

Kaposi's sarcoma: a cancer of the walls of blood or lymphatic vessels that appears as purple or brown skin lesions (blotches). It is a common AIDS-related cancer, especially in gay men.

LAV: an early name for HIV; no longer in use.

Monogamy: being married to one person, or having sex with only one person of the opposite or same sex during an extended relationship.

Needle exchange: a program/practice instituted by many cities to reduce the risk of AIDS among injecting drug users who are at high risk for becoming infected by sharing, or transferring, needles and syringes. Injecting drug users turn in their used needles for clean ones, eliminating the chance of infecting other people or becoming infected themselves by reusing needles that other injectors have already used.

Nonoxynol-9: a spermicide that has been shown to kill HIV in laboratory tests.

Opportunistic infection (OI): an infection caused by a microorganism that normally occurs in the environment and poses no threat to healthy individuals, but causes disease in persons with weakened or compromised immune systems.

Pandemic: an epidemic that is spread over an especially wide geographic area.

Partner notification: a controversial issue regarding whether there is an obligation to inform the partner(s) of an HIV-infected individual that they, too, might be at risk.

Pentamidine: a drug used to treat *Pneumocystis carinii* pneumonia (PCP), a very common opportunistic infection.

Persistent generalized lymphadenopathy: prolonged swelling of the lymph glands. A common symptom of HIV infection; often an early symptom.

Placebo controlled trial: a study in which half of the test subjects are given a placebo (a pill containing an inactive nonmedicinal substance, such as sugar) to test the effectiveness of a new drug.

Pneumocystis carinii **pneumonia (PCP)**: a form of pneumonia caused by a protozoan parasite that grows rapidly in the lungs of people with AIDS. It is the leading specific cause of death in AIDS patients in the United States.

Prostitute: a male or female commercial sex worker who performs sex acts in exchange for money or drugs.

PWA (person with AIDS): a person who has been infected with HIV, whose immune system has been severely damaged by HIV, and who has been diagnosed with AIDS. Also referred to as a PLWA (person living with AIDS).

Quarantine: isolation of people with communicable diseases in order to prevent their spread. Most people who are placed in quarantine have a disease that is communicable through the air or casual (not sexual) contact of a very limited duration. The quarantine of people with AIDS and HIV has become a social rights and legal issue.

Retrovirus: a virus that contains the genetic material RNA and reproduces itself using the reverse of the usual process. It copies its RNA into the DNA inside an infected cell, resulting in the incorporation of altered DNA into the genetic structure of that cell. The defective DNA is then replicated in each new cell created by the original infected cell.

Risk factor: any personal or environmental condition or activity that increases an individual's probability of getting a disease.

Safer sex: sexual activity that allows no semen or vaginal fluids to pass from one person to another. It often involves the use of condoms and spermicide containing nonoxynol-9 to provide protection from HIV infection, or practicing nonpenetrative sex (such as mutual masturbation or sex between the legs of the partner).

Seroconversion: the development of antibodies in the blood as a result of infection.

Seronegative: the condition in which antibodies to HIV are not found in the blood.

Seropositive: the condition in which antibodies to HIV are found in the blood.

Seroprevalence: the proportion of the population that is infected, as measured through serological (blood-related) research.

Sexually active: engaging in sexual activity on a regular basis with one or more partners.

Sexually transmitted diseases (STDs): diseases, such as syphilis, chlamydia, genital herpes, chancroid, granuloma inguinale, lymphogranuloma venereum, hepatitis, and gonorrhea, that are transmitted primarily by penetrative sexual behavior.

SIV (simian immunodeficiency virus): a virus found in monkeys that is similar to the HIV-2 found in humans.

Surveillance: the monitoring of such public health conditions as epidemics.

Syphilis: a sexually transmitted disease that causes sores on the body and, if left untreated, can cause serious health problems, including neurosyphilis (which results in insanity).

T4 lymphocytes (T4 cells): the cells that help the other immune system cells to activate. These cells appear to be the primary targets of HIV infection.

Thrush: a fungal infection of the mouth and throat characterized by white eruptions on the tongue or in the throat cavity.

Toxoplasmosis: a disease caused by infection with *Toxoplasma gondii*, a protozoan parasite. In people with AIDS or other immunosuppressive disorders, it causes inflammation of the brain, and may affect other organs.

Vaccine: a substance of inactivated microorganisms (viruses or bacteria) that causes an immune reaction against the antigen and protects the body against future infection by that organism.

Western blot test: a more accurate procedure than the Elisa test for identifying antibodies against specific protein molecules. While it is more specific and sensitive in antibody detection, it is also more difficult to perform and is more costly.

Resource Directory

The following is a selected list of national organizations providing HIV/AIDS services. For more detailed information, see *National Organizations Providing HIV/AIDS Services: A Directory for Community-Based Organizations* (Rockville, Md.: CDC National AIDS Clearinghouse, October 1995).

Advocates for Youth, 1025 Vermont Avenue NW, Suite 200, Washington, DC 20005; (202) 347–5700; fax (202) 347–2263.

AIDS Action Council (AAC), 1875 Connecticut Avenue NW, Suite 700, Washington, DC 20009; (202) 986–1300; fax (202) 986–1345.

AIDS Clinical Trials Information Service (ACTIS), P.O. Box 6421, Rockville, MD 20849–6421; toll-free (800) 874–2572; fax (301) 738–6616.

AIDS Coalition to Unleash Power, New York (ACT-UP), 135 W. 29th Street, 10th Floor, New York, NY 10001; (212) 564–2437; fax (212) 594-5441.

AIDS National Interfaith Network (ANIN), 110 Maryland Avenue NE, Suite 504, Washington, DC 20002; (202) 546–0807; toll-free (800) 288–9619; fax (202) 546–5103.

American Foundation for AIDS Research (AmFAR), Public Policy Office, 1828 L Street NW, Suite 802, Washington, DC 20036; (202) 331–8600; fax (202) 331–8606.

American Institute for Teen AIDS Prevention, P.O. Box 136116, Fort Worth, TX 76136; (817) 237–0230; fax (817) 238–2048.

American Red Cross, National Headquarters, Office of HIV/AIDS Education, 8111 Gatehouse Road, Falls Church, VA 22042; toll-free (800) 375–2040; fax (703) 206–7754.

Athletes and Entertainers for Kids, 381 Van Ness, Suite 1507, Torrance, CA 90501; (310) 783–0575; toll-free (800) 933-KIDS; fax (310) 783–0585.

Gay and Lesbian Medical Association (GLMA), 211 Church Street, Suite C, San Francisco, CA 94114; (415) 255–4547; fax (415) 255–4784.

Gay Men's Health Crisis (GMHC), 129 W. 20th Street, New York, NY 10011–3629; (212) 337–3553; hotline (212) 807–6655; fax (212) 337–3656.

Girls, Inc., Keeping Healthy Keeping Safe AIDS/HIV Project, 441 W. Michigan Street, Indianapolis, IN 46202; (317) 634–7546; fax (317) 634-3024.

Metro TeenAIDS, Teen AIDS Youth Coalition, The Jubilee Center, 651 Pennsylvania Avenue SE, Washington, DC 20003–5577; mail: P.O. Box 15577, Washington, DC 20003–5577; (202) 543–3963 or (202) 792–9355; fax (202) 543–3343.

NAMES Project Foundation, AIDS Memorial Quilt, 310 Townsend, Suite 310, San Francisco, CA 94107; (415) 882–5500; fax (415) 882–6200.

National AIDS Fund, 1400 Eye Street NW, Suite 1220, Washington, DC 20005–2208; (202) 408–4848; fax (202) 429–1818.

National Association of People with AIDS (NAPWA), 1413 K Street NW, 8th Floor, Washington, DC 20005–3476; (202) 898–0414; fax (202) 898–0435.

National Hemophilia Foundation, Hemophilia and AIDS/HIV Network for Dissemination of Information (HANDI), 110 Greene Street, Suite 303, Soho Building, New York, NY 10012; (212) 431–8541; fax (212) 431–0906.

National Minority AIDS Council (NMAC), 1931 13th Street NW, Washington, DC 20009–4432; (202) 483–6622; fax (202) 483–1135.

National Network for Youth, Safe Choices Project, 1319 F Street NW, Suite 401, Washington, DC 20004; (202) 783–7949; toll-free (800) 878–2437; fax (202) 793–7955.

Pediatric AIDS Foundation (PAF), 1311 Colorado Avenue, Santa Monica, CA 90404; (310) 395–9051; fax (310) 395–5149.

Project Inform, HIV Treatment Hotline, 1965 Market Street, Suite 220, San Francisco, CA 94103; (415) 558–8669; hotline (415) 558–9051; toll-free (800) 822–7422; fax (415) 558–0684.

StandUP, National Office, P.O. Box 461292, Aurora, CO 80046–1292; (303) 699–4KID; toll-free (800) 365–4543.

U.S. Department of Health and Human Services, Public Health Service, Centers for Disease Control and Prevention, National AIDS Clearinghouse (CDC NAC), P.O. Box 6003, Rockville, MD 20849–6003; toll-free (English and Spanish) (800) 458–5231; fax (301) 738–6616.

U.S. Department of Health and Human Services, Public Health Service, Centers for Disease Control and Prevention, National AIDS Hotline (CDC NAH), P.O. Box 13827, Research Triangle Park, NC 27709–3827; toll-free (English) (800) 342–2437; toll-free (Spanish) (800) 344–7432; fax (919) 361–4855.

Index

About the Editors

DOUGLAS A. FELDMAN is a medical and applied anthropologist, a specialist in international and domestic AIDS social research since 1982, and the President of D. A. Feldman & Associates, a health research organization based in Fort Lauderdale, Florida. He is a Research Associate Professor, University of Miami School of Medicine. Dr. Feldman is the editor of *Global AIDS Policy* (Bergin & Garvey, 1994), *Culture and AIDS* (Praeger, 1990), and co-editor (with Thomas M. Johnson) of *The Social Dimensions of AIDS: Method and Theory* (Praeger, 1986), and has written many articles on anthropological research on AIDS. He received the prestigious Kimball Award in 1996 for his contributions in advancing the anthropology of AIDS, and is currently conducting funded AIDS social research in South Florida and Central Africa.

JULIA WANG MILLER is a sociologist who has worked extensively in public health on the AIDS issue.